PRIMARY BILIARY CIRRHOSIS

Published by
West End Studios Ltd
10 Grange Gardens, Eastbourne BN20 7DA, UK

Typeset in 8pt on 11pt Gill Sans by
West End Studios Ltd
10 Grange Gardens, Eastbourne BN20 7DA, UK

ISBN 0 9535570 0 6

Printed and bound in the United Kingdom by
Dunnsprint Ltd, Clarence Road, Eastbourne BN22 8HJ

Produced as a service to gastroenterology by
Falk Foundation eV

CONTENTS

CONTENTS

INTRODUCTION

Primary Biliary Cirrhosis (PBC) remains an enigmatic and fascinating disease. In the last decade there have been major advances in the understanding of the epidemiology, pathogenesis and treatment of the disease. There still remains very many unanswered questions: the cause of PBC has not yet been identified and treatment remains largely symptomatic. Ursodeoxycholic Acid is the only drug currently licensed for the treatment of the disease and liver transplantation is the only therapeutic option for end-stage patients.

The contributions in this volume are based on a meeting held in Grantham, England in 1998. The meeting was sponsored by the Falk Foundation and Cortecs Laboratory. Many people have contributed to making the meeting a great success and in particular I must thank the members of the Scientific Committee, Professor David Adams and Professor Gustav Paumgartner. I would also like to thank particularly Dr Herbert Falk and Mr Mark Keeling for sponsoring the meeting.

I am delighted that so many people have contribution to this volume. I am aware that there is a degree of overlap between chapters and in editing this volume I have intentionally left these in place. Few people will read the book from cover-to-cover and each chapter, therefore, is complete in itself. On occasion, conflicting views are given and again I have not edited these. It seems more important for the reader to appreciate the controversy rather than present the reader with bland uniformity.

I would like to express my thanks to all the authors for their contributions. I hope it will not be too long before another edition of this volume can be produced in which the pathogenesis can be clearly defined and definitive treatment suggested.

James Neuberger

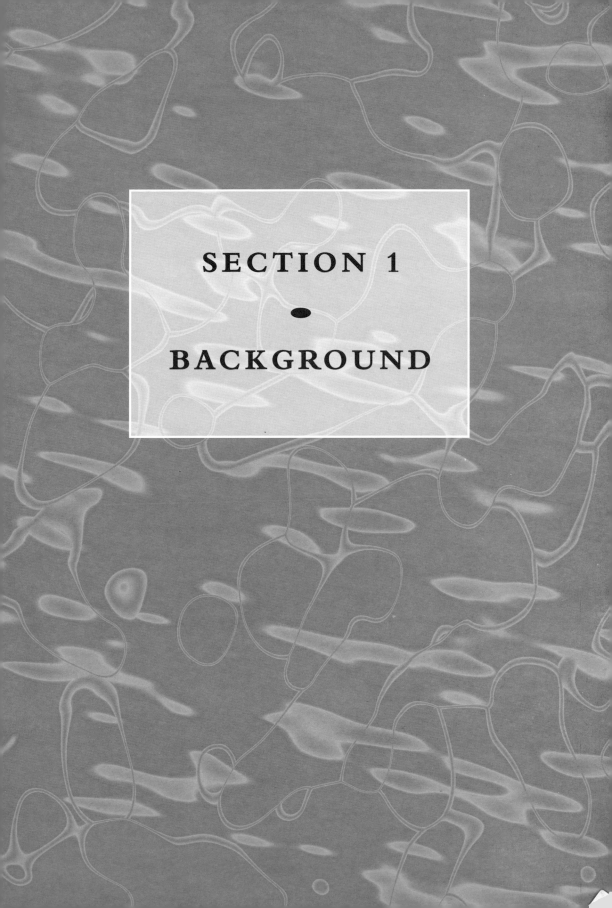

SECTION 1

—•—

BACKGROUND

PRIMARY BILIARY CIRRHOSIS: A HISTORICAL PERSPECTIVE

Jenny Heathcote

Department of Medicine, The Toronto Hospital,
University of Toronto, Toronto Ontario Canada.

In 1851, Addison and Gull described six patients with jaundice, vitiligo and xanthomas[1]. However, the term 'primary biliary cirrhosis (PBC)' was first used by Ahrens in 1950 indicating that the disease originated within the liver[2]. The term PBC is often a misnomer, as cirrhosis is not always present. However, the more appropriate descriptive term, 'chronic nonsuppurative granulomatous cholangitis', has never come into popular use. In 1966, the clear association of a non-organ, non-species specific antibody present in serum and directed towards mitochondria (identified using immunofluorescence techniques employing rat kidney and stomach) was described by Doniach et al[3]. Serum testing showed that patients with extrahepatic biliary obstruction were consistently AMA negative. At much the same, the histopathological features and stages of PBC were first clearly described by Scheuer[4]. By the mid-1960's a confident diagnosis of PBC could be made in a patient with a compatible clinical history, physical examination and biochemical tests who tested AMA positive and had a confirmatory or diagnostic liver biopsy. The introduction of ultrasound and endoscopic retrograde cholangiopancreatography in the mid 1970's did not really assist in the diagnosis of PBC, rather these tests were able to exclude other chronic biliary disorders such as primary sclerosing cholangitis.

The reported association of many autoimmune diseases in patients diagnosed with PBC prompted the suggestion that the pathogenesis of PBC was autoimmune[5,6]. But the inciting antigen(s) remain elusive. In the 1980's Fussey et al. described the substrates to which mitochondrial antibodies were directed[7]. These are a family of enzymes (the 2-oxo acid dehydrogenase family) located on the inner membrane of mitochondria. Once the substrates were identified, more specific testing for AMA using ELISA and immunoblotting were developed. The sensitivity of these tests to diagnose patients with PBC remains at about 95%. Some patients with otherwise obvious PBC never have detectable antibodies to these mitochondrial antigens in their sera[8].

Other immunologic irregularities have been reported with PBC. Increased complement consumption was noted by Potter et al[9]. A relatively weak HLA class II association of PBC with DR8 has been described by many authors, but Manns et al. noted that the relative risk of patients with PBC carrying both HLA Class II DR8 and C4A-QA0 alleles was 183.75[10]. This observation would suggest that an autoimmune process and specific involvement of the complement system may play a role in the pathogenesis of PBC

More recently, studies have concentrated on the aberrant distribution of the inner mitochondrial membrane enzymes in the cytoplasm and on the apical membrane of biliary epithelial cells taken from patients with PBC, with or without AMA testing positive in sera[11]. It remains unclear whether this biliary epithelial cell staining is due to earlier bile duct injury, possibly induced by upregulated apoptosis, causing exposure to native mitochondrial membrane enzymes or due to 'molecular mimicry'[12]. Evidence of lymphocyte sensitisation to mitochondrial antigens has been found in peripheral circulating lymphocytes taken from patients with PBC[13].

The first asymptomatic cases of PBC were described in the English literature by Long et al.[14] who noted that of twenty patients who were asymptomatic, less than half became symptomatic in a follow-up of ten years. A decade later, Mitchison et al. identified patients who had the histologic findings of PBC but were not only asymptomatic but who had normal liver biochemistry, their only serum marker being a positive AMA in a titre of >1:40 by immunofluorescence[15]. In the 1990's it became apparent that patients could have clinical, biochemical and histological manifestations of PBC but remain AMA negative[8].

The first randomised controlled trial of therapy in PBC was initiated twenty years ago when it appeared that PBC was an autoimmune disease. Immunosuppressive therapy in the form of azathioprine, was thought to be appropriate, but two trials showed the drug to be relatively safe but ineffective. Subsequently, there have been several trials employing other immunosuppressive agents, namely cyclosporine, chlorambucil, methotrexate, and prednisolone, and none to date has shown a beneficial effect on the survival of patients with PBC. Many of these drugs have been associated with severe side effects so that their use is controversial in a disease whose natural history suggests a median survival of 12 years for symptomatic patients and 17 years for asymptomatic subjects.

Other modes of therapy thought to slow the progression of fibrosis and cholestasis have been tried. Both colchicine and D-penicillamine have been assessed in several randomised controlled trials. D-penicillamine therapy was associated with a very high rate of side-effects and no benefit was seen. Colchicine would appear to improve some aspects of liver function but none of the studies have been large enough to assess any potential benefit on survival. More recently, the hydrophilic bile acid, ursodeoxycholic acid (UDCA), shown to increase the transport of endogenous bile acids across the liver cell and the canalicular membrane thereby reducing the concentration of retained hydrophobic membrane-damaging bile acids[16,17], has been assessed in 10 different randomised controlled trials. The combined raw data from three of the largest trials employing 13-15 mg/kg/day UDCA has shown that this drug significantly delays the time to liver transplantation in patients with PBC[18]. However, liver transplantation still remains the only definitive treatment for this disease even though the disease has been shown to recur in the liver allograft in some patients despite the ongoing use of immunosuppressive therapy[19].

One hundred and fifty years have passed since the first recognition of PBC as a specific disease of the liver. Over the last 30 years, the likely autoimmune origin of PBC has been realised, but the exact pathogenesis remains obscure and currently no drug therapy has been shown to reverse the disease, only liver transplantation is curative.

REFERENCES

1. Addison T, Gull W. On a certain affection of the skin, vitiligoidea - a plana, b tuberosa. *Guy's Hosp Rep* 1851; **7**: 265-276.

2. Ahrens EH, Rayne MA, Kunkle HG, Eisenmenger WH, Blondeim SH. Primary biliary cirrhosis. *Medicine* 1950; **29**: 299-364.

3. Doniach D, Roitt IM, Walker JG, et al. Tissue antibodies in primary biliary cirrhosis, active chronic (lupoid) hepatitis, cryptogenic cirrhosis and other liver diseases and their clinical implications. *Clin Exp Immunol* 1966; **1**: 237-262.

4. Scheuer PJ. Primary biliary cirrhosis. *Proc R Soc Med* 1967; **60**: 1257-1260.

5. Golding PL, Brown R, Mason AMS, Taylor E. "Sicca complex" in liver disease. *Br Med J* 1970; **4**: 340-342.

6. Culp KS, Fleming CR, Duffy J, et al. Autoimmune associations in primary biliary cirrhosis. *Mayo Clin Proc* 1982; **57**: 365-370.

7. Fussey S, Guest JR, James O, et al. Identification and analysis of the major M2 autoantigens in primary biliary cirrhosis. *Proc Natl Acad Sci* 1988; **85**: 8654-8658.

8. Michieletti P, Wanless IR, Katz A, et al. Antimitochondrial antibody negative primary biliary cirrhosis: a distinct syndrome of autoimmune cholangitis. *Gut* 1994; **35**: 260-265.

9. Potter BJ, Elias E, Jones A. Hypercatabolism of the third component of complement in patients with primary biliary cirrhosis. *J Lab Clin Med* 1976; **88**: 427-439.

10. Manns MP, Bremm A, Schneider PM, et al. HLA Drw8 and complement C4 deficiency as risk factors in primary biliary cirrhosis. *Gastroenterology* 1991; **101**: 1367-1373.

11. Tsuneyama K, Van de Water J, Van Thiel D, Coppel R, Ruebner B, Nakanuma Y, Dickson ER, Gershwin ME. Abnormal expression of PDC-E2 on the apical surface of biliary epithelial cells in patients with antimitochondrial antibody-negative primary biliary cirrhosis. *Hepatology* 1995; **22**: 1440-6.

12. Burroughs AK, Butler P, Sternberg MJE, Baum H. Molecular mimicry in liver disease. *Nature* 1992; **358**: 377-378.

13. Jones DEJ, Palmer JM, Yeaman SJ, Bassendine MF, Diamond AG. T-cell responses to natural human proteins in primary biliary cirrhosis. *Clin Exp Immunol* 1997; **107**: 562-568.

14. Long RG, Scheuer PJ, Sherlock S. Presentation and course of asymptomatic primary biliary cirrhosis. *Gastroenterology* 1977; **72**: 1204-1207.

15. Mitchison HC, Bassendine MF, Hendrick A, Bennett MK, Bird G, Watson AJ, James OFW. Positive antimitochondrial antibody but normal alkaline phosphatase: is this primary biliary cirrhosis? *Hepatology* 1986; **6**: 1279-1284.

16. Jazrawi RP, Caestecker JS, Goggin PM, Britten AJ, Joseph AEA, Maxwell JD, Northfield TC. Kinetics of hepatic bile acid handling in cholestatic liver disease: Effect of ursodeoxycholic acid. *Gastroenterology* 1994; **106**: 134-142.

17. Setchell KDR, Rodrigues CMP, Clerici C, et al. Bile acid concentrations in human and rat liver tissue and in hepatocyte nuclei. *Gastroenterology* 1997; **112**: 226-235.

18. Poupon RE, Lindor KD, Cauch-Dudek K, Dickson ER, Poupon R, Heathcote EJ. Combined analysis of randomised controlled trials of ursodeoxycholic acid in primary biliary cirrhosis. *Gastroenterology* 1997; **113**: 884-890.

19. Dmitrewski J, Hübscher SG, Mayer AD, Neuberger JM. Recurrence of primary biliary cirrhosis in the liver allograft: the effect of immunosuppression. *J Hepatol* 1996; **24**: 253-257.

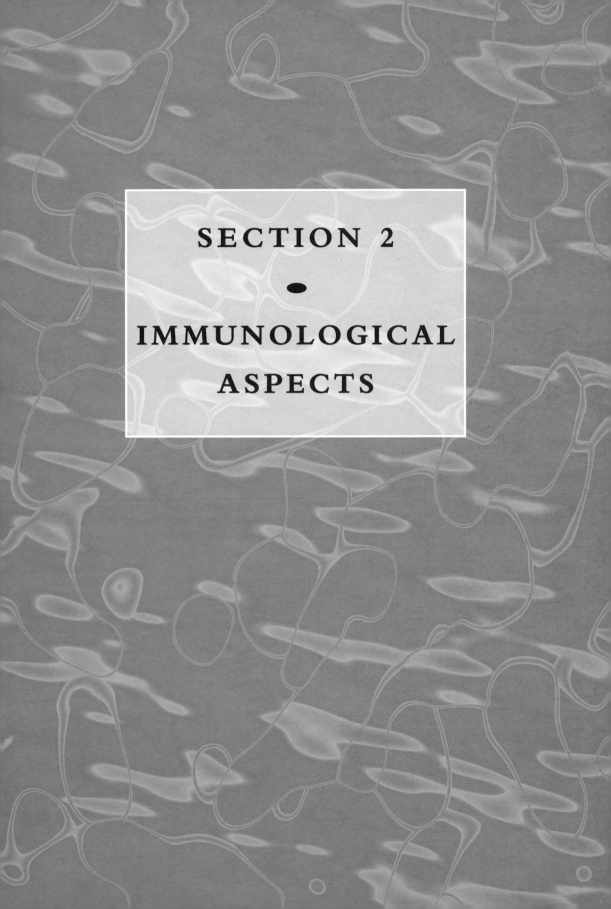

SECTION 2

•

IMMUNOLOGICAL ASPECTS

BILIARY EPITHELIAL CELLS IN PRIMARY BILIARY CIRRHOSIS

Ruth Joplin, Adrian Keogh, James Neuberger

Liver Research Laboratories, University Hospital,
Birmingham, B15 2TH.

SUMMARY

A continuing question in primary biliary cirrhosis (PBC) is the extent to which biliary epithelial cells (BEC) abnormality might contribute to the progressive damage to the intrahepatic biliary ducts. Many potential mechanisms exist which could account for destruction of portions of the biliary tree. Interruption of the peribiliary plexus by which the biliary tract receives it's blood supply is just one such possibility. Other possibilities include mechanical blockage of biliary ducts of a certain diameter or reaction to potentially toxic factors in bile. Thus it is conceivable to account for the heterogeneous disappearance of biliary ducts in PBC without invoking a primary mechanism involving BEC. Nonetheless, in recent years BEC have been shown increasingly not to be a simple inert lining to the biliary ducts but to have important functions such as modulation of bile. They also form an important immunological barrier at the interface between liver and gastro-intestinal tract. BEC are increasingly recognised as immunologically active; they respond actively to cytokine stimulation by expression and secretion of a number of immunological molecules. BEC in sections of PBC liver have been shown to express molecules requisite for immune recognition including MHC Class II, ICAM-1 and B7 co-stimulatory factors. In addition enhanced expression of specific mitochondrial autoantigen is also present on BEC in PBC. That expression of B7 is relatively weak suggests that BEC may not be important antigen presenting cells but this does not exclude them from being targets for CD8+ cytotoxic T-cells. Alternatively, they may present antigen via other co-stimulatory routes which do not utilize the B7/CD28 system. The availability of human BEC *in vitro* will permit better definition of such characteristics and may ultimately contribute new understanding to the part played by BEC in generation of NSDC in PBC.

Primary biliary cirrhosis (PBC) is characterised by non-suppurative destructive cholangitis (NSDC), specifically involving small to medium sized interlobular biliary ducts. A histologically similar lesion characterizes graft versus host disease (GVHD), the result of a well defined allo-immune reaction. It is thus, generally considered that the biliary tract damage in PBC is also immune-mediated and parallels with organ-specific autoimmune conditions are apparent. However there are also paradoxes. Firstly, a major autoimmune feature associated with PBC is the presence of disease specific but tissue non-specific autoantibodies. It is difficult to envisage that immune reaction to widely distributed antigens can induce damage so highly focused that only a minor population of cells is destroyed; in the case of PBC, the biliary epithelial cells (BEC). Secondly, the major PBC autoantibodies recognise mitochondrial antigens. Such antigens are normally shielded from the immune system by virtue of their intracellular location. Study of the biliary tract which might shed light on these paradoxes has been hampered by lack of an appropriate experimental model with which to study autoimmune recognition of biliary ductules. If BEC are destroyed by

autoimmunological mechanisms in PBC they must differ antigenically from other epithelial populations that escape damage; immunohistochemical studies of BEC in tissue sections support this contention. However, there are difficulties associated with interpreting results of such studies. BEC are sparsely distributed in liver sections and there can be problems with obtaining an adequate representative sample. This is particularly relevant in PBC as there is considerable heterogeneity in extent of disease within individual organs. Recently, new methods of studying BEC have been developed which allow analysis of a larger sample of cells. Such studies are enhancing our understanding of the normal and patho-biology of BEC, including their role in PBC.

The normal biliary tree

The normal intrahepatic biliary tree is a system of branching ductules and ducts which ramify throughout the parenchyma and drain bile toward the hilum of the liver for excretion. Conventionally biliary ducts are classified according to their diameter (see Table 1). The luminal surface of the biliary ducts is lined by a simple epithelium, the biliary epithelium. In common with other

TABLE 1: CLASSIFICATION OF BILIARY DUCTS IN THE NORMAL BILIARY TRACT

Classification	Diameter
Biliary ductules (BD)	<15μm
Interlobular ducts (ILD)	>15μm <100μm
*Septal ducts (SD)	>100μm <400μm
*Segmental ducts	>400μm <800μm
*Main R and L hepatic ducts	800μm
*Extrahepatic biliary ducts	

*Few bile ducts >100μm are involved in PBC and will not be considered further here. For review see Desmet[1]

epithelia, BEC are situated on a basement membrane and demonstrate polarity; the nucleus is situated toward the basal pole while the luminal aspect possesses numerous microvilli. Junctional complexes between adjacent cells create a barrier which is impermeable to bile. Organelles are scant. Considerable morphological, phenotypic and functional homogeneity is apparent between BEC in different regions of the normal biliary tract although some minor heterogeneity between different BEC populations has been reported (Table 2).

Morphological heterogeneity relates mostly to the size and shape of the cells. Cells lining ductules are cuboidal and have a high nucleo-cytoplasmic ratio but become taller and the nucleo-cytoplasmic ratio decreases with increasing duct diameter[1]. In the rat, secretin receptors (secretin R), chloride/bicarbonate anion exchanger-2 (AE-2) and cystic fibrosis transductance regulator (CFTR) are present on the apical plasma membrane of BEC lining medium and large ducts but not small ductules[2]. However, the evidence for heterogeneity between BEC from ducts of different sizes in normal human liver is less certain. Housset et al, found little heterogeneity between BEC lining the differing classes of ducts and ductules in normal human liver[5]. AE-2 was

found on canaliculi and all classes of intrahepatic biliary ducts except large, segmental ducts indicating a species difference in the expression of this antigen. Much more heterogeneity between bile duct cell populations is seen in diseased liver as will be considered later (Table 3). It is noteworthy however, that in studies using rat liver, the bile ductular population is frequently expanded by bile duct ligation, a situation analogous to biliary obstruction in humans. Thus the heterogeneities reported in rats may be a reflection of liver pathology due to biliary obstruction by the ligature.

The biliary tract in primary biliary cirrhosis

Morphologically, PBC is classified by histological staging of the granulomatous cholangitis. Pre-cirrhotic PBC is characterised by NSDC. Dense accumulations of immune cells are present adjacent to biliary ducts, and mononuclear cells infiltrate the duct walls. The biliary epithelium lining is irregular and desquamated. Fibrosis produces focal breaks of continuity in the ducts localized to points of inflammatory reaction. Various ultrastructural abnormalities have been reported in BEC in PBC including mitochondrial anomalies paralleling the presence of mitochondrial antibodies. Mitochondria appear variably enlarged, edematous, increased in number and excessively branching[8-9].

Mechanisms involved in disruption of the biliary epithelium in PBC remain poorly understood. A number of phenotypic heterogeneities have been reported suggesting that some BEC are antigenically distinct; well documented are molecules associated with immune recognition of targets including lymphocyte adhesion molecules, major histocompatibility complex (MHC) antigens and lymphocyte co-stimulatory molecules (Table 3). However these molecules are commonly induced in liver disease and are not specific for PBC. A few studies have reported antigens which appear to be altered specifically in PBC. These include anion

TABLE 2: HETEROGENEITY WITHIN THE NORMAL HUMAN BILIARY TRACT

	BD	ILD	SD	S/EHD	Ref
Morphology	small cuboidal	cuboidal	columnar	columnar	1
Phenotype					
*egp34	+	+	+	+	3
*CK-19	+	+	+	+	4
CFTR	+	+	+	+	5
AE-2	+	+	+	-	5
BGA(ABH)	-	-	+	ND	6
Clones 14 + 26	-	-	+	ND	7

S/EHD= segmental and extrahepatic ducts, * Homogenous distribution of antigen on ducts and ductules of all sizes exchanger-2 (AE-2), a chloride bicarbonate exchanger present on the apical membrane of all BEC except for those lining segmental ducts[18]. Expression of AE-2 is reduced in PBC BEC relative to normal and other liver disease controls[19]. It is not known how AE-2 could be involved in either the pathogenesis or progression of PBC but abnormal anion exchange could contribute to cholestasis and extrahepatic manifestations such as the polyglandular features frequently seen in PBC. It could also render BEC susceptible to changes in autoantigens.

TABLE 3: PHENOTYPIC CHANGES TO BILIARY EPITHELIUM IN PBC-				
	Normal	PBC	OLD	Ref
No change				
egp34	+	+	+	10
CK-19	+	+	+	10
MHC Class I	+	+	+	11
MCA151A	+	+	+	12
PBC non-specific				
MHC Class II	-	+/-	+/-	13-14
ICAM-1	-	+/-	+/-	15
B7	-	+/-	+/-	16-17
PBC specific				
AE-2	+	-/+	+	18-19
PDC-E2	+	+++	+	20-21
PDC-E3bp	+	+++	+	22

Key: MCA151A antigen of the mitochondrial inner membrane   +/- heterogeneous induction of positivity
      +   homogenous positivity   -/+ decrease in positivity
      -        negative   +++ heterogeneous increase in positivity

TABLE 4: EXPERIMENTAL MODELS OF PRIMARY BILIARY CIRRHOSIS			
	AMA	NSDC	Ref
(PBC)	+	+	
AMA + NSDC -			
Immunization with r-PDC-E2	+	-	24
AMA - NSDC +			
Mdr2 knockout	-	+	25
Il2 knockout	-	+	26
Bacterial LPS	-	+	27
Freunds complete adjuvent	-	+	27
Mycoplasma	-	+/-	28
SCID mice	-	+	29
AMA +/- NSDC +/-			
GVHD	+/-	+	30
Immunization of rats with BEC	a-BEC	+	31
Immunization of mice with BEC	+/-	+/-	32
Spontaneous (rabbit/mouse)	+/-/a-BEC	+/-	33-34
Immunization with n-PDC-E2	+	ND	35

Key: a-BEC   BECspecific mitochondrial non-specific antibodies   NSDC non supportive destructive cholongitis
      r-PDC-E2   recombinant human PDC-E2   AMA   Antimitochondrial antibody generated
      n-PDC-E2   natural human PDC-E2

The major autoantigens in PBC, pyruvate dehydrogenase-E2 (PDC-E2) and E3 binding protein (PDC-E3bp, previously known as PDC-X) are up-regulated in BEC in PBC[20-22]. Furthermore, this up-regulation is present early in the natural history of PBC[16] and is also present in BEC in allografts of patients with recurrent PBC following liver transplantation[23], suggesting a role for these antigens in the pathogenesis and/or progression of PBC.

Experimental models of primary biliary cirrhosis

A wide range of potential animal models of PBC have been reported but as yet, none fully reflects the range of features which characterize PBC (Table 4). In theory autoimmunity should be inducible by immunizing experimental animals with autoantigen. However,

immunization of a wide range of laboratory animals (rats, rabbits, mice, guinea-pigs and monkeys) with recombinant human PDC-E2 resulted in generation of antimitochondrial antibodies (AMA) but not NSDC or extrahepatic, polyglandular manifestations (EHM) found in PBC[24]. More recently, Bassendine et al, used natural human PDC-E2 in Freund's complete adjuvant to immunize autoimmune susceptible inbred female mice. All five of the mouse strains tested produced AMA and in one, NSDC was observed, although no data was available regarding EHM[35]. However, Freund's complete adjuvant alone can produce granulomatous lesions of the portal tracts in susceptible strains[27]. In other

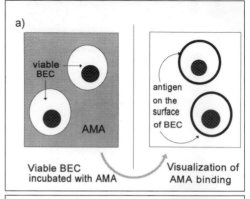

a)

viable BEC

AMA

Viable BEC incubated with AMA

antigen on the surface of BEC

Visualization of AMA binding

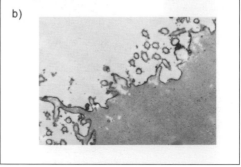

b)

Figure 2. **Detection of plasma membrane antigen on biliary epithelial cells**[38]
The scheme (a) illustrates differential staining of the plasma membrane. Viable BEC purified from patients with PBC and controls were attached to glass cover slips and incubated with anti-E2/E3bp (1:10) for 30 minutes at 4°C. After washing in PBS, the cells were incubated with biotinylated goat anti-human IgG (30 mins at 4°C). The cells were washed x 3 in PBS before fixing in 2.5% glutaraldehyde for 30 mins. After further washes the fixed cells were incubated with streptavidin horseradish peroxidase for 30 mins at room temperature. Sites of primary antibody binding were visualized using 3,3'-diaminobenzidine substrate. The specimens were osmicated with 4% osmium tetroxide and processed for transmission electron microscopy. Ultra-thin sections (70nm) were observed using a Jeol 100 electron microscope. BEC isolated from patients with PBC, but not controls showed staining associated with the plasma membrane. The figure (b) shows anti-E2/E3bp binding to the plasma membrane of a BEC purified from the liver of a patient with PBC. Positive staining appears as a black precipitate and is limited to the plasma membrane; antibody has not penetrated into the interior of the cell.

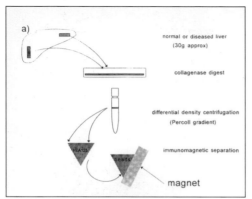

a)

normal or diseased liver (30g approx)

collagenase digest

differential density centrifugation (Percoll gradient)

immunomagnetic separation

magnet

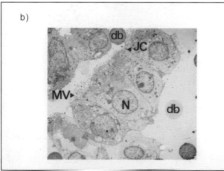

b)

Figure 1. **Isolation of biliary epithelial cells from normal and diseased human liver**[37]
The scheme (a) illustrates immunomagnetic purification of BEC from normal and diseased human liver. Liver is finely diced and digested with collagenase Type 1A (37°C for 2-3 hours). BEC are purified by centrifugation on a Percoll gradient (equal volumes of 1.04g/ml and 1.09g/ml Percoll at 800g for 30 mins). The semi pure cells which equilibrate at the interphase between 1.04 and 1.09 g/ml Percoll are incubated with mouse monoclonal antibody to egp[34] (HEA125) followed by magnetic extraction using antibody coated magnetic beads (10^7 sheep anti-mouse IgG coated dynabeads). The freshly isolated cells show typical epithelial cell morphology and ultrastructure being polar cells with nucleus (N) toward the basal pole and microvilli (MV) at the apical surface. The cells purify as aggregates and junctional complexes are evident between adjacent cells (JC). The figure (b) shows BEC purified from the liver of a patient with PBC. (db = dynabeads).

studies, immunization of severe combined immuno-deficient (SCID) mice with peripheral blood lymphocytes from patients with PBC resulted in both AMA and NSDC but this could have been through a GVHD mechanism[29]. Attempts to use GVHD as a model for PBC resulted in NSDC and EHM but not consistently, AMA and immunization with allogeneic or xenogeneic BEC or a range of infectious organisms variably

induced NSDC, AMA or other BEC specific antibody (see Table 4 for detail).

Because of difficulties in obtaining the full spectrum of features associated with PBC in an animal model we have developed a model using human BEC *in vitro* (correlated wherever practical with observation of cells *in vivo*).

Biliary epithelial cells in primary biliary cirrhosis: an in vitro model

BEC are purified immunomagnetically using the mouse monoclonal antibody HEA125 which recognises a

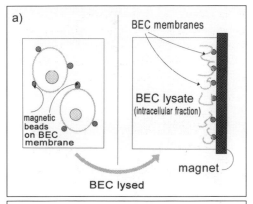

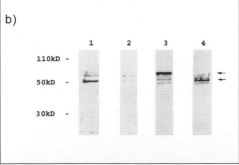

Figure 3. **Characterisation of BEC mitochondrial and plasma membrane antigens**[39].

The scheme (a) shows how BEC plasma membranes were prepared free from contamination by mitochondrial membranes. Viable BEC were incubated with HEA125 and sheep anti-mouse IgG coated dynabeads. The cells were then lysed and the beads with adherent plasma membranes were harvested using a magnetic particle concentrator. The lysate constituted the intracellular fraction which contained mitochondrial antigen. The bead/plasma membrane complexes were washed x3 in PBS and harvested magnetically. The separate plasma membrane and intracellular fractions were subjected to PAGE and western blotting with anti-E2/E3bp. In controls in which no separation of plasma membrane from mitochondrial protein was performed, two bands were seen corresponding to PDC-E2 and PDC-E3bp. The intensity of PDC-E3bp was higher in BEC from patients with PBC than controls. When the separate sub-cellular fractions were analyzed the mitochondrial fraction contained both PDC-E2 and PDC-E3bp (albeit at relatively lower concentration than in unfractionated samples). When the plasma membrane fraction was analyzed, a band which fractionated with PDC-E3bp was detected but not PDC-E2. The figure (b) shows - lane 1, BEC with a patient with PBC (membrane and intracellular fractions combined); lane 2, normal BEC; lane 3, intracellular fraction of BEC from a patient with PBC; lane 4, plasma membrane fraction of BEC from a patient with PBC. In lanes 1-3, two bands are present representing PDC-E2 and PDC-E3bp (upper and lower arrows respectively). In lane 4 only one band is present which fractionates with PDC-E3bp.

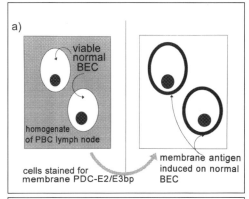

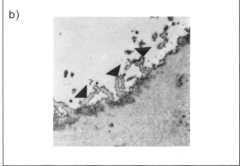

Figure 4. **Induction of plasma membrane PDC-E2/E3bp on normal biliary epithelial cells**[40]

In previous studies we demonstrated high intensity of PDC-E2 in portal lymph nodes of patients with PBC but not controls[20]. To see whether normal BEC could be induced to show the characteristic membrane antigen seen previously on PBC BEC we incubated BEC purified from normal livers with homogenates of portal lymph nodes taken from the hilum of livers of patients with PBC and controls. The lymph nodes were homogenized at 0.5g/ml in distilled water and the osmolarity was adjusted by addition of an equal volume of 2x PBS. The homogenates were diluted 1:10 in BEC culture medium before addition to viable BEC (scheme a). BEC were cultured with homogenates for 18 hours before washing and addition of fresh medium. Culture was continued for a further 7 days after which cells were stained for the presence of plasma membrane antigen as described in figure 2 (see above). BEC cultured with PBC lymph node homogenates, but not control nodes, showed plasma membrane staining in a pattern similar to that previously seen only in PBC. The figure (b) shows a BEC from a normal subject which had been incubated with PBC lymph node homogenate and stained for plasma membrane antigen. A linear pattern of staining was detected (arrows) similar to the pattern seen on PBC BEC (compare figs 2 and 4).

34kD epithelial glycoprotein (egp34) present on the surface of BEC but not other cells in liver[37]. The freshly isolated cells are predominantly cuboidal/columnar and demonstrate polarity (Figure 1). Yield is approximately 10[4] BEC per gram of liver and up to 50-100 grams can be used to generate a larger, more representative sample of cells than is available in tissue sections. The availability of PBC BEC *in vitro* has permitted a number of studies which were impossible using tissue sections, including studies to localize the sub-cellular distribution of autoantigen, to characterize BEC antigens and to explore mechanisms involved in induction and recognition of autoantigen.

Studies using purified BEC

1) Sub-cellular distribution of PDC-E2/PDC-E3bp; AMA bind to the plasma membrane of PBC BEC[38]

High precision sub-cellular localization of antigens can be undertaken using purified BEC. To determine the presence of plasma membrane antigen, viable BEC were incubated with antibody to PDC-E2 and PDC-E3bp (anti-E2/E3bp) (see Figure 2 for detail). Under these conditions antibody is excluded from the cell interior and can only access antigen associated with the external aspect of the cells. This technique revealed that anti-E2/E3bp bound to the external aspect of BEC from patients with PBC but not controls. The results suggest that altered sub-cellular distribution of PDC-E2/E3bp may participate in immune recognition of BEC.

2) Characterisation of mitochondrial and plasma membrane antigen; a PBC BEC plasma membrane antigen has features consistent with PDC-E3bp[39]

Separate preparations of BEC membrane and cytoplasmic antigens (including mitochondrial antigen) were prepared and subjected to polyacrylamide gel electrophoresis and Western blotting using anti-E2/E3bp (see Figure 3 for detail). Both PDC-E2 and PDCE3bp were detected in the cytoplasmic fraction. In PBC BEC a 50kD antigen was detected in the plasma membrane fraction. The results suggest firstly that the plasma membrane antigen may be PDC-E3bp and secondly that no other cross-reactive antigen is involved although the possibility exists that additional,

conformational epitopes may have been missed by Western blotting.

3) Induction of PDC-E2/E3bp; the PBC plasma membrane antigen can be induced on normal BEC[40]

Normal BEC were incubated with homogenates of lymph node from patients with PBC (see Figure 4 for detail). The normal BEC were induced to show a membrane distribution of antigen. This distribution had been observed previously only on BEC from patients with PBC. These results suggest that PBC tissue contains a transmissible factor which is able to induce normal BEC to behave as PBC BEC.

4) MHC Class II can be induced on biliary epithelial cells in vitro by incubation with pro-inflammatory cytokine[41-43]

A number of studies have been undertaken in which the ability of cytokines to induce MHC Class II on BEC has been studied. Results parallel observations of BEC in tissue sections. BEC from normal liver can be induced to express MHC Class II by addition of interferon gamma (gIFN) or interleukin 1 (IL1) to the culture medium41-42. BEC from patients with PBC appear more sensitive to gIFN and IL1 than BEC from normal subjects; MHC Class II can be induced with as little as 0.1 U/ml gIFN in PBC BEC compared with 10 U/ml in normal BEC[43].

5) Lymphocytes from patients with PBC are cytotoxic for autologous BEC[44]

BEC were incubated with autologous lymphocytes and cytotoxicity was determined by lactate dehydrogenase release. Lymphocytes from patients with PBC were more cytotoxic for autologous BEC than controls.

6) Functional studies

In a number of other studies function[45], adhesion[46] and cytokine production[47] were studied. Functional studies of AE-2 in normal BEC demonstrated species difference in regulation of bicarbonate secretion between humans and rodents[45] reflecting previous studies[2,5,18] which demonstrated species difference in the distribution of this and other antigens. Further immunological aspects relating to lymphocyte recognition and adhesion to BEC will be considered more fully by Adams and Shields.

REFERENCES

1. Desmet VJ, Roskams T & De Vos R. Gallbladder and bile ducts: normal anatomy. In: Gastroenterology and hepatology: the comprehensive visual reference. Feldman M, Ed. Volume "Gallbladder and bile ducts", La Russo N, Ed. Philadelphia: Current Medicine G, Glaser.

2. Alpini G, Roberts S, Kuntz SM et al. Morphological, molecular and functional heterogeneity of cholangiocytes from normal rat liver. *Gastroenterol* 1996; **110**: 1636-43.

3. Momburg F, Moldenhauer G, Hammerling GH et al. Immunohistochemical study of the surface expression of a Mr 34,000 human epithelium-specific glycoprotein in normal and malignant tissues. *Cancer Res* 1987; **47**: 2883-91.

4. van Eyken P, Sciot R, van Damme B et al. Keratin immunohistochemistry in normal liver. Cytokeratin pattern of hepatocytes, bile ducts and acinar gradient. *Virchows Archives* 1987; **412**: 63-72.

5. Scoazec JY, Bringuier AF, Medina JF et al. The plasma membrane polarity of human biliary epithelial cells: in situ immunohistochemical analysis and functional implications. *J Hepatol* 1997; **26**: 543-53.

6. Okada Y, Jinnon K, Shousuke M et al. Blood group antigens in the intra-hepatic biliary tree. 1. Distribution in normal liver. *J Hepatol* 1988; **6**: 63-70.

7. Ayres RCS, Hübscher SG, Shaw J et al. New monoclonal antibodies reacting with bile ducts: further insights into the pathogenesis of bile ductular proliferation in biliary disease. *J Pathol* 1991; **165**: 153-61.

8. Bernuau D, Feldmann G, Degott C et al. Ultrastructural lesions of bile ducts in primary biliary cirrhosis. Human Pathol 1981; 12: 782-93.

9. Tobe K. Electron microscopy of liver lesions in primary biliary cirrhosis. Acta Pathol Jpn 1982; 32: 57-70.

10. Joplin R, Strain AJ & Neuberger JM. Biliary epithelial cells from the liver of patients with primary biliary cirrhosis: isolation, characterisation and short-term culture. J Pathol 1990; 162: 255-60.

11. Barbatis C, Woods J, Morton JA et al. Immunohistochemical analysis of HLA (A,B,C) antigens in liver disease using a monoclonal antibody. Gut 1981; 22: 985-91.

12. Joplin R, Johnson GD, Matthews JB et al. Distribution of pyruvate dehydrogenase dihydrolipoamide acetyltransferase (PDC-E2) and another mitochondrial marker in salivary gland and biliary epithelium from patients with primary biliary cirrhosis. Hepatol 1994; 19: 1375-80.

13. Ballardini G, Mirikian R, Bianchi RB et al. Aberrant expression of HLA-DR antigens on bile duct epithelium in primary biliary cirrhosis. Lancet 1984; 2: 1009-13.

14. van den Oord J, Sciot R & Desmet VJ. Expression of MHC products by normal and abnormal bile duct epithelium. J Hepatol 1986; 3: 310-17.

15. Adams DH, Hübscher SG, Shaw J et al. Increased expression of intercellular adhesion molecule-1 (ICAM-1) on bile ducts in primary biliary cirrhosis and primary sclerosing cholangitis. Hepatol 1991; 14: 426-31.

16. Tsuneyama K, Van de Water J, Leung PSC et al. Abnormal expression of the E2 component of the pyruvate dehydrogenase complex on the luminal surface of biliary epithelium occurs before major histocompatibility complex Class-II and BB1/B7 expression. Hepatol 1995; 21: 1031-7.

17. Spengler U, Leifeld L, Braunschweiger I et al. Anomalous expression of costimulatory molecules B7-1, B7-2 and CD28 in primary biliary cirrhosis. J Hepatol 1997; 26: 31-6.

18. Martinez-Anso E, Castillo JE, Diez J et al. Immunohistochemical detection of chloride/bicarbonate anion-exchangers in human liver. Hepatol 1994; 19: 1400-6.

19. Medina JF, Martinez-Anso E, Vasquez JJ et al. Decreased anion exchanger 2 Immunoreactivity in the liver of patients with primary biliary cirrhosis. Hepatol 1997; 25: 12-17.

20. Joplin R, Lindsay JG, Hübscher SG et al. Distribution of dihydrolipoamide acetyltransferase (E2) in the liver and portal lymph nodes of patients with primary biliary cirrhosis: an immunohistochemical study. Hepatol 1991; 14: 442-7.

21. Van de Water J, Ansari A, Surh CD et al. Evidence for targeting by 2-oxo-dehydrogenase enzymes in the T-cell response of primary biliary cirrhosis. J Immunol 1991; 146: 89-94.

22. Joplin R, Wallace LL, Johnson GD et al. Distribution of component X of pyruvate dehydrogenase dihydrolipoamide acetyltransferase complex (PDC-X) in liver and salivary gland of patients with primary biliary cirrhosis (PBC) and controls. Hepatol 1994; 20: 150A/213.

23. Van de Water J, Gerson LB, Ferrell LD et al. Immunohistochemical evidence of disease recurrence after liver transplantation for primary biliary cirrhosis. Hepatology 1996; 24: 1079-84.

24. Krams SM, Surh CD, Coppel RL et al. Immunization of experimental animals with dihydrolipoamide acetyltransferase, as a purified recombinant polypeptide, generates mitochondrial antibodies but not primary biliary cirrhosis. Hepatol 1989; 9: 411-16.

25. Howell CD, Yoder T, Clanman HN et al. Hepatic homing of mononuclear inflammatory cells isolated during murine chronic graft-vs-host disease. J Immunol 1989; 143: 476-83.

26. Smit JJM, Schinkel AH, Oude Elferink RPJ et al. Homozygous disruption of the murine mdr2 p-glycoprotein gene leads to a complete absence of phospholipid from bile and to liver disease. Cell 1994; 460.

27. Sadlack B, Lohler J, Schorle H et al. Generalized autoimmune disease in interleukin-2-deficient mice is triggered by an uncontrolled activation and proliferation of CD4+ T-cells. Eur J Immunol 1995; 25: 3053-9.

28. Ide T, Sata M, Suzuki H et al. An experimental model of primary biliary cirrhosis induced by lipopolysaccharide and pyruvate dehydrogenase. Kurume Med J. 1996; 43: 185-8.

29. Johnson L, Wirostko E & Wirostko W. Primary biliary cirrhosis in the mouse: induction by human mycoplasma-like organisms. Int J Exp Pathol 1990; 71: 701-12.

30. Krams SM, Dorshkind K & Gershwin ME. Generation of biliary lesions after transfer of human lymphocytes into severe combined immunodeficient (SCID) mice. J Exp Med 1989; 170: 1919-30.

31. Ueno Y, Phillips JO, Ludwig J et al. Development and characterisation of a rodent model of immune-mediated cholangitis. Proc Natl Acad Sci USA 1996; 93: 216-20.

32. Kobayashi H, Yamamoto K, Yoshioka T et al. Nonsuppurative cholangitis is induced in neonatally thymectomized mice: a possible animal model of primary biliary cirrhosis. Hepatol 1994; 19: 1424-30.

33. Tison V, Callea F, Morisi C et al. Spontaneous "primary biliary cirrhosis" in rabbits. Liver 1982; 2: 152-61.

34. Hayashi Y, Utuyama M, Kurashima C et al. Spontaneous development of organ specific autoimmune lesions in aged C57BL/6 mice. Clin Exp Immunol 1989; 78: 120-6.

35. Bassendine MF, Palmer JM, Decruz D et al. Approaches to a murine model of AMA positive non-suppurative destructive cholangitis (NSDC). J Hepatol. 1998; 28: 59.

36. Joplin R, Strain AJ & Neuberger JM. Immuno-isolation and culture of biliary epithelial cells from normal human liver. in vitro Dev Cell Biol 1989; 25: 1189-92.

37. Joplin R, Wallace LL, Johnson GD et al. Subcellular localization of pyruvate dehydrogenase dihydrolipoamide acetyltransferase in human intrahepatic biliary epithelial cells. J Pathol 1995; 176: 381-90.

38. Joplin R, Wallace LL, Lindsay JG et al. The human biliary epithelial cell plasma membrane antigen in primary biliary cirrhosis: pyruvate dehydrogenase X? Gastroenterol 1997; 113: 1727-33.

39. Sadamoto T, Joplin R, Keogh A et al. Expression of pyruvate dehydrogenase complex PDC-E2 on biliary epithelial cells induced by lymph nodes from primary biliary cirrhosis. Lancet 1998; 352: 1595-6.

40. Ayres RCS, Neuberger JM, Shaw J et al. Intercellular adhesion molecule-1 and MHC antigens on human intrahepatic biliary epithelial cells: effect of pro-inflammatory cytokines. Gut 1993; 34: 125-9.

41. Demetris AJ, Markus B, Saidman S et al. Establishment of primary cultures of human biliary epithelium and induction of Class II major histocompatibility complex antigens by interferon gamma. Trans Proc 1988; XX(1): 728-30.

42. Sadamoto T, Neuberger JM & Joplin R. Effect of pro-inflammatory cytokines on human biliary epithelial cells (BEC): interleukin 1 up-regulates pyruvate dehydrogenase E2/X (PDC-E2/X). Hepatol 1997; 26: 444A/1264.

43. Joplin R, Blake SMS, Wallace LL et al. Cytotoxicity of lymphocytes for autologous intrahepatic biliary epithelial cells in primary biliary cirrhosis. J Hepatol 1996; 25: 69.

44. Strazzabosco M, Joplin R, Zsembery A et al. Na+-dependent and -independent Cl-/HCO3- exchange mediate cellular HCO3 transport in cultured human intrahepatic bile duct cells. Hepatol 1997; 25: 976-85.

45. Leon MP, Bassendine MF, Gibbs P et al. Immunogenicity of biliary epithelium: study of adhesive interaction with lymphocytes. Gastroenterol 1997; 112: 968-77.

46. Morland C, Fear J, Joplin R et al. Human biliary epithelial cells express chemokines interleukin-8 and monocyte chemotactic protein-1 in response to inflammatory cytokine stimulation. Proc Association Am Physicians 1997; 109: 372-82.

LYMPHOCYTE RECRUITMENT & ACTIVATION IN PRIMARY BILIARY CIRRHOSIS

David H Adams, Philip L Shields

Liver Research Laboratories, University of Birmingham and
MRC Centre for Immune Regulation, Queen Elizabeth Hospital, Edgbaston, Birmingham, England

SUMMARY

Primary biliary cirrhosis is characterised by a chronic inflammatory infiltrate of the liver comprising predominantly T-lymphocytes associated with damage to intrahepatic bile ducts. The establishment of chronic inflammation depends upon the recruitment of lymphocytes from the circulation into the target tissue where they are then activated by exposure to antigen and retained by as yet poorly defined mechanisms. Factors in the local microenvironment will determine whether chronic inflammation is established and maintained and whether the recruited lymphocytes damage or destroy target structures. This article will concentrate on the mechanisms responsible for the recruitment and retention of lymphocytes in the liver in PBC and on mechanisms that may target this response to the intrahepatic bile ducts. The autoantigens involved are discussed elsewhere.

Extrathymic activation and differentiation of T-lymphocytes

During their maturation in the thymus lymphocytes are programmed to respond to specific peptide antigens. On leaving the thymus these naïve or virgin lymphocytes enter the circulation and are carried throughout the body. They express cell surface receptors that allow them to enter secondary lymphatic organs via specialized postcapillary venules, called high endothelial venules (HEV). Antigens are concentrated in lymphatic tissue were they are presented to lymphocytes by specialised dendritic cells, which migrate into the lymph node from tissues via the afferent lymphatics.[1] In the case of the liver hepatic dendritic cells are activated by antigen and migrate via the hepatic sinusoids to the lymphatics before accumulating selectively in the hepatic lymph nodes in the porta hepatis.[2] On entering lymph node, dendritic cells activate naïve T-cells to undergo clonal expansion into immunoblasts. During this activation the lymphocyte undergoes differentiation resulting in the expression of adhesion molecules that allow it to selectively home back to the tissue in which it was activated.[3,4] If the original antigen persists in the tissue infiltrating lymphocytes will be retained and activated and inflammation established. This results in the release of local cytokines which upregulate endothelial adhesion molecule and cytokine expression thereby providing signals that broaden leukocyte recruitment and retention.[5] Once the antigen has been removed the signal for lymphocyte activation will be removed and a complex series of events lead to the resolution of inflammation. During this quiescent phase lymphocytes will not be retained in the tissue and return via the lymphatics to the circulation where they exist as long-lived memory T-cells (Figure 1). The homing molecules induced on naïve cells during their activation persists on memory T-cells allowing these cells to subsequently migrate preferentially back to the tissue in which they were activated thereby enhancing their chances of encountering antigen again in the future.[6] It has been demonstrated that peripheral lymph nodes and mucosa-associated lymphoid tissues in the gut represent functionally distinct recirculation routes for immunoblast homing and recent evidence suggests that the liver also has the potential to recruit distinct subsets of lymphocytes.[7]

Molecular regulation of lymphocyte recruitment

In general terms lymphocyte recruitment into tissue is regulated by a complex cascade of adhesive interactions with the endothelium that allow a lymphocyte flowing at up to 500 micrometers/sec in the vessel lumen to be attracted and recruited across the endothelium (Figure 2).[6] Under conditions of shear stress, members of the selectin superfamily (P-, E- and L-selectin) and their mucin-type glycoprotein ligands (PSGL-1, MAdCAM-1 and PNAd) are the predominant molecules involved in initiating contacts between the lymphocyte and endothelial cell[1]. This initial transient, reversible binding causes the cells to roll on the vessel wall at a greatly reduced velocity thereby allowing it to be activated by local factors. The most important stimuli that activate rolling leukocytes are signals triggered by a special class of chemotactic cytokines

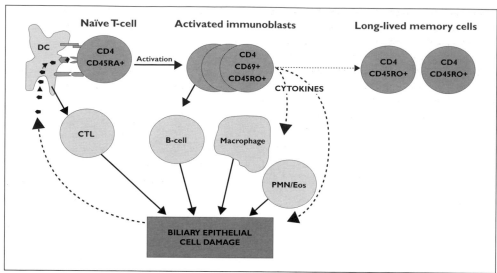

Figure 1. **Differentiation and activation of peripheral T-cells**

During their maturation in the thymus lymphocytes are programmed to respond to specific peptide antigens. On leaving the thymus these naïve lymphocytes circulate between blood and secondary lymphatic organs where antigens are concentrated and presented by specialised dendritic cells (DC). After activation by antigen in the liver DCs migrate into portal lymph node from the liver via the hepatic sinusoids and afferent lymphatics. DCs activate naïve T-cells to undergo clonal expansion into immunoblasts that subsequently selectivity home back to the liver and orchestrate the range of effector mechanisms mediated by cytotoxic lymphocytes (CTLs), antibodies, and other effector cells which results in damage to the biliary epithelium. In addition lymphocyte activation results in the generation of long-lived circulating memory T-cells.

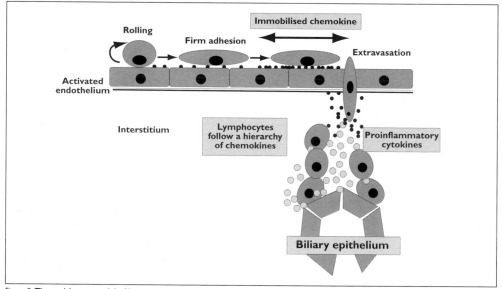

Figure 2. **The multi-step model of leucocyte-endothelial interactions and subsequent migration into and through tissue**

(1) Leucocytes are initially induced to roll on the endothelium by activation-independent primary adhesion (classically mediated by adhesion molecules called selectins).

(2) Firm adhesion is triggered when rolling leukocytes encounter chemokines present at the endothelial surface that engage specific G-protein binding, 7-transmembrane-spanning receptors on the leukocyte. This results in conformational activation of leukocyte adhesion molecules called integrins from a low-affinity to a high affinity state allowing them to bind strongly to endothelial counter-receptors such as ICAM-1 or VCAM-1 which brings the cell to a halt.

(3) Extravasation through the endothelium into tissue occurs in response to a gradient of chemokines and adhesion ligands.

(4) In tissue the leukocyte migrates along a hierarchy of different chemokines that direct it towards the inflammatory site where it is retained and effector functions activated resulting in either killing of invading pathogens, in an appropriate protective response, or the destruction of local tissues such as the biliary epithelium in primary biliary cirrhosis. Tissue inflammation results in the release of more chemokines and cytokines that then amplify and perpetuate leukocyte recruitment.

called chemokines that bind to specific g-protein-linked seven-pass transmembrane receptors on subsets of leukocytes. Activation of chemokine receptors on leukocytes triggers a conformational change in leukocyte integrins that promotes binding to endothelial counter-receptors such as ICAM-1, -2 and BCAm-1 resulting in strong, stationary adhesion which is followed by cell spreading and migration to intercellular endothelial junctions, through which it migrates into tissue in response to an immobilised gradient of chemokine.[8-10] The cell subsequently migrates through the extracellular matrix by a poorly understood process that requires regulated integrin function and a gradient of chemokine until it reaches the antigen-bearing target T-cell. There it will become activated if it expresses the appropriate antigen receptor. Activated T-cells are retained at the site of inflammation where they either destroy target cells after recognising antigen in the context of MHC antigens (cytotoxic cells) or secrete further cytokines and chemokines which can perpetuate the inflammatory response (helper cells).

Lymphocyte recruitment to the liver

Many adhesion molecules are constituitively expressed on certain cell types, whereas others can be induced and/or up-regulated upon inflammation.[5] The selectivity of the adhesion process is controlled, not only by selective expression of functionally active adhesion molecules but also by the requirement for several sequential adhesive events. Successful emigration into tissue requires at least four successive receptor-ligand interactions and if any of these are absent, recruitment into tissue will fail. The nature of the molecules involved in these steps in the liver is only beginning to be understood[1] (Table 1). Because the liver is a major site of antigen exposure, with its own lymphatic supply and resident lymphocyte population, it seems probable that specific mechanisms will have evolved to regulate hepatic lymphocyte homing and recruitment. The complex vascular anatomy of the liver means that there are different portals of entry for circulating leucocytes entering the liver via either the portal vein or the hepatic artery. These vessels enter the portal tracts where their terminal branches empty into the hepatic sinusoids that run between the liver cell plates, before emptying into the hepatic veins and returning to the inferior vena cava. The nature of an inflammatory response in the liver will be determined, at least in part, by where in this system lymphocytes bind to endothelium and leave the blood to enter liver tissue.[11] If this occurs in the sinusoids, lymphocytes will enter the parenchyma whereas extravasation across portal vessels will result in infiltration of the portal tracts.[7,12]

Hepatic lymphocyte-endothelial interactions take place in sinusoidal vessels under conditions of low-velocity blood flow. Leukocyte interactions with sinusoidal endothelium differ from those involved with post-capillary venules in several important aspects. The characteristic rolling phase of primary adhesion that is seen in interactions with post-capillary venules is not observed and adhesion to sinusoidal endothelium is unaffected in animals lacking endothelial selectins.[13] Retention of leukocytes in the hepatic sinusoids is, however, adhesion dependent because it is greatly reduced, although not abolished, in animals that lack ICAM-1 or in those treated with antibodies against ICAM-1. Antibodies to ICAM-1 also reduce binding of lymphocytes to human sinusoids in tissue section.[13,14] The paradigm of lymphocyte homing has emerged mainly from studies of continuous vascular endothelium in high-velocity vascular beds and the unique observations made from studies of the hepatic sinusoidal bed argues against generalization of the results obtained in more easily accessible model systems. The nature of putative tissue-specific activation signal(s) in the liver is unknown. None of the 50 plus chemokines identified to date appear to be truly tissue-specific and the exact mechanisms of lymphocyte recruitment through hepatic endothelium during both physiological homing and hepatic inflammation have only recently begun to be studied.

TABLE 1: EXAMPLES OF MOLECULES INVOLVED AT EACH STAGE IN THE INTERACTION OF LYMPHOCYTES WITH HEPATIC ENDOTHELIUM. SEVERAL OPTIONS ARE AVAILABLE AND THE PRECISE HIERACHY IS NOT YET KNOWN FOR MOST OF THE INTERACTIONS

	Tether	Trigger	Strong adhesion	Migration
Endothelium	VAP-1	IP-10	ICAM-1	RANTES
T-cell	VAP-1r	CXCR3	LFA-1	CCR5
Endothelium	?VCAM-1	RANTES	VCAM-1	MIP-1a
T-cell	VLA-4	CCR5	VLA-4	CCR5
Endothelium	–	MIP-1a	–	IP-10
T-cell		CCR5		CXCR3

Lymphocytes in human liver
Normal liver

The normal liver sinusoids contain large granular lymphocytes (Pit-cells), that are intimately associated with sinusoidal cells. These have natural killer cell activity and enter the liver from the circulation by a process involving adhesion to the sinusoidal endothelium.[15] In addition, the normal human liver contains significant numbers of T-lymphocytes in the portal tracts and scattered through the parenchyma. It has been suggested that some of these lymphocytes are activated T-cells that are removed by the liver and induced to undergo apoptosis. However in normal human liver relatively few liver-infiltrating lymphocytes express apoptotic markers and many are presumably patrolling the liver as part of the process of immune surveillance.[16]

Inflamed liver

Pathological infiltration of the liver by lymphocytes occurs in response to infectious agents, most notably the hepatitis viruses and in several autoimmune and inflammatory disorders including primary biliary cirrhosis. Liver-infiltrating lymphocytes in primary biliary cirrhosis are predominantly memory T-cells (i.e., cells that have been previously primed by antigen in lymph node) as defined by high levels of CD45RO and low levels on CD45RA on the cell surface when compared with autologous peripheral blood T-cells

(Figure 3)[17,18]. The liver-infiltrating cells are also highly activated as determined by high levels of expression of the activation antigens CD69 and HLA-DR low level expression of the differentiation antigen CD45RB suggests they are terminally differentiated.[18] These cells also express low levels of the growth factor receptors CD25 and CD71 suggesting that proliferation occurs at low levels within the liver. Functional defects in in vitro T-cell proliferation have also been described in PBC[19]. The distribution of hepatic infiltration can take several forms depending on the inflammatory stimulus. In primary biliary cirrhosis lymphocytic infiltration is localised predominantly to the portal tracts although lobular inflammation and infiltration of the parenchyma can be seen (see chapter by SG Hübscher elsewhere in this book). In addition many lymphocytes are seen in characteristic lymphoid aggregates and these structures have several features in common with classical lymph node follicles suggesting that they develop to promote the recruitment[5] and retention of lymphocytes at sites of chronic inflammation[20] (see Figure 4). Thus, lymphocytes can enter hepatic tissue by different routes. Although the factors that determine the distribution of hepatic infiltration in any given situation are poorly understood, the recognition that hepatic endothelium is heterogeneous with respect to adhesion molecule expression provides a molecular explanation for the distinct distribution and composition of lymphocytic infiltration in liver disease (Table 2).

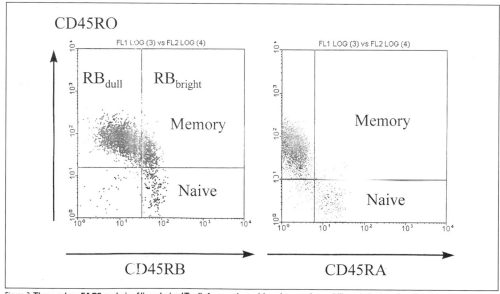

Figure 3. **Three-colour FACS analysis of liver derived T-cells from patient with endstage primary biliary cirrhosis undergoing liver transplantation**
Cells have been gated for size by their forward and side scatter characteristics and also by positivity for CD3. T-cells within the liver are mainly primed cells expressing low levels of the RB isoform of CD45 (CD45RB dull) suggesting they are terminally differentiated, activated T-cells. They also express high levels of the memory T-cell marker CD45RO. There is a small population of naïve (CD45RA+ve) T-cells within the liver that may represent either a population capable of local differentiation within the liver or memory T-cell revertants.

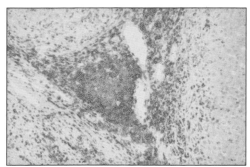

Figure 4. Lymphoid aggregates in PBC may represent secondary lymphoid tissue within the liver
T-cells within the portal tract form aggregates that resemble germinal centres with a central B-cell core surrounded by T-cells of the CD4 and CD8 phenotypes. Structures resembling high endothelial venules are seen within lymphoid aggregates and these may represent accessory pathways for T-cell recruitment to the inflamed liver.

Lymphocyte recruitment though the sinusoids

In vivo studies have demonstrated that leukocyte recruitment to the hepatic parenchyma occurs via the sinusoids and involves adhesive interactions with sinusoidal endothelium that is fenestrated and lacks a basement membrane. There is evidence for hetero-geneity within the sinusoidal bed and it is possible that recruitment through the perivenular and periportal sinusoidal endothelium might be differentially regulated.[21]

The minimal role of endothelial selectins and absence of rolling in sinusoidal vessels in the mouse[13] is consistent with previous human studies reporting a lack of selectin expression on sinusoidal endothelium when compared with vascular endothelium in portal tracts

and central veins.[22,23] Hepatic sinusoidal endothelium, however, is one of the few endothelial cell types other than the lymph node high endothelial venule that expresses the novel adhesion molecule vascular adhesion protein-1, constituitively. VAP-1 has been shown to support shear-dependent adhesion to lymph node HEVs and recent evidence shows that is also supports shear-dependent adhesion of T-cells to human sinusoidal endothelium *in vitro* and to endothelium in non-inflamed liver sections.[7,12,14] Thus, VAP-1 might support the initial adhesion of lymphocytes to sinusoidal endothelium prior to secondary integrin-mediated adhesion via ICAM-1 or ICAM-2, both of which are expressed on non-inflamed sinusoidal endothelium.[22]

The expression of endothelial adhesion molecules increases on hepatic sinusoidal endothelium during inflammation thus broadening the potential molecular interactions with circulating lymphocytes.[11,22,24] The expression of ICAM-1 and LFA-3 are increased and VCAM-1 and CD31 are induced. Furthermore, in chronic inflammatory diseases, including primary biliary cirrhosis, sinusoidal endothelium adjacent to areas of active inflammation and fibrosis undergoes capillarization[25] and expresses CD34 and CD36.[26] The expression of VAP-1, however, remains constant and the sinusoids are notable for a lack of E- and P-selectin expression, even in conditions in which these molecules are induced on adjacent hepatic veins and portal endothelium.[22,23] In the absence of selectins primary adhesion to activated sinusoidal endothelium could be mediated by VAP-1 or alternatively via

	Normal Sinusoids	PBC Sinusoids	Normal Vascular	PBC Vascular	PBC Neovessels
CD31	+	++	+++	++	++
LFA-3	+	+	±	+	++
ICAM-1	++	++	−	+++	+++
VCAM-1	−	±	−	++	+
CD62E	−	−	−	++	−
CD62P	−	−	−	+++	+
CD34	−	+	++	++	+++
Heca-452	−	+	−	+	++
VAP-1	+++	+++	++	++	++

TABLE 2: EXPRESSION OF ENDOTHELIAL ADHESION MOLECULES AS DETERMINED BY IMMUNOHISTOCHEMISTRY ON TISSUE SECTIONS FROM ORGAN DONORS (NORMAL) OR PATIENTS WITH PBC. DISTRIBUTION OF MOLECULES ON VASCULAR ENDOTHELIUM IN PORTAL TRACTS, SINUSOIDS AND NEOVESSELS ASSOCIATED WITH LYMPHOID AGGREGATES IS SHOWN

interactions between $\alpha 4$ integrins and VCAM-1 with subsequent secondary adhesion involving LFA-1 and ICAM-1.[13,14,27] Liver-infiltrating T-cells express higher levels of VLA-4 and LFA-1 compared with peripheral blood T-cells which would support a role for these pathways.[14,26] The lack of MadCam-1 expression on hepatic endothelium in primary biliary cirrhosis and the low numbers of $\alpha 4\beta 7$ positive lymphocytes in the liver suggests that, in contrast to the gut, $\alpha 4\beta 7$ plays little role in the liver.[26,28]

Lymphocyte infiltration via the portal tact

Lymphocytes are seen in portal tracts in normal liver and infiltration is massively increased as part of the chronic inflammation that characterises primary biliary cirrhosis. The exact route of entry for lymphocytes into portal tracts is unclear. The portal vessels include hepatic arteries and their portal tract capillaries and portal veins, which do not have classical post-capillary venules but instead empty into the sinusoids.[21] During chronic inflammation new microvessels develop in portal tracts.[26] These vessels, which are associated with lymphocytic infiltrates in primary biliary cirrhosis, have morphological and phenotypic similarities with the secondary high endothelial venules that have been described in the inflamed synovium[26] and their development during inflammation is likely to facilitate and perpetuate the recruitment of lymphocytes.

In chronic inflammatory conditions portal vessels express P-selectin, E-selectin and VCAM-1 (none of which are detected on non-inflamed portal endothelium), and high levels of ICAM-1. Assuming that recruitment occurs via a multi-step process the selectins induced on inflamed portal vessels could promote primary adhesion and tethering of lymphocytes with subsequent secondary adhesion occurring via lymphocyte integrins and endothelial VCAM-1 and ICAM-1. There is increased expression of both VLA-4 and LFA-1 on lymphocytes infiltrating inflamed portal tracts when compared to peripheral blood T-cells.[14,26] However, very few lymphocytes in inflamed liver express either L-selectin or E-selectin ligands[23] arguing against a role for L-selectin and E-selectin. VAP-1 is also expressed on portal vessels and could again play a role in regulating recruitment of lymphocytes to the portal tract.

The expression of several chemokines is also increased in the liver in chronic inflammation including primary biliary cirrhosis[29,30] (Table 3). These chemokines are secreted by liver cells, including liver endothelium and biliary epithelium as well as by the infiltrating leucocytes.[31,32] It has been difficult to determine which of these chemokines is functionally significant for recruitment. Recent, unpublished data from our group shows that liver infiltrating T-cells in PBC express high levels of two chemokine receptors, CXCR3 and CCR5, that bind the chemokines IP-10 (CXCR3) and MIP-1α, MIP-1ß and RANTES (CCR5) (Figure 5). In contrast very few T-cells expressed the MCP-1 receptor CCR2 or the IL-8 receptors CXCR1 and CXCR2 suggesting that CXCR3 and CCR5 may be particularly important for lymphocyte recruitment. A novel chemokine LARC is preferentially, although not exclusively, expressed in the liver and its receptor CCR6 is restricted to lymphocytes suggesting it may also be important.[33]

Retention of lymphocytes within the liver in PBC

Under normal conditions inflammation will resolve once the foreign antigen that initiates the response has been removed by the immune system. The reasons why

TABLE 3:			
	Receptor	**Distribution**	**Source**
IP-10	CXCR3	Sinusoids	Endothelium Leukocytes
MIP-1α, MIP-1β	CCR5	Vascular endothelial cells Sinusoids	Leukocytes Endothelium
RANTES	CCR5	Vascular endothelial cells Biliary cells	Endothelium Leukocytes Biliary cells
LARC	CCR6	?	?
MCP-1	CCR2	Vascular endothelial cells Biliary cells	Leukocytes Endothelium Biliary cells

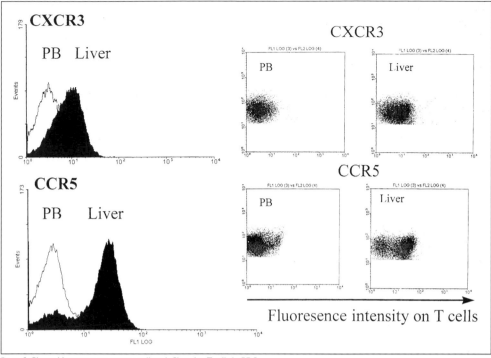

CXCR3

CCR5

Fluoresence intensity on T cells

Figure 5. **Chemokine receptor usage on liver infiltrating T-cells in PBC**
Chemokine receptor CXCR3 (for IP-10) and CCR5 (for MIP-1α, MIP-1ß and RANTES) expression was measured on both peripheral blood (PB) T-cells and PBC liver derived T-cells by two-colour FACS analysis. T-cells were selected by forward and side scatter characteristics and by their expression of CD3. CXCR3 was expressed at only low levels on PBT-cells but was upregulated on LDL with increased median channel fluorescence intensity. CCR5 was present on a small percentage of PB T-cells but on most liver derived T-cells. Upregulation of these chemokine receptors on LDL and the expression of their chemokine ligands within the liver provides a potential mechanism for the selective recruitment of these cells to inflamed liver in PBC.

this fails to happen in chronic inflammatory conditions such as PBC is poorly understood. Several mechanisms might be involved. Firstly, persistence of the autoantigen may provide a continuing signal for lymphocyte activation; the expression and role of various autoantigens at different stages of the disease will be discussed in more detail elsewhere (see chapters by Gershwin, Joplin and Bassendine). However, other factors are likely to play a role in the persistence of inflammation. Firstly, as mentioned above, chronic inflammation causes angiogenesis in and around the portal tracts resulting in the appearance of neovessels that have some of the characteristics of high endothelial venules in lymph nodes.[26] In PBC these vessels are prominent and are associated with structured lymphoid aggregates, suggesting that they facilitate lymphocyte recruitment (Figure 4). Once such structures have become established they may be able to perpetuate lymphocyte recruitment. Secondly, the ability of biliary epithelium to secrete high levels of functional chemokines in response to proinflammatory cytokines suggests that the liver itself could be producing signals that perpetuate lymphocyte recruitment in PBC.[31] We have unpublished studies showing that corticosteroids

fail to suppress chemokine secretion from biliary epithelial cells and this might explain in part why PBC responds so poorly to steroid therapy. Thirdly, it is possible that PBC is associated with a failure of the mechanisms responsible for down-regulating lymphocyte responses. These mechanisms involve the induction of apoptosis in highly differentiated and activated T-cells via receptors such as Fas and CTLA-4 that are expressed at high levels on these cells. A role for another cell surface molecule, CD40, in the chronic inflammation of PBC is suggested by the intriguing findings of Hayward et al.[34] They described bile duct damage and inflammation in patients with sex linked hyper-IgM syndrome, in whom there is a deficiency of the CD40 ligand CD154. The binding of CD40, which is expressed on B cells, with CD154 on T-cells has many consequences, including immunoglobulin class switching from IgM to IgG. This provides a molecular explanation for the high levels of IgM in these patients who are characterised by persistent infections with herpes viruses and cryptosporidiosis that lead to a chronic cholangiopathy. The defect in CD40L/CD40 signalling is probably responsible for the inability of the immune system to clear these organisms efficiently. The fact that this disease is associated with high levels of IgM and a cholangiopathy suggests that defects in CD40/CD40L signalling could be involved in the pathogenesis of PBC. This is an intriguing hypothesis for which at present there are no published supporting data and it should also be noted that the affected patients with hyper IgM are males and the cholangiopathy has more features of PSC than PBC.

Lymphocyte interactions with liver cells

Lymphocyte interactions with liver cells may take several forms and have distinct consequences (Figure 6). Interactions between lymphocytes and stromal cells have been shown to prevent apoptosis of terminally differentiated activated T-cells by as yet poorly understood mechanisms.[35] Activated T-cells in primary biliary cirrhosis are found in the periseptal areas closely related

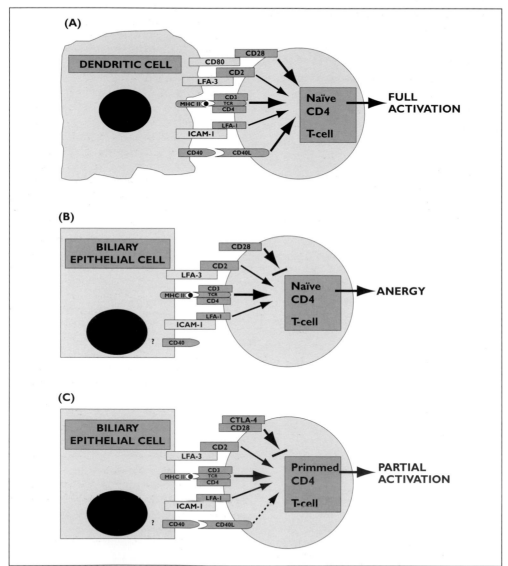

Figure 6. **The potential role of biliary epithelial cells in antigen presentation to CD4+ T-cells**

(a) Optimal T-cell activation is provided by activated dendritic cells that present antigenic peptides in the context MHC KK antigens in the presence of the required adhesion and costimulatory signals, particularly CD80 which activates a signal via CD28 on the T-cells surface to prevent the induction of apoptosis.

(b) CD28 activation is particularly important for activation of naïve T-cells and lack of CD28 ligands on biliary epithelial cells means that although they might interact with CD4 T-cells through other pathways the likely outcome will be anergy.

(c) Most liver-infiltrating lymphocytes are memory T-cells that have been primed by DCs in draining lymph node and these cells may respond differently when they encounter antigen and MHC II on biliary epithelial cells. The outcome of such interaction is not known at present but the ability of biliary epithelial cells to express costimulatory molecules such as CD40 and ICAM-1 might be sufficient for at least partial activation of memory T-cells.

to fibroblasts and associated with active fibrosis. Interactions between the two cell types might be important both for the activation of fibrosis as well as providing important signals that prolong lymphocyte survival and promote persistent inflammation. However, the lymphocytic infiltrate is centred on portal tracts where the biliary epithelium is the major target of immune-mediated attack and it is thus important to understand how biliary epithelial cells might interact with lymphocytes.

Lymphocyte biliary epithelial cell interactions may be important during both the afferent and effector arms of the immune response.[36] Lymphocyte activation by stimulating cells has strict requirements[37]: the cells must be able to present antigenic peptides in association with MHC class II molecules in order to interact with CD4 T-cells, or MHC class I to interact with CD8 T-cells. In addition the cell must provide an adhesive signal to an opposing lymphocyte to allow the cells to interact closely and an additional co-stimulatory signal if the lymphocyte is to be fully activated.[38,39] It was demonstrated by several groups that intrahepatic bile ducts express both MHC II and MHC I antigens in inflammatory conditions and work with isolated human biliary epithelial cells in vitro has demonstrated that MHC molecules are induced on these cells in response to pro-inflammatory cytokines[40-43] (see Figure 7). Furthermore biliary epithelial cells also express high levels of several adhesion molecules, including ICAM-1 and LFA-3 that are important for mediating adhesion to lymphocytes.[44,45] Thus the cells can be induced to express molecules that will promote interactions with lymphocytes.

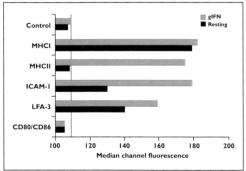

Figure 7. Induction of costimulatory molecules on human biliary epithelial cells
Human biliary epithelial cells were analysed by flow cytometry for their expression of MHC antigens and adhesion molecules before and after five days activation with g IFN. Activated biliary epithelial cells expressed high levels of MHC II antigens, ICAM-1 and LFA-3 but failed to express either CD80 or CD86 as determined by binding of specific mAb and binding of a CTLA-4-Ig fusion protein.

Biliary epithelial cell interactions with CD4 T-cells

CD4 T-cells require a costimulatory signal provided by activation of CD28 on the lymphocyte cell surface to allow them to be fully activated and to prevent them undergoing apoptosis after T-cell receptor engagement. Activation of CD28 occurs when it binds to one of two molecules, CD80 or CD86, on the antigen-presenting cell. The expression of CD80 and CD86 is largely restricted to professional antigen presenting cells such as dendritic cells. This prevents lymphocytes being activated by other cell types and reduces the chance of developing unwanted responses to self-antigens. Thus the ability of biliary epithelial cells to express either of the CD28 ligands CD80 or CD86 would allow them to act as antigen presenting cells and thereby to provoke and maintain a T-cell-mediated response. There is controversy about the ability of biliary epithelial cells to express CD28 ligands. Most of the studies suggest that they do not, and the most comprehensive studies by Leon and colleagues have failed to demonstrate CD80 or CD86 protein or mRNA in biliary cells.[46] However, one study does suggest that CD80 appears on biliary epithelial cells late in the course of PBC,[47] although even if it can be confirmed it is doubtful whether expression late in the disease course has any relevance for pathogenesis. Leon et al. also studied functional lymphocyte responses to biliary epithelial cells. Interferon-activated biliary epithelial cells failed to support either IL-2 production or proliferation of allogenic CD4 T-cells unless additional costimulation through CD28 was provided.[48] Thus biliary epithelial cells are unlikely to promote the activation of unprimed CD4 T-cells. In fact it is likely that naïve T-cells will be tolerized by such interactions. Very few naïve T-cell enter liver tissue and most liver-infiltrating lymphocytes are memory T-cells that have been primed by DCs in draining lymph node. These memory cells may respond differently when they encounter their antigen presented by MHC II high biliary epithelial cells. The outcome of such interactions is not known at present but the ability of biliary epithelial cells to express costimulatory molecules such as CD40 and ICAM-1 might be sufficient for at least partial activation of memory T-cells.

Biliary epithelial cell interactions with cytotoxic T-cells

The ability of biliary epithelial cells to act as targets for lymphocyte cytotoxicity is less controversial. They are susceptible to lysis by lymphokine-activated natural killer cells[45] and recent work from Joplin and colleagues suggests that liver-derived T-cells in PBC can kill E2 expressing biliary epithelial cells. The cytotoxic lymphocyte must interact closely with a putative target

T-cell in order to recognise peptide in association with MHC class I and this is facilitated by adhesion to ICAM-1 and LFA-3, both of which are increased on inflamed biliary cells in PBC. After adhering to the cell and recognising antigen/MHC I CTL use several mechanisms to kill target cells by apoptosis. These include the injection of proteases, such as granzymes and perforins that activate caspases and apoptosis in the target cell[49] and the engagement of Fas on the surface of the target cell which activates downstream signalling events resulting in apoptosis[50] (Figure 8). There is evidence that biliary epithelial cells undergo apoptosis in PBC but the mechanisms responsible are not clear.[51] Studies have shown increased expression of perforin and granzymes in PBC[52] and Fas is upregulated on the biliary epithelial cell membrane so it is possible that both of these pathways are involved.

The role of T-cell cytokines in determining persistent liver inflammation; the Th1/Th2 paradigm

After activation by antigen, T-cells proliferate and secrete cytokines and depending on which cytokines they produce can be divided functionally into either T-helper Th1 cells that secrete IL-2, gIFN TNF and IL-12 or Th2 cells that secrete IL-4, IL10 and IL-13. Th1 cells promote a cell-mediated response whereas Th2 responses are associated with antibody secretion, chronic inflammation and downregulation of the Th1 effector mechanisms[53] (Figure 9). In chronic schistosomiasis the development of hepatic granulomata is associated with the local secretion of Th2 cytokines[54] suggesting that a predominantly Th2 response is responsible for their development and the persistence of chronic

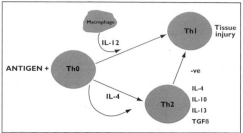

Figure 9. **The role of T-cell cytokines in regulating chronic inflammation** Activation of naïve T-cells by antigen presenting cells can lead to the differentiation of distinct functional subsets determined by their ability to secret particular cytokines. Th1 cells differentiate in the presence of certain cytokines, particularly IL-12 from macrophages and secrete cytokines that promote a cell-mediated response to infection or antigen. In contrast Th2 cells develop in the absence of IL-12 and the presence of IL-4 and secrete cytokines that promote a predominantly humoral response. In addition some Th2 cytokines, i.e., IL-10, can act to downregulate Th1 responses.

inflammation. Th2 cytokines have also been proposed as playing a role in the establishment and persistence of inflammation in a variety of autoimmune disorders[53] and recent evidence suggests that a failure to develop a peripheral Th1 response might be responsible for the persistence of viral infection in chronic viral hepatitis. Although these findings suggest that PBC would be associated with a predominantly Th2 cytokine profile, a recent paper shows that it is fact associated predominately with intrahepatic Th1 cytokines.[55] This study reported Th1 cells, as determined by gIFN expression, in association with damaged bile ducts and these findings are consistent with the development of CTLs. Another study has shown an association with gIFN expression and liver damage in PBC, supporting the association with ongoing cell damage. However, PBC is also associated with eosinophilic infiltration and increased expression of IL-5, a Th2 cytokine[52] and the relative roles of Th1/Th2 cytokines in PBC remain unclear. Furthermore, the high levels of IL-10 found in normal liver suggest that complex networks of cytokines will be involved in regulating the development of liver cell damage and chronic persistent inflammation.[56]

REFERENCES

1. Butcher EC, Picker LJ. Lymphocyte homing and homeostasis. *Science* 1996; **272**: 60-66.

2. Kudo S, Matsuno K, Ezaki T, Ogawa M. A novel pathway for rat dendritic cells from the blood: hepatic sinusoids-lymph translocation. *J Exp Med* 1997; **185**: 777-784.

3. Picker LJ, Treer JR, Ferguson-Darnell B, Collins PA, Buck D, Terstappen LW. Control of lymphocyte recirculation in man. I. Differential regulation of peripheral lymph node homing receptor L-selectin on T-cells during the virgin to memory cell transition. *J Immunol* 1993; **150**: 1105-1121.

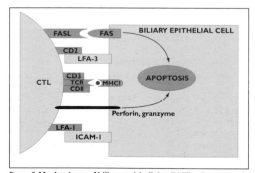

Figure 8. **Mechanisms of biliary epithelial cell killing by cytotoxic T-lymphocytes**
The ability of biliary epithelial cells to express MHC I antigens and to upregulate adhesion ligands such as ICAM-1 and LFA-3 allows them to interact with CTLs. If the CTL recognises antigen in the context of MHC I on the biliary epithelial cell it can kill the biliary epithelial cell either by injecting perforin or granzymes into the target T-cells or by activating Fas on the biliary epithelial cell surface. The result of both of these pathways is induction of apoptosis.

4. Picker LJ, Treer JR, Ferguson-Darnell B, Collins PA, Bergstresser PR, Terstappen LW. Control of lymphocyte recirculation in man. II. Differential regulation of the cutaneous lymphocyte-associated antigen, a tissue-selective homing receptor for skin-homing T-cells. J Immunol 1993; **1500**: 1122-1136.

5. Bevilacqua MP. Endothelial-leukocyte adhesion molecules. Annu Rev Immunol 1993; **11**: 767-784.

6. Adams DH, Shaw S. Leucocyte endothelial interactions and regulation of leucocyte migration. Lancet 1994; **343**: 831-836.

7. Salmi M, Adams Dh, Jalkanen S. Lymphocyte trafficking in the intestine and liver. Am J Physiol 1998; **274**: G1-G6.

8. Tanaka Y, Kimata K, Adams Dh, Eto S. Modulation of cytoline function by proteoglycans: sophisticated models for the regulation of cellular responses to cytokines. Proceedings of the Association of American Physicians 1998; **110**: 118-125.

9. Tanaka Y, Adams DH, Hübscher S, Hirano H, Siebenlist U, Shaw S. T-cell adhesion induced by proteoglycan-immobilized cytokine MIP-1ß. Nature 1993; **361**: 79-82.

10 Adams DH, Harvath L, Bottaro DP, et al. Hepatocyte growth factor and macrophage inflammatory protein-1?: structurally distinct cytokines that induce rapid cytoskeletal changes and subset-preferential migration in T-cell. Proc Nati Acad Sci USA 1994; **91**: 7144-7148.

11. Jaeschke H. Cellular adhesion molecules: regulation and functional significance in the pathogenesis of liver disease. American Journal of Physiology 1998; **273**: G602-G611.

12. Adams DH. Lymphocyte-endothelial interactions in hepatic inflammation. Hepatogastroenterology 1996; **43**: 32-43.

13. Wong J, Johnston B, Lee SS, et al. A minimal role for seletins in the recruitment of leukocytes into the inflamed liver microvasculature. Journal of Clinical Investigation 1997; **99**: 2782-2790.

14. Yoong KF, Hübscher SG, Adams DH. Vascular adhesion protein-1 and ICAM-1 support the adhesion of tumor infiltrating lymphocytes to tumor endothelium in human hepatocellular carcinoma. Journal of Immunology 1998; **160**: 3978-3988.

15. Winnock M, Barcina MG, Lukomska B, Bioulac-Sage P, Balabaud C. Liver-associated lymphocytes: role in tumour defence. Seminars in Liver Disease 1993; **13**: 81-92.

16. Crispe NI, Mehal WZ. Strange brew: T-cells in the liver. Immunol Today 1996; **17**: 522-525.

17. Van de Water J, Shimoda S, Niho Y, Coppel R, Ansari A, Gershwin ME. The role of T-cells in primary biliary cirrhosis (Review) (60 refs). Seminars in Liver Disease 1997; **17**: 105-113.

18. Leon MP, Spickett G, Jones DJ, Bassendine MF. CD4+ T-cell subsets defined by isoforms of CD45 in primary biliary- cirrhosis. Clincial and Experimental Immunology 1995; **99**: 233-239.

19. Jones DE, Palmer JM, Leon MP, Yeaman SJ, Bassendine MF. T-cell responses to tuberculin purified protein derivative in primary biliary cirrhosis. Gut 1997; **40**: 227-283.

20. Berlin C, Bargatze RF, Campbell JJ, et al. Alpha-4 integrins mediate lymphocyte attachment and rolling under physiological flow. Cell 1995; **80**: 413-422.

21. Vidal- Vanaclocha F, Rocha MA, Asumendi A, Barbera-Guillem E. Role of periportal and perivenous sinusoidal endothelial cells in hepatic homing of blood and metastatic cancer cells. Seminars in Liver Disease 1993; **13**: 60-71.

22. Steinhoff G, Behrend M, Schrader B, Duijvestijn AM, Wonigeit K. Expression patterns of leukocyte adhesion ligand molecules on human liver endothelia – lack of ELAM-1 and CD62 inducibility on sinusoidal endothelia and distinct distribution of VCAM-1, ICAM-1, ICAM-2 and LFA-3. American Journal of Pathology 1993; **142**: 481-488.

23. Adams DH, Hübscher SG, Fisher NC, Williams A, Robinson M. Expression of E-selectin (CD62E) and E-selectin ligands in human liver inflammation. Hepatology 1996; **24**: 533-538.

24. Scoazec J, Feldman G. The cell adhesion molecules of hepatic sinusoidal endothelial cells. J Hepatol 1994; **20**: 296-300.

25. Babbs C, Haboubi NY, Mellor JM, Smith A, Rowan BP, Warnes TW. Endothelial cell transformation in primary biliary cirrhosis – a morphological and biochemical study. Hepatology 1990; **11**: 723-729.

26. Garcia-Monzon C, Sanchez-Madrid F, Garcia-Buey L, Garcia-Arroyo A, Garcia-Sanchez A, Moreno-Otero R. Enhanced expression of vascular adhesion molecules in chronic viral hepatitis. Evidence of neoangiogenesis in portal tracts. Gastroenterology 1995; **108**: 231-241.

27. Lalor PE, Clements JM, Pigott R, Humphries MJ, Spragg JH, Nash GB. Association between receptor density. Cellular activation, and transformation of adhesive behaviour of flowing lymphocytes binding to VCAM-1. European. European Journal of Immunology 1997; **27**: 1422-1426.

28. Briskin M, Winsor-Hines D, Shyjan A, et al. Human mucosal addressin cell adhesion molecule-1 is preferentially expressed in intestinal tract and associated lymphoid tissue. Am J Pathol 1997; **151**: 97-110.

29. Afford SC, Fisher NC, Neil DAH, et al. Distinct patterns of chemokine expression are associated with leucocyte recruitment in alcoholic hepatitis & alcoholic cirrhosis. Journal of Pathology 1998; (in press).

30. Adams DH, Fear J, Shaw S, Hübscher SG, Afford S. Hepatic expression of macrophage inflammatory protein-1a and macrophage inflammatory protein-1β after liver transplantation. Transplantation 1996; **61**: 817-825.

31. McNab G, Afford SC, Morland CM, Strain AJ, Joplin R, Adams DH. Cultured human hepatic sinusoidal endothelial cells express and secrete adhesion molecules and chemokines that are important for leukocyte recruitment to the liver. In: Wisse E, Knook DL, Dalabaud C, eds. Cells of the hepatic sinusoid, Leiden: The Kupffer Cell Foundation, 1997; 123-127.

32. Morland CM, Fear J, McNab G, Joplin R, Adams DH. Promotion of leukocyte transendothelial cell migration by chemokines derived from human biliary epithelial cells in vitro. Proceedings of the Association of American Physicans 1997; **109**: 372-382.

33. Baba M, Imai T, Mishimura M, et al. Identification of CCR6, the specific receptor for a novel lymphocyte-directed chemokine LARC. Journal of Biological Chemistry 1997; **272**: 14893-14898.

34. Hayward AR, Levy J, Facchetti F, et al. Cholangiopathy and tumors of the pancreas, liver and biliary tree in boys with X-linked immunodeficiency and hyper-IgM. J Immunol 1997; **158**: 977-983.

35. Akbar AN, Salmon M. Cellular environments and apoptosis: Tissue microenvironments control activated T-cell death. Immunol Today 1997; **18**: 72-76.

36. Adams DH. Biliary epithelial cells: active participants in immune-mediated liver disease? Journal of Laboratory and Clinical Medicine 1996; **128**: 528-530.

37. Schwartz RH. Costimulation of T-lymphocytes: The role of CD28, CTLA-4, and B7/BB1 in interleukin-2 production and immunotherapy. Cell 1992; **71**: 1065-1068.

38. Liu Y, Wenger RH, Zhao M, Nielsen PJ. Distinct costimulatory molecules are required for the induction of effector and memory cytotoxic t lymphocytes. Journal of Experimental Medicine 1997; **185**: 251-262.

39. Boussiotis VA, Gribben JG, Freeman GJ, Nadler LM. Blockage of the CD28 co-stimulatory pathway: a means to induce tolerance. Curr-Opin-Immunol 1994; **6**: 797-807.

40. Lautenschlager I, Taskinene E, Inkinen K, Lehto VP, Hayry P. Distribution of the MHC antigens on different cellular components of human liver. Cell Immunol 1984; **85**: 191-200.

41. Daar AS, Fuggle SV, Fabre JW, Ting A, Morris PJ. The detailed distribution of MHC class II antigens in normal human organs. Transplantation 1984; **38**: 293-298.

42. Hübscher SG, Adams DH, Elias E. Changes in the expression of MHC class II antigens in liver allograft rejection. J Pathol 1990; **162**: 165-171.

43. Ayres R, Neuberger JM, Shaw J, Adams DH. Intercellular adhesion molecule-1 and MHC antigens on human intrahepatic bile ducT-cells: effect of pro-inflammatory cytokines. Gut 1993; **34**: 1245-1249.

44. Adams DH, Hubshcer SG, Shaw J, et al. Increased expression of ICAM-1 on bile ducts in primary biliary cirrhosis and primary sclerosing cholangitis. Hepatology 1991; **14**: 426-432.

45. Leon MP, Bassendine MF, Gibbs P, Thick M, Kirby JA. Immunogenicity of biliary epithelium: study of the adhesive interaction with lymphocytes. Gastroenterology 1997; **112**: 968-977.

46. Leon MP, Kirby JA, Gibbs P, Burt AD, Bassendine MF. Immunogenicity of biliary epithelial-cells – study of the expression of B7 molecules. *J Hepatol* 1995; **22**: 591-595.

47. Tsuneyama K, Van de Water J, Leung PS, *et al.* Abnormal expression of the E2 component of the pyruvate dehydrogenasecomplex on the luminal surface of biliary epithelium occurs before major histocompatiblity complex class II and BB1/B7 expression. *Hepatology* 1995; **21**: 1031-1037.

48. Leon MP, Bassendine MF, Wilson JL, Ali S, Thick M, Kirby JA. Immunogenicity of biliary epithelium: investigation of antigen presentation to CD4+ T-cells. *Hepatology* 1996; **24**: 561-567.

49. Sarin A, Adams DH, Henkart PA. Protease inhibits selectively block T-cell receptor-triggered programmed cell-death in a murine T-cell hybridoma and activated peripheral T-cells. *Journal of Experimental Medicine* 1993; **178**: 1693-1700.

50. Nagata S, Goldstein P. The Fas death factor. *Science* 195; **267**: 1449-1456.

51. Harada K, Ozaki S, Gershwin ME, Nakanuma Y. Enhanced apoptosis relates to bile duct loss in primary biliary cirrhosis. *Hepatology* 1997; **27**: 1399-1405.

52. Martinez OM, Villanueva JC, Gershwin ME, Krams SM. Cytokine patterns and cytotoxic mediators in primary biliary cirrhosis. *Hepatology* 1995; **21**: 113-119.

53. Charlton B, Lafferty KJ. The Th1/Th2 balance in autoimmunity. *Current Opinion in Immunology* 1995; **7**: 793-798.

54. Lukacs NW. Chensue SW, Smith RE, *et al.* Production of monocyte chemoattractant protein-1 and macrophage inflammatory protein-1-alpha by inflammatory granuloma fibroblasts. *American Journal of Pathology* 1994; **144**: 711-718.

55. Harada K, Van de Water J, Lleung PS, *et al.* In situ hybridization of cytokines in primary biliary cirrhosis: predominance of the Th1 subset. *Hepatology* 1995; **25**: 791-796.

56. Dumoulin FL, Bach A, Leifld L, *et al.* Semiquantitative analysis of intrahepatic cytokines mRNA in chronic hepatitis C. *J Infect Dis* 1997; **175**: 681-685.

51. Afford SC, Randhawa S, Eliopoulos AG, Hübscher SG, Young LS, Adams DH. CD40 activation induces apoptosis in cultured human hepatocytes via induction of Fas ligand expression and amplifies Fas mediated Hepatocyte death diving allograft rejection. *J Exp Med* 1999 (in press).

ETIOLOGICAL CONSIDERATIONS OF PRIMARY BILIARY CIRRHOSIS

Atsushi Tanaka[1], Santiago Munoz[2], Judy Van De Water[1],
Ross L Coppel[3], Aftab Ansari[4], M Eric Gershwin[1]

[1] Division of Rheumatology, Allergy and Clinical Immunology, School of Medicine,
University of California at Davis, Davis, CA 95616.
[2] Center for Liver Disease, Albert Einstein Medical Center, Philadelphia, PA 19141.
[3] Department of Microbiology, Monash University, Clayton, Victoria 3168, Australia.
[4] Department of Pathology, Emory University School of Medicine, Atlanta, GA 30322.

SUMMARY

The basis for the selective destruction of biliary epithelial cells in PBC remains unknown. The identification of mitochondrial autoantigens has been a great help in the investigation of PBC. It is possible to postulate that PDC-E2 derived from bacteria and/or often microrganisms are a key in breaking tolerance against human PDC-E2. It will be crucial to determine if tissue-specific bile duct antigens are found in patients with PBC. In addition, there has been no information about the promoter to determine if PDC-E2 is overexpressed in biliary epithelial cells. We would also like to emphasize the significance of the clinical paradoxes and/or paradigms of PBC. Important clinical questions should not be overlooked. Why is there a high female predominance in patients with PBC? Has the ratio of female to males changed in recent years? Why does PBC not develop in or before adolescence? What is the reason for the large geographical and ethnic variations in the prevalence of PBC? Are bone diseases found in PBC different, or similar to those in patients without PBC? Data on these fundamental questions will be of great help to us to refine the understanding of PBC. In this review we attempt to discuss some of these issues.

INTRODUCTION

In this decade there have been great advances in the immunophathogenesis of primary biliary cirrhosis (PBC), primarily due to progress in basic immunology and molecular biology. The break-through was the identification of a cDNA for the 74kD mitochondrial autoantigen, leading to the identification of the major PBC autoantigen as the E2 component of the mitochondrial pyruvate dehydrogenase complex (PDC)[1-3]. Nonetheless, as additional studies followed, it became clear that these findings are just the prelude to other questions and that the precise molecular mechanisms, in particular, those that are involved in the induction of disease remain a challenge for the future. For instance, we still cannot answer four basic questions:

- How does the immune system recognise mitochondrial proteins that exist inside cells?

- Why are the biliary epithelial cells the only (or primarily the only) targets for autoimmune reaction, even though mitochondrial proteins are present throughout the body?

- Are anti-mitochondrial autoantibodies (AMA) primary or secondary products in PBC?

- Why are the autoantibodies primarily directed against a number of mitochondrial proteins (subcellular specificity)?

Mitochondrial Autoantigens

PBC, specifically affecting intrahepatic small bile ducts, is considered an autoimmune disease because of several reasons. First, a variety of autoantibodies are found in the sera of patients with PBC. Moreover, AMA are so specific in patients with PBC that these antibodies are clinically used as a diagnostic tool of PBC. It is now well recognised that the targets of AMA are members of the 2-oxoacid dehydrogenase complex (2-OADC), including the E2 subunit of the pyruvate dehydrogenase complex (PDC-E2), the E2 subunit of branched chain 2-oxoacid dehydrogenase complex (BCOADC-E2), and the E2 subunit of the 2-oxoglutarate dehydrogenase complex (OGDC-E2). Other AMA recognise the E1α subunit of PDC and dehydrolipoamide dehydrogenase-binding protein (E3BP), once termed protein X (Table I). These molecules are all mitochondrial enzymes.

All mitochondria have a basic two-membrane structure: an outer membrane enclosing an inner membrane, which is highly folded. It is the inner membrane where 2-OADC is located. Structurally, the three enzymes, PDC, BCOADC and OGDC are similar, each containing E2, E2 and E3 subunits[4-6]. The E2 subunits of PDC, BCOADC and OGDC are conserved. All of them have a lipoyl domain near the N-terminal, an E3 binding region in the middle and the catalytic site near the

TABLE 1. CHARACTERISTICS OF ANTIMITOCHONDRIAL AUTOANTIBODIES AND MITOCHONDRIAL ANTIGENS IN PBC

Antigen	M.W. (kD)[1]	Frequency (%) in PBC[2]	Lipoyl Domain	B-cell epitopes	Major Ig isotype	Inhibition of function by AMA
PDC-E2	74	95	+	Outer and inner lipoyl domain	IgG3, IgM	+
BCOADC-E2	52	53-55	+	Lipoyl domain	NR	+
OGDC-E2	48	39-88	+	Lipoyl domain	IgG2, IgM	+
PDC-E1α	41	41-66	+	TFP binding & phosphorylation sites	NR	+
E3 binding protein	55	95	+	NR	NR	+

[1] Determined by SDS-PAGE and immunoblotting against PBC sera.
[2] Determined by immunoblotting or ELISA against recombinant proteins.
NR: not reported.

C-terminal which are interconnected by an alanine-proline-rich region (Figure 1). The number of lipoyl domains for each of these enzymes, however, differs. Thus, PDC-E2 has 2 lipoyl domains and both BCOADC and OGDC each have a single lipoyl domain (Figure 1). Information on the three-dimensional structure of bacterial PDC-E2 has been clarified using X-ray crystallography and 2-dimensional nuclear magnetic resonance (NMR)[7-9]. According to the three-dimensional structure, each lipoate binding domain consists of approximately 80 amino acids with the lipoyl-lysine being found with a DKA motif[10]. A core of hydrophobic residues is present with two four-stranded β sheets forming a β-barrel; the lipoyl-lysine residue occupies an exposed position at the tip of a β-turn in one of the sheets[10].

Recently, dehydrolipoamide dehydrogenase-binding protein (E3BP) of the human pyruvate dehydrogenase complex, which was once called protein X, has been cloned and sequenced[6]. The protein has a multi-domain structure analogous to that of the E2 component of the complex, with the exception of only a single lipoyl domain (Figure 1). While it seems that the only function of E3BP may be to anchor E3 to the complex, it still remains unclear whether E3BP has an intrinsic catalytic activity of its own.

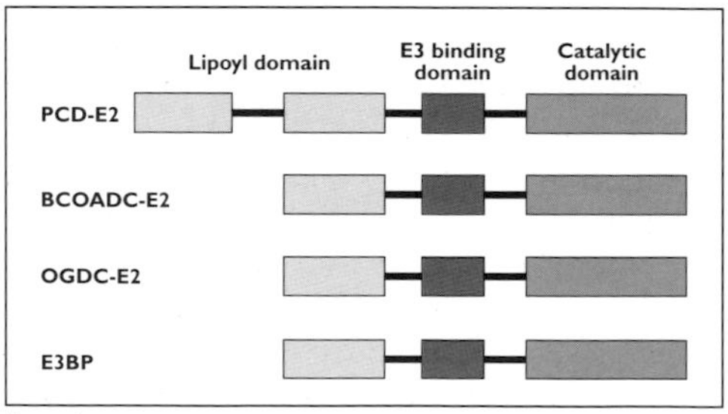

B Cell and T-cell Epitopes of Mitochondrial Autoantigens

The availability of powerful techniques, including the in vitro expression of recombinant human mitochondrial autoantigens by E.coli, has greatly facilitated the mapping of B cell epitopes of the 2-oxoacid dehydrogenase complexes. Several studies, using either oligopeptides[2] or recombinant fusion proteins[11], have shown that the predominant epitope of PDC-E2 is located within the lipoyl domain of PDC-E2. The AMA also react with the outer domain, but at a 100-fold lower dilution, and only 1/26 PBC sera react weakly to the E1/E3 binding region[11]. To map the B cell epitope more precisely, truncated constructs of PDC-E2 were generated by using convenient restriction sites at the amino and the carboxyl termini of the epitopic region. Sera from PBC patients strongly reacted with the 93 amino acid peptide (residues 128-221), and weakly react with the 75 amino acid peptide (residues 146-221). This pattern of reactivity was abolished when further truncated peptides, such as residues 160-227, were used. This observation suggests that anti-PDC-E2 autoantibodies most likely recognise a conformational epitope, including the conformation encoded by the inner lipoyl domain. These findings were confirmed[12], using similar truncated peptides of PDC-E2 and combinatorial human autoantibodies derived from an immunoglobulin library of patients with PBC. The combinatorial

Figure 1.
Diagrammatic representation of the structural and functional domains of 2-OADC E2 subunits and E3 binding protein and their corresponding B-cell epitopes.

autoantibodies showed the strongest reactivity with residues 128-227, but did not show detectable reactivity against 146-227. Interestingly, the antibodies demonstrated substantial heterogeneity in the recognition of different recombinant PDC-E2 constructs.

Using recombinant BCOADC-E2, Leung et al. reported that the autoantibodies recognise a conformational epitope[13]. Truncated peptides of BCOADC-E2 were generated according to appropriate restriction sites, and the immunoreactivity of patient sera against the peptides determined. The results demonstrated that residues 1–227, consisting of the lipoic domain and part of the E2 core region, was the B cell epitope of BCOADC-E2. The absorption of anti-BCOADC-E2 antibodies by a full-length cDNA spanning residues 1–421 removed all reactivity, whereas the combination of peptides prepared from expression clones, such as 1 to 115 and 115 to 421, or 1 to 84, 84 to 227 and 115 to 421, were not capable of abolishing the reactivity, suggesting that the epitope is dependent on the conformation of the BCOADC-E2. Moteki et al. mapped the AMA epitope of OGDC-E2 within an 81 amino acid polypeptide (residues 67–147) corresponding to the lipoyl domain of OGDC-E2. Taken together, it appears that the reactive AMA to PDC-E2, BCOADC-E2 and OGDC-E2 each recognise conformational epitopes, and the lipoic acid domain is necessary for strong antibody binding. Although the B cell epitope of E3BP has not been determined, similar results are expected, based on the homology of amino acid sequences between E3BP and the other 2-oxoacid dehydrogenase complex proteins.

The T-cell autoepitope of PDC-E2 was identified by Shimoda et al.[14]. They established six PDC-E2 specific T-cell clones using various peptides from PDC-E2 as a clone-selecting antigens. The minimal autoepitopes recognised by these T-cell clones were all located within the same region of PDC-E2 peptide 163-176 (GDLLAEIETDKATI), which also is contained within the inner lipoyl domain of human PDC-E2. Of interest was the finding that each of the 6 T-cell clones also reacted to the PDC-E2 peptide 36-49 (GDLIAEVETDKATD), which corresponds to the outer lipoyl domain. Interestingly, the T-cell autoepitope of human PDC-E2, peptide 163-176, located in the inner lipoyl domain not only almost completely overlaps the B cell epitope described above, including the lipoyl-lysine residue at aa174, but also overlaps with the structurally exposed region of the human PDC-E2 molecule determined by X-ray crystallography or 2-D NMR[7-9].

One may consider that lipoic acid plays a role in AMA or T-cell recognition of PDC-E2, since the lipoyl-lysine residue is located within the autoepitope of B- and T-cells. Although there have been no data on lipoate attachment and antigen processing towards T-cell recognition, the role of lipoic acid in AMA binding appears controversial. Leung et al. showed that AMA are capable of binding to both lipoylated and unlipoylated PDC-E2[15], whereas Quinn et al. demonstrated the importance of lipoate attachment to PDC-E2 in AMA binding[16]. The three-dimensional structure, however, clearly shows that this region is exposed on the surface of the complex molecules and relatively mobile. It thus seems plausible that AMA would recognise this exposed region.

T-cell recognition of the peptide 163-176, located within the inner lipoyl domain, would be also affected by the tertiary structure of human PDC-E2. Recently, Landry indicated that differential antigen processing in the APC would exert a strong effect on immuno-dominance pattern of the T-cell epitope of a given peptide, and that immunodominant epitopes correlate with nearby structurally unstable segments[17]. The inner lipoyl domains of human PDC-E2 are flexible despite the large size of the PDC, and are preferentially cleaved by proteases. The identification of the tertiary structure of other mitochondrial autoantigens, BCOADC-E2 or OGDC-E3, by X-ray crystallography or 2-D NMR would be of great help in the determination of T-cell autoepitopes of the molecules.

Putative Molecular Mimicry Between PDC-E2 and Bacterial Components – Implications In Tolerance Breakdown

Mitochondrial autoantigens intracellularly are located within the inner membrane of mitochondria and are thus sequestered from immune system of the host. It is therefore highly unlikely that autoreactive T-cell clones specific for the mitochondrial autoantigens are completely deleted by apoptosis during negative selection within the thymus. Rather, it is well established that self-reactive T-cells exist in the peripheral T-cell pool even in healthy individuals or a variety of normal animals[18]. However, the frequency of these cloned populations of PDC-E2 specific T-cells detected in these healthy individuals is relatively very low[14]. This could occur if mitochondrial autoantigens are not presented to thymocytes, or are generated at subthreshold levels for acting as T-cell epitopes in the thymus[19-21]. Instead, it may be possible that while thymocytes specific for mitochondrial autoantigens with high affinity are deleted by negative selection, and that thymocytes with relatively lower affinity for the autoantigens would be positively selected and peripheralize with the circulation[22,23]. All mitochondrial autoantigens are coded by nuclear DNA, and the resulting mRNA is transcribed in the nucleus and transported into the cytoplasm. MRNA for these proteins contain mitochondrial targeting sequences (MTS) in the 5' region, which leads to the selective transport of the synthesized protein from the cytosol into the mitochondria across the mitochondrial outer and inner membrane[24]. By contrast, HLA class I or class II molecules, which are required for the presentation of autoantigens to the immune system, are synthesized in the cytosol and transferred to the endoplasmic reticulum. HLA class II molecules have to be transported to the endocytic compartment via the Golgi apparatus where they get loaded with peptides predominantly from exogenous antigen[25,26].

One thesis that explains the recognition of self molecules is the concept of molecular mimicry. The concept of molecular mimicry is based on the fact that there is a close similarity between a protein of infectious agents such as bacteria, virus, parasites or yeast and an autologous host protein exposure to the infectious agent source of the protein. In particular, the peptide processed from this protein may be significantly distinct but cross reactive with a self peptide. The cross-reactive T or B cell is then able to induce a pathogenic autoimmune response that leads to disease[27-29]. Indeed, it is well know that molecular mimicry plays a role in the pathogenesis of rheumatic fever, where streptococcal cell wall proteins crossreact with myocardial proteins[30]. In Guillain-Barre syndrome (GBS), there is an association between intestinal infection with Campylobacter jejuni and the onset of GBS[31]. Davies also proposed that molecular mimicry between proteins/peptides from infectious organisms and self proteins/peptides may be involved in the immunopathogenesis of Lyme disease, myasthenia gravis, viral myocarditis, peripheral demyelinating neuropathy, ankylosing spondylitis, and systemic lupus erythematosus[32].

PDC-E2 is critical in the respiratory chain. Evolutionary, it is well conserved among various species, from eubacteria to mammals[33]. Although PDC-E2 is present in mitochondria, several lines of evidences suggest that one component of the 2-oxoacid dehydrogenase complex, dihydrolipoamide dehydrogenase, PDC, OGDC and BCOADC, are detectable in the membrane fraction of E.coli[34], Neisseria meningitidis[35], and Trypanosoma brucei[36]. It is also reported that the protein located in the membrane of Neisseria meningitidis consists of 11 amino acid residues highly homologous with that of the lipoyl domain of E2 component[35]. Since it is believed that the origin of mitochondria in mammalian cells are intracellular organisms, it may be reasonable that mitochondrial components, usually located in the mitochondrial inner membrane, are detected in the membrane of the organisms. The presence of these displayed proteins on the cell surface of bacteria may help tolerance breakdown.

There are several lines of evidence to support the concept that molecular mimicry may operate in PBC. It is believed that there is a high prevalence of bacteruria with a very high recurrence rate in females with PBC compared to other forms of chronic liver disease[37]. Patients with recurrent urinary tract infections, all of whom have normal liver functions, are reported to have weak AMA reactivity (69%)[38]. This (if true) suggests an association between E.coli or other bacteria causing urinary tract infection and the etiology of PBC. In fact, several lines of evidence demonstrate cross-reactivity of AMA against prokaryotic antigens, including E.coli, Klebsiella pneumoniae, Proteus mirabilis, Staphylococcus aureas, and Salmonella minnesota, although the target components of AMA in the bacteria have not been fully determined[39]. Furthermore, the sera from patients with PBC have been shown to react with both human PDC-E2 and E.coli PDC-E2, and the epitope of E.coli PDC-E2 also maps to similar lipoyl domains[40]. Vilagut et al. demonstrated that the sera from patients with PBC react with an extracts of Mycobacterium gordonae[41], and that antibodies to the M. gordonae 65 kD heat-shock protein weakly cross-react with the mitochondrial autoantigens, PDC-E2 and BCOADC-E2[42], implicating M. gordonae in the etiology of PBC. In contrast, the presence of reactivity of patients sera against M. gordonae was not supported by another group[43]. Klein et al. demonstrated that sera from 12 out of 28 patients (43%) with active pulmonary tuberculosis reacted to the PDC-E2 subunit, whereas only two of 82 patients with other bacterial and viral infections including 25 patients with E.coli infections reacted with the PBC-specific autoepitopes[44], also implicating mycobacterial infection in PBC. These cross-reactivities are not surprising, in view of the conserved structure of the PDC-E2 among many organisms (Table 2).

It is critical, however, to realize that T-cell mediated immune responses specific for the autoantigen needs to be present to initiate the immune response by providing appropriate helper T-cell function for the B cell to make antibodies. By reason, therefore, cross-reactivity at the T-cell level is required to break self-tolerance. Shimoda et al.[14] demonstrated cross-reactivity between human PDC-E2 and E.coli PDC-E2. One of their T-cell clones cross-reacts with the exogenous peptide derived from the lipoic acid binding domain of E.coli PDC-E2 (EQSLITVEGDKASM). From a human PDC-E2 study, the amino acids E, D, and K, at

TABLE 2. ALIGNMENT OF THE INNER LIPOYL DOMAIN OF PDC-E2 (AMINO ACID RESIDUES 135-190) OF HUMAN, *M. TUBERCULOSIS* AND *E. COLI*

human	135	V L L P A L S P T M T M G T V Q R W E K K V G E K L S E G	163
E. coli		K E V N V P D I G G D E V E V T E V M V K V G D K V A A E	
M. tuberculosis		V Q M P A L G E S V T E G T V T R W L K Q E G D T V E L D	
human	164	D L L A E I E T D K A T I G F E V Q E E G Y L A K I L	190
E. coli		Q S L I T V E G D K A S M E V P A P F A G V V K E L K	
M. tuberculosis		E P L V E V S T D K V D T E I P S P A A G V L T K I I	

The identical amino acid residue with human PDC-E2 are shown in bold letters. The underlined letters indicate closely related amino acid residues with human PDC-E2.

positions 170, 172, and 173 respectively, are found to be essential amino acid residues for the T-cell epitope. The T-cell epitope of *E.coli* PDC-E2 also contains this EXDK sequences. These results indicate that molecular mimicry between human PDC-E2 and *E.coli* PDC-E2 could be operative at the T-cell clonal level in PBC. However, none of the T-cell clones reacted to the *Pseudomonas putida* BCOADC peptide 104-117 (DELLATIETDKIDI), which also has EXDK sequences, and non of T-cell clones cross-react to self-peptides derived from human glycogen phosphylase β (LVDLERMDWDKAWD) or the HLA DR α chain (QGALANIAVDKANL), both of which contain some amino acid homology with human PDC-E2 163-176 but do not contain EXDK sequences.

This result, showing no cross-reactivity with HLA DR α chain in the T-cell level, should be noted in understanding the molecular mimicry in PBC, MHC linkage to autoimmune disease is well known and, in some cases, can be considered as the cross-reactivity between MHC molecules and infectious agents, as described elsewhere[45]. Baum et al. thus proposed the 'MHC-mimicry' model for explaining the induction of autoimmunity[46]. According to his model, MHC-derived peptides are prominent in selecting the repertoire of CD4+ T-cell reactivity. In the periphery, 'mimicking' foreign peptides activate positively-selected autoreactive CD4+ T-cells, resulting in autoimmune disease. They described the striking similarity between nuclear autoantigen SP-100 (SHDLQRMFTED), which is detected in PBC, and a peptide of HLA-Bw47 (SHTLQRMFGCD)[46]. However, the fact that there is not a strong homology of mitochondrial autoantigens with HLA molecules and that there is no cross-reactivity with the HLA DR α chain at the T-cell level makes it unlikely that this model is operational in human PBC. Rather, we propose that peripheral tolerance might be directly arrogated by microbial infections, leading to the clonal expansion of cross-reactive T-cell clones specific for mitochondrial autoantigens, which have not been deleted in the thymus.

Why Only Biliary Duct? – The Significance of Tissue-Specific Antigens

However, even if human PDC-E2 specific T-cell clones are once activated by exogenous bacterial antigens secondary to urinary tract infections, autoimmune reactions, such as AMA production to tissue damage, would not normally occur, since human mitochondrial autoantigens are intracellular proteins and are not normally exposed to autoreactive T-cell clones. Moreover, human PDC-E2 is present in every mitochondrion in the human body. In PBC, there must be a reason why only biliary epithelial cells would be chosen as a target of autoimmune reaction after T-cell clones specific for human PDC-E2 are activated. In some organ-specific autoimmune diseases, tissue-specific autoantigens recognised by autoantibodies or autoepitope-specific T-cells have been identified. Myocardial proteins, which are the target of autoantibodies in rheumatic fever[30], or ganglioside GM1 in Guillain-Barre syndrome[31], are good examples of tissue-specific antigens. One of the best characterized autoantigens is the nicotinic acetylcholine receptor (AChR), which is the target of the pathogenic autoantibodies in myasthenia gravis (MG) which leads to reduced AChR levels and subsequent muscle weakness. T-cell clones specific for human AChR have also been established[47]. Another good example of tissue-specific antigens is thyroglobulin (Tg), which is a major autoantigen in autoimmune thyroiditis; B cell and T-cell pathogenic autoepitopes of Tg have been mapped[48]. In autoimmune thyroid disease, thyroptropin receptor (TSHR) is also known to be a target of an autoantibody response. In general, Hashimoto's disease is due to T-cell responses directed against Tg, and Graves' disease is mediated by autoantibodies to the TSHR[49]. Therefore, it is not atypical that disease-specific antigens would be also expressed exclusively on biliary epithelial cells in patients with PBC, and that antigen-specific autoimmune reaction would be directed against the antigens.

We previously reported the development and characterisation of PDC-E2 specific murine monoclonal antibodies[50]. Among these, there are eight monoclonal antibodies that have been mapped to four different regions of PDC-E2 by studies utilizing ELISA and immunoblotting with overlapping recombinant fragments. All produced intense immunofluorescence of mitochondria when used to stain Hep-2 cells. We used these eight murine monoclonal antibodies against PDC-E2 to investigate the localization of PDC-E2 in PBC liver. In addition, we also used a human Fab combinatorial antibody termed LC5 specific for PDC-E2, derived from a PBC lymph node Fab combinatorial library. This Fab recombinant antibody reacts with PDC-E2 and protein X but not BCOADC-E2, OGDC-E2 or PDC-E1α by immunoblotting. It is also specific for the lipoyl domain of PDC-E2.

Using this panel of eight mouse monoclonal antibodies and a human combinatorial antibody specific for PDC-E2, we examined by indirect immunofluorescence and confocal microscopy sections of liver from patients with PBC, and progressive sclerosing cholangitis (PSC) and hepatocellular carcinoma as controls[51]. The monoclonal antibodies gave typical mitochondrial immuno-fluorescence on biliary epithelium and on hepatocytes from patients with either PBC, PSC or hepatocarcinoma. However, one of the eight mouse monoclonal antibodies, C355.1, and the human combinatorial antibody reacted with great intensity and specificity with the luminal region of biliary epithelial cells from patients with PBC. The selective reactivity of some anti-PDC-E2 monoclonal antibodies may be interpreted as indicating the presence of tissue-specific autoantigens, which are cross-reactive with PDC-E2 or, less likely, PDC-E2 itself, in the luminal region of biliary epithelial cells in PBC.

We believe that the tissue-specific antigens on biliary epithelium in PBC would be the targets of T-cells as well as B cells. CD4+ T-cells specific for human PDC-E2, even if activated by the cross-reactivity with bacterial components, must recognise the tissue-specific antigens on the biliary epithelial cells in the context of HLA molecules and be clonally expanded to help the production of high-titer AMA. Several line of evidences have shown that HLA class I and II molecules are aberrantly expressed on biliary epithelial cells[52]. Biliary epithelial cells, however, are "non-professional" antigen presenting cells, and the expression of the co-stimulatory molecules is crucially important for antigen presentation to naive T-cells. It is generally accepted that T-cells recognizing the peptide bound within the HLA groove would become anergic without the second

signal delivered from co-stimulatory molecules[53]. Therefore, the expression of co-stimulatory molecules on biliary epithelial cells would be necessary to act as antigen presenting cells. However, the results on the expression of co-stimulatory molecules are somewhat contradictory. Leon et al.[54] failed to demonstrate the expression of the CD50/CD86 molecules on damaged bile ducts expressing HLA class II in PBC. By contrast, Nakanuma et al. found that CD86 was faintly expressed on epithelial cells in half the bile ducts in PBC using formalin-fixed and paraffin-embedded sections after antigen retrieval by microwave treatment[52]. The capability of biliary epithelial cells for antigen presentation, in terms of the expression of co-stimulatory molecules, is an important issue and needs to be resolved.

Aberrant ductal expression of PDC-E2?

If PDC-E2 itself is differentially expressed on the surface of biliary epithelial cells in patients with PBC, it may be easily recognised by the host and by yet an unknown mechanism lead to a breakdown of self-tolerance against PDC-E2. Several hypothesis can be considered to explain the ductular overexpression of PDC-E2. The first possibility of overexpression of PDC-E2 in biliary epithelial cells. In situ hybridization of PDC-E2, however, showed that there were no significant differences in PDC-E2 expression between PBC and other liver diseases. Second, mutant or tissue-specific variants of PDC-E2 may cause an abnormal turnover of the molecule, leading to the accumulation of PDC-E2 in the cells. In this case, it is unlikely that mutations would take place in genomic DNA of the host, because PDC-E2 is a crucial molecule in metabolism of a cell and the host would not survive if all PDC-E2 molecules are affected. Rather, transcription of PDC-E2 would be abnormal and altered PDC-E2 mRNA would be locally produced.

It is also possible that the leader sequences of PDC-E2 becomes changed or altered and leads to abnormality subcellular distribution, from mitochondria to plasma membrane[24]. PDC-E2 will remain in the mitochondria without any modification in the leader sequence even if overexpressed or accumulated. PDC-E2 are coded by nuclear DNA And imported from the nucleus into the mitochondria by a mitochondrial targeting sequence (MTS). PDC-E2 has to be delivered into the endoplasmic reticulum (ER) and Golgi apparatus via a secretory route to be expressed on the cell surface of biliary ducts, and the whole leader sequence of PDC-E2 must be replaced by an ER-targeting signal instead of MTS. This might occur by abnormal splicing during synthesis of mRNA coding for PDC-E2.

In addition, if the molecules which anti-PDC-E2 recognises on the apical surface of biliary ducts are human PDC-E2 itself, peptides generated from human PDC-E2 must be presented in association with HLA molecules to be recognised by T-cells, otherwise biliary epithelial cells cannot be a target for PDC-E2 specific T-cells. In normal conditions PDC-E2 never enters the processing route of intracellular antigens which, following processing into peptides, are bound to HLA class I molecules. The leader sequences of PDC-E2 must be modified by antibody binding or mutations which may lead to intracellular degradation by non-classical antigen processing enzymes which leads to the generation of peptides being presented on the cell surface in the context of HLA class I molecules. It is also possible that PDC-E2 is released into the bile fluid and extracellular proteases, reduced peptides which because of their relative higher affinity replace the existing peptides bound to the MHC class I molecules in the biliary epithelial cells.

Do biliary duct-specific novel antigens cross react with PDC-E2?

Alternatively, the molecules on the ductular surface of biliary epithelial cells which are recognised by anti-PDC-E2 monoclonal antibodies may not be PDC-E2 itself. Rather, it may be molecules which "look like" PDC-E2 and crossreact with human PDC-E2. One possibility for a source of this molecule is infectious agents, such as an intracellular bacteria or virus, or an endogenous retrovirus.

Although the biliary tract is believed to be aseptic in normal conditions, bacteria may infect bile ducts and biliary epithelial cells in some pathological conditions, such as those seen with gallstones or chronic cholecystitis, in which a number of bacteria are found in bile acid. As previously described, PDC-E2 are well conserved between human and bacteria, and it is likely that bacterial PDC-E2 from any intracellular bacterium would be recognised by anti-PDC-E2 antibodies. Alternatively, bacterial infection may result in auto-antibody formation against self components, including mitochondrial proteins. Infection with Helicobacter pylori, known to be a cause for gastric inflammation, ulcers, and carcinoma, induces autoantibodies reactive with the protein located in gastric parietal cell canaliculi, H^+K^+-ATPase[55]. Infected patients develop antibodies to H. pylori lipopolysaccharide (LPS) and native H^+K^+-ATPase. Since H^+K^+-ATPase is also the major autoantigen in autoimmune gastritis and pernicious anaemia, the initiating role of H. pylori in these diseases has been proposed. We are impressed by recent findings that Helicobacter species, such as

H. Bilis, Flexispira rappini, or H. Pullorum, are detected in bile in patients with chronic cholecystitis by PCR[56]. Another group also identified a high prevalence (65.2%), of autoantibodies against the CagA protein of H. pylori, in infected patients[57].

Viruses are often cited as possible causative factors in autoimmune diseases. Indeed, Epstein-Barr virus (EBV), cytomegalovirus (CMV), and enteroviruses are frequently indicated as candidates of environmental triggers for the induction of autoimmunity. Furthermore, two human retroviruses, human immune deficiency virus (HIV) and human T-cell leukemia virus type-I (HTLV-I), can induce conditions that resemble classic autoimmune diseases, and the pathological mechanisms of diseases induced by these agents may have important autoimmune components. HIV infections may lead to a wide array of autoimmune diseases or autoimmune disease-like conditions, including hematological disorders (thrombocytopenia and anaemia), Sjögren's syndrome-like disease, systemic lupus erythematosus (SLE), polymyositis, and vasculitis[58], whereas HTLV-I is well known to be associated with tropical spastic paraparesis (TSP)/HTLV-I associated myelopathy. HTLV-I transgenic mice expressive the HTLV-I tax gene develop symptoms similar to Sjögren's syndrome, and transgenic mice expressing parts of the HTLV-I env and tax gene develop an arthropathy resembling rheumatoid arthritis[59].

Several other mechanisms by which virus infection results in autoimmune diseases have also been proposed[58,60,61]. First, as previously described, molecular mimicry between viral components and host proteins may occur. Second, virus-induced alteration of autoantigens, or of their presentation to the immune system, may be possible. As proposed elsewhere[61], cytolytic viruses might also contribute to the development of autoimmunity by exposing intracellular antigens generally not accessible to immune cells. Retroviruses, like several other viruses, may also induce the synthesis of immunogenic proteins, such as heat shock proteins. Alternatively, viral determinants are often expressed in cell surface and elicit antiviral host responses that might trigger autoimmune reactions against autoantigens in close proximity to the viral antigens[61]. Third, autoimmunity may be elicited through transcriptional factors derived from viruses. The long terminal repeats (LTR) found at both ends of an integrated retroviral provirus contains potent transcriptional promoters than can respond to various transcriptional control mechanisms. For example, mouse mammalian tumor virus (MMTV) and related endogenous retro elements are activated in female mice by estrogens because of hormone response elements in the TLR. Some HERV are also activated by sex hormones. This could explain the female predominance in most autoimmune diseases, including PBV. Retroviruses are known to produce powerful transcriptional activators, Tax of HTLV or Tat of HIV, which may induce the overexpression of other autoantigens.

There is no known structural similarity of viral proteins with human mitochondrial autoantigens. Nevertheless, the possibility of viral infection, or activation of HERV, as a trigger for the onset of PBC should not be underestimated. Still it is an attractive hypothesis to assume the presence of an endogenous retrovirus-like element which is specifically expressed in biliary epithelial cells in patients with PBC under the influence of female hormones, and is highly homologous with human PDC-E2.

Alternatively, the tissue-specific autoantigens cross-reactive with mitochondrial protein may not be infectious agents. They may be self-antigens, i.e. cell surface proteins. Infection by bacteria or virus may alter the antigenicity of self proteins, leading to the presentation to the immune system with HLA molecules and recognition by PDC-E2 specific T-cells. Self proteins would immunologically behave in a different manner if (a) the amino acid residues are replaced and/or (b) the change of proteolytic pattern would result in the presentation of cryptic epitope, and/or (c) the amino acid sequence of T-cell epitope would be altered. It is well accepted that the quality of the T-cell response evoked by so-called altered peptide ligands (APL) can be very different[62]. Thus, APL derived from self protein might be cross-reactive with PDC-E2 specific T-cells clones which escaped peripheral tolerance, resulting in autoimmune cascade. If this is the case, however, the infectious agents will be present in the epithelial cells only in the initial step of the induction of the disease, and it seems impossible to detect them at the ductal stage in liver with patients diagnosed as having PBC.

Difficulty In Predicting a Molecular Mimic

One difficulty in determining targets of anti-PDC-E2 antibodies on biliary epithelial cells is that these antibodies recognise conformational epitopes. Although the epitope of AMA has been mapped to the inner lipoyl domain of PDC-E2, several lines of data suggest that AMA instead recognise a conformational epitope on PDC-E2[11], as described. This fact implicates that molecular mimicry at the B cell level cannot be predicted by a homology search of the amino acid

sequences. It is possible that two molecules which are quite different in their primary structure might have a similar conformation and are recognised by the identical antibody.

The T-cell epitope, on the other hand, is believed to be more simple. Linear amino acids, even though the length of them vary, are bound to the groove of HLA class I or class II molecules and are recognised by the T-cell receptor (TCR). Thus, it is considered that molecular mimicry between microbial peptides and self-antigens at the T-cell level is expected by the sequence homology, based on the assumption that the identity of the primary sequences of amino acids would lead to such crossreactivity[27,28]. However, growing evidence demonstrate that antigen recognition of T-cells are me complex and degenerate than expected. It has been reported that an antigen-specific T-cell could cross-react with peptides sharing only a few homologous amino acid residues which are critical for binding to the appropriate HLA groove[63,64]. Moreover, Hemmer et al. recently demonstrated that human CDR+ autoreactive T-cell clones specific for myelin basic protein (MBP) 87-99, VHFFKNIVTPRTP, showed a proliferative response to the agonist peptide, GGLLAHVISAKKA, which had no sequence homology with the original MBP 87-99 peptide[65], although they claimed that the sequence of the agonist was able to be predicted by the relative influence of each amino acid residue of the original and substituted sequences[66-68]. This implicates the extreme difficulty of the prediction of the unrelated molecules which cross-react with PDC-E2 by homology search. Nevertheless, as Roudier et al. suggested[66], protein databases have been growing fast, and there has been considerable improvement in the computer software used to explore them. PDC-E2 specific T-cells might be activated by an unexpected molecule in patients with PBC.

Th1 and Th2 Balance

As previously described, it is crucial to elucidate how antigen-specific autoimmune reactions against disease-specific antigens take place in biliary epithelial cells in patients with PBC. The disease-specific antigens, however, might be also expressed even in healthy individuals. Although it is true that autoreactive T-cells specific for the autoantigens are responsible for the development of disease, the expression of autoantigens might not be enough to develop the disease. The importance of non-specific factors, with antigen-specific responses, should not be overlooked.

The concept of the Th1/Th2 paradigm has gained importance[69]. Th1 cells are known to secrete IL-2 or

IFN-γ and believed to play a role in delayed-type hypersensitivity (DTH) and cellular immunity. On the other hand, Th2 cells secrete IL-4, IL-5, IL-6 or IL-13 which influence humoral immunity, including activation of B cells and class switching. Th2 cells are important in allergy reactions via enhancing IgE secretion and activation of mast cells or eosinophils. Since IFN-γ from Th1 cells suppresses the secretion of cytokines from Th2, and, in contrast, IL-10 from Th2 cells suppresses Th1 cytokines, the two prototype subsets, Th1 and Th2, counteract each other. Therefore, the balance of Th1 and Th2 cells are crucial for maintenance of normal immunological status. The predominance of either Th1 or Th2 may lead to the development of autoimmune diseases.

In organ-specific autoimmune diseases, Th1 cells are believed to be more important in developing disease. In fact, in mice with experimental autoimmune encephalitis (EAE), Th1 cells are dominant in infiltrating lymphocytes around the lesions when the disease is exacerbated[70-72]. In non-obese diabetic (NOD) mice, which is a murine model for human type I diabetes, Th1 cells have been shown to play an important role for islet cell destruction[73-75].

In PBC, several lines of studies suggest the dominance of Th1 cells. Shindo et al. demonstrated IFN-γ was the major cytokine in the liver of patients with PBC by RT-PCR[76]. Tsai also detected Il-2 and IFN-γ in the liver by RT-PCR but failed to detect IL-4[77]. Berg et al. investigated the cytokine profiles in supernatants of nonstimulated PBMC from 50 anti-M2 positive PBC patients and 20 healthy controls in order to define whether Th1 or Th2 response predominate in PBC. The results showed there was a shift in the Th2/Th1 ratio towards Th1 (1:1) as compared to the healthy controls (ratio 3:1), indicating the Th1 dominance[78]. Van de Water et al. also found that T-cell clones specific for PDC-E2 derived from PBC livers secreted mainly either IL-2 or IFN-γ, but not Th2 cytokines, such as IL-4[79]. Moreover, by in situ hybridization, Harada et al. showed that IFN-γ mRNA expression was more commonly detected than IL-4 expression in PBC livers[80]. Taken together, it is very likely that Th1 cells predominance, and the cytokines secreted from Th1 cells, have a great influence on the immunopathogenesis of PBC.

Then why are the Th1 cells predominant in PBC or other tissue-specific autoimmune diseases? One possibility for the polarization of Th1/Th2 is that this is due to an infectious process due to microorganisms. It is well known that T-cell subsets will determine susceptibility against Leishmania infections in mice[81]. For example, as described elsewhere, experimental infections with L. major in genetically susceptible mice results in a disseminated, lethal disease. The infected animal responds to the invading parasite with CD4+ Th2 cells secreting IL-4, IL-5, IL-6 and IL-10. However, in genetically resistant strains, a predominant CD4+ Th1 response occurs, with secretion of IFN-γ, IL-2 and tumor necrosis factor β (TNF-β), leading to spontaneous recovery. It has been proposed that natural killer (NK) cells, which promptly react to infection, are responsible for IFN-γ secretion and thus may participate in the initiation of a human, Th1-like T-cell response in Leishmania infections. Also, Mycobacterium leprae infections in humans are associated with strong cell-mediated, delayed-type hypersensitivity (DTH) responses to mycobacterial antigens with the infection results in a subclinical or localized form. Disseminated (lepromatous) leprosy is associated with a lack of DTH reaction and increased production of antibodies. Thus, the Th1-dominant reaction is favourable in terms of the eradication of M. leprae.[82]. While it seems that a Th1 response elicited by NK cells, as a first-line defence against micro-organisms, is necessary to cease the infection as localized and subclinical form, the polarization of Th1 reaction may be of importance in the induction of tissue-specific autoimmune diseases, which would be triggered by microorganisms.

The Th1/Th2 balance may also be affected by the stimulus from environmental infectious agents, or even vaccinations[83]. For instance, mycobacteria infections are no longer epidemic in the developed countries. Since mycobacteria induces a predominant TH1-like reaction in the infected host, it may be one of the reasons for the increasing incidence of allergy, one of the Th2 diseases, in modern countries. Indeed, Shirakawa et al. demonstrated a strong inverse association between delayed hypersensitivity to Mycobacterium tuberculosis and atopy, known to be Th2-disease, indicating that the exposure to mycobacteria may inhibit atopic disorders by inverting the Th1/Th2 balance[84]. Also, bacterial flora may influence the Th1/Th2 balance. The human intestinal flora is a very complex system, consisting of 1.5kg bacterial mass, over 400 different species of microorganisms[85]. These facts have led to the concept that there is a very close connection between resident bacteria and the mucosal immune system. Continuous stimulation from resident bacteria would be required to maintain an appropriate Th1/Th2 balance. In humans, involvement of bacterial flora in the bowel in the pathogenesis of rheumatoid arthritis has been frequently proposed[86-90]. The incidence of autoimmune diseases, including PBC, is higher in more developed countries where sanitary system and a clean water supply are provided. These "clean" environments which inhibit the growth of conventional bacterial flora may play a significant role in the change of the polarization of Th1/Th2 balance. Another candidate which may determine Th1/Th2 balance is NK1.1* T-cells. These cells constitute a unique subset among mature CD4⁻CD8⁻ and CD4⁺CD8⁻ T lymphocytes that co-express the NK1.1 antigen[91-93]. Strikingly, NK1.1⁺ T-cells express a single invariant T-cell receptor α chain encoded by the Vα14 and Jα281 segments, mostly in association with Vβ8[94-96]. The implication of NK1.1⁺ T-cells in Th1/Th2 deviation has been suggested by the fact that NK1.1⁺ T-cells secrete a large amount of IL-4 promptly after CD3 stimulation[97,98], and that the failure to produce IL-4 and IgE in response to anti IgD antibody injection in SJL mice and β2-microglobulin-deficient mice was linked to their deficiency in IL-4 producing NK1.1⁺ T-cells[99,100]. In addition, the role of NK1.1⁺ T-cells in Th1 immune

response has been also demonstrated; they produce IFN-γ as well as macrophage inflammatory protein-1 $\alpha\beta$ and lymphotactin[93,101,102]. Interestingly, Makino et al. reported that Vα14⁺ NK1.1⁺ T-cells was selectively reduced along with the development of autoimmune disease in 1pr mice[103]. In human, it was demonstrated that T-cells bearing an invariant Vα24JαQ, the human counterpart of Vα14Jα281 NK1.1⁺ T-cells in mice, was selectively reduced in peripheral blood of patients with systemic sclerosis[104]. Thus, it has been proposed that NK1.1⁺ T-cells would operate as regulatory cells in the immune system, and be in part responsible for the development of autoimmune diseases. It should also be noted that NK1.1⁺ T-cells differentiate at extrathymic sites, including the liver, through contact with CD1d molecules. Recently, the ligand of this TCR/CD1d complex has been determined as glycosylceramides, which are also detected in certain bacteria[105].

REFERENCES

1. Gershwin M, Mackay I, Sturgess A, et al. 1987. Identification and specificity of a cDNA encoding the 70kd mitochondrial antigen recognised in primary biliary cirrhosis. J Immunol 138: 3525-3531.

2. Van de Water J, Gershwin M, Leung P. 1988. The autoeptiope of the 74-kD mitochondrial autoantigen of primary biliary cirrhosis corresponds to the functional site of dihydrolipoamide acetyltransferase. J Exp Med 167: 1791-1799.

3. Coppel R, McNeilage L, Surh C. 1988. Primary structure of the human M2 mitochondrial autoantigen of primary biliary cirrhosis: dihydrolipoamide acetyltransferase. Proc Natl Acad Sci USA 85: 7317-7321.

4. Yeaman S. 1986. The mammalian 2-oxoacid dehydrogenase: a complex family. Trends Biochem Sci 11: 293-296.

5. Bassendine M, Fusey S, Mutimer D, et al. 1989. Identification and characterization of four M2 mitochondrial autoantigens in primary biliary cirrhosis. Semin Liver Dis 9: 124-131.

6. Harris R, Bowker-Kinley M, Wu P, et al. 1997. Dihydrolipoamide dehydrogensase-binding protein of the human pyruvate dehydrogenase complex. DNA-derived amino acid sequence, expression, and reconstitution of the pyruvate dehydrogenase complex. J Biol Chem 272: 6361-6369.

7. Mattevi A, Obmolova G, Schulze E. 1992. Atomic structure of the cubic core of the pyruvate dehydrogenase multienzyme complex. Science 255: 1544-1550.

8. Davis A, Laue E, Perham R. 1995. Three-dimensional structure of the lipoyl domain from Baccilus sterothemophilus pyruvate dehydrogenase multienzyme complex. J Mol Biol 229: 1037-1048.

9. Green J, Laue E, Perham R. 1995. Three-dimensional structure of a lipoyl domain from the dihydrolipoyl acetyltransferase component of the pyruvate dehydrogenase multienzyme complex of Escherichia coli. J Mol Biol 248: 328-343.

10. Bassendine M, Jones D, Yeaman S. 1997. Biochemistry and autoimmune response to the x-oxoacid dehydrogenase complexes in primary biliary cirrhosis. Semin Liver Dis 17: 49-60.

11. Surh C, Coppel R, Gershwin M. 1990. Structural requirement for autoreactivity on human pyruvate dehydrogenase-E2, the major autoantigen of primary biliary cirrhosis. Implication for a conformational autoepitope. J Immunol 144: 1321-1328.

12. Cha S, Leung P, Coppel R, et al. 1994. Heterogeneity of combinatorial human autoantibodies against PDC-E2 and biliary epithelial cells in patients with primary biliary cirrhosos. Hepatology 20: 574-583.

13. Leung S, Chuang D, Wynn R, et al. 1995. Autoantibodies to BCOADC-E2 in patients with primary biliary cirrhosis recognize a conformational epitope. Hepatology 22: 505-513.

14. Shimoda S, Nakamura M, Ishibashi H. 1995. HLA DRB4 0101-restricted immunodominant T-cell autoeptiope of pyruvate dehydrogenase complex in primary biliary cirrhosis: evidence of molecular mimicry in human autoimmune disease. J Exp Med 181: 1835-1845.

15. Leung P, Iwayama T Coppel, R, et al. 1990. Site-directed mutagenesis of lysine within the immunodominant autoepitope of PDC-E2. Hepatology 12: 1321-1328.

16. Quinn J, Diamond A, Palmer J, et al. 1993. Lipoylated and unlipoylated domains of human PDC-E2 as autoantigens in primary biliary cirrhosis: significance of lipate attachment. Hepatology 18: 1384-1391.

17. Landry S. 1997. Local protein instability predictive of helper T-cell eiptopes. Immunology Today 18: 527-532.

18. Wekerle H, Bradl M, Linington C, et al. 1996. The shaping of the grain-specific T lyphocyte repertoire in the thymus. Immunol Rev 149: 231-243.

19. Sercarz E, Lehemann P, Ametani A, et al. 1993. Dominance and crypticity of T-cell antigenic determinants. Annu Rev Immunol 11: 729-766.

20. Lanzavecchia A. 1995. How can cryptic epitopes trigger autoimmunity? J Exp Med 181: 1945-1948.

21. Barnaba V. 1996. Viruses, hidden self-epitopes and autoimmunity. Immunol Rev 152: 47-66.

22. Fairchild P, Wraith D. 1996. Lowering the tone: mechanisms of immunodominance among eoptopes with low affinity for MHC. Immunology Today 17: 80-85.

23. Barnaba V, Sinigaglia F. 1997. Molecular mimicry and T-cell-mediated autoimmune disease. J Exp Med 185: 1529-1531.

24. Kieber M, Becker K, Pfanner N, et al. 1993. Mitochondrial protein import: specific recognition membrane translocation of preproteins. J Membrane Biology 135: 191-207.

25. Neefjes J, Momburg F. 1993. Cell biology of antigen presentation. Curr Opin Immunol 5: 27-34.

26. Rammensee H, Falk K, Rotzchke O. 1993. MHC molecules as peptide receptors. Curr Opin Immunol 5: 35-44.

27. Anderson D, Van Schooten W, Barry M, et al. 1988. A Mycobacterium leprae-specific human T-cell epitope crossreacts with an HLA-DR2 peptide. Science 242: 259-261.

28. Fujinami R, Oldstone M. 1985. Amino acid homology between the encephalitogenic site of myelin basic protein and virus: mechanism for autoimmunity. Science 230: 1043-1045.

29. Wraith D, Brunn B, Fairchild P. 1992. Cross-reactive antigen recognition by an encephalitogenic T-cell receptor: implication for T-child biology and autoimmunity. *J Immunol* **149**: 3765-3770.

30. Froude J, Gibofsky A, Buskirk D, *et al.* 1989. Cross-reactivity between streptococcus and human tissue: a model of molecular mimicry and autoimmunity. *Curr Top Microbiol Immunol* **145**: 5-26.

31. Yuki N, Taki T, Imagaki M. 1993. A bacterium lipopolysaccharide that elicits Guillain-Barre syndrome has a GM_l gaglioside-like structure. *J Exp Med* **178**: 1771-1775.

32. Davies J. 1997. Molecular mimicry: Can epitope mimicry induce autoimmune disease? *Immunol Cell Biol* **75**: 113-126.

33. Yeaman S, Fussey S, Danner D. 1988. Primary biliary cirrhosis: identification of two major M2 mitochondrial auroantigens. *Lancet* **i**: 1067-1070.

34. Owen P, Kaback H, Grame-cook K. 1980. Identification of antigen 19/27 as dihydrolipoyl dehydrongenase and its probable involvement in ubiquinone-mediated NADH-dependent transport phenomena in membrane vesicles of *Escherichia coli*. *FEMS Microbiology Letters* **7**: 345-348.

35. de al Sierra I, Pernot L, Prange T, *et al.* 1997. Molecular structure of the lipoamide dehydrogenase domain of a surface antigen from *Niesseria meningitidis*. *J Mol Biol* **269**: 129-141.

36. Danson M, Conroy K, McQuattie A, *et al.* 1987. Dihydrolipoamide dehydrogenase from *Trypanosoma brucei*: characterization and cellular location. *Biochem J* **243**: 661-665.

37. Burroughs A, Rosenstein I, Epstein O, *et al.* 1984. Bacteuria and primary biliary cirrhosis. *Gut* **25**: 133-137.

38. Butler P, Valle F, Hamilton-Miller J, *et al.* 1993. M2 mitochondrial antibodies and urinary rough mutant bacteria in patients with primary biliary cirrhosis and in patients with recurrent bacteriuria. *J Hepatol* **17**: 408-414.

39. Baum H. 1995. Mitochondrial antigens, molecular mimicry and autoimmune disease. *Biochem Biophys Acta* **1271**: 111-121.

40. Fussey S, Ali S, Guest J. 1990. Reactivity of primary biliary cirrhosis sera with *Escherichia coli* dihydrolipoamide acetyltransferase (E2p): characterization of the main immunogenic region. *Proc Natl Acad Sci USA* **87**: 3987-3991.

41. Vilagut L, Vila J, Vinas O, *et al.* 1993. *Mycobacterium gordonae* in primary biliary cirrhosis: possible etiology for the disease. *J Hepatol* **18**(Suppl 1): S7.

42. Vilagut L, Pares A, Vinas O, *et al.* 1997. Antibodies to mycobacterial 65-kD heat shock protein cross-react with the main mitochondrial antigens in patients with primary biliary cirrhosis. *Eur J Clin Invest* **27**: 667-672.

43. O'Donohue J, McFarlane B, Bomford A, *et al.* 1994. Antibodies to atypical mycobacteria in primary biliary cirrhosis. *J Hepatol* **21**: 887-889.

44. Klein R, Wiebel M, Engelhart S, *et al.* 1993. Sera from patients with tuberculosis recognize the M2a-epitope (E2-subunit of pyruvate dehydrogenase) specific for primary biliary cirrhosis. *Clin Exp Immunol* **92**: 308-316.

45. Ebringer A. 1992. Ankylosing spondylitis is caused by *Klebsiella*. Evidence from immunogenetic, microbiologic, and serologic studies. *Rheum Dis Clin North Am* **18**: 105-121.

46. Baum H, Davies H, Peakman M. 1996. Molecular mimicry in the MHC: hidden clues to autoimmunity? *Immunology Today* **17**: 64-70.

47. Hawke S, Matsuo H, Nicolle M, *et al.* 1996. Autoimmune T-cells in myasthenia gravis: heterogeneity and potential for specific immunotargetting. *Immunology Today* **17**: 307-311.

48. Carayannoitis G, Rao V. 1997. Searching for pathogenic epitopes in thyroglobulin: parameters and caveats. *Immunology Today* **18**: 83-88.

49. Prabhaker B, Fan J, Seatharamaish G. 1997. Thyrotropin-receptor-mediated diseases: a paradigm for receptor autoimmunity. *Immunology Today* **18**: 437-442.

50. Surh C, Coppel R, Gershwin M. 1990. Comparative epitope mapping of murine monoclonal and human autoantibodies to human PDH-E2, the major mitochondrial autoantigen of primary biliary cirrhosis. *J Immunol* **144**: 2647-2652.

51. Van de Water J, Turchany J, Leung P, *et al.* 1993. Molecular mimicry in primary biliary cirrhosis: evidence for biliary epithelial expression of a molecule cross-reactive with pyruvate dehydrogenase complex-E2. *J Clin Invest* **91**: 2653-2664.

52. Nakanuma Y, Yashoshima M, Tsuneyama K, *et al.* 1997. Histopathology of primary biliary cirrhosis with emphasis on expression of adhesion molecules. *Semin Liver Dis* **17**: 35-47.

53. Schwartz R 1992. Costimulation of T lymphocytes: the role of CD28, CTLA-4, and B7/BB1 in interleukin-2 production and immunotherapy. *Cell* **71**: 1065-1068.

54. Leon M, Kirby J, Gibbs P. 1995. Immunogenicity of biliary epithelial cels: study of the expression of B7 molecules. *J Hepatol* **22**: 591-595.

55. Appelmark B, Faller G, Claeys D, *et al.* 1998. Bugs in trial: the case of *Helicobacter pylori* and autoimmunity. *Immunology Today* **19**: 296-299.

56. Fox J, Dewhirst F, Shen Z, *et al.* 1998. Hepatic *Helicobacter* species identified in bile and gallbladder tissue from Chileans with choronic cholecystitis. *Gastroenterology* **114**: 755-763.

57. Figura N, Cetta F, Angelico M, *et al.* 1998. Most *Helicobacter pylori*-infected patients have specific antibodies, and some also have *H. pylori* antigens and genomic material in bile: is it a risk factor for gallstone formation? *Dig Dis Sci* **43**: 854-862.

58. Garry R, Krieg A, Cheevers W, *et al.* 1995. Retroviruses and their roles in chronic inflammatory diseases and autoimmunity. In *The Retroviridae, vol. 4*. J Levy, ed. Plenum Press, New York, p. 491-602.

59. Iwakura Y, Tosu M, Yoshida E. 1991. Induction of inflammatory arthropathy resembling rheumatoid arthritis in mice transgenic for HTLV-I. *Science* **253**: 1026-1028.

60. Wilkinson D, Mager D, Leong J. 1995. Endogenous human retroviruses. In *The Retroviridae, vol. 4*. J Levy, ed. Plenum Press, New York, p. 465-533.

61. McFarlane I, Path M. 1991. Autoimmunity and hepatotropic viruses. *Semin Liver Dis* **11**: 223-233.

62. Evavold B, Sloan-Lancaster J, Wilson K, *et al.* 1995. Specific T-cell recognition of minimally homologous peptides: evidence for endogenous ligands. *Immunity* **2**: 655-663.

63. Bhardwaj B, Kumar V, Geysen H, *et al.* 1993. Degenerate recognition of a dissimilar antigenic peptide by myelin-bacis protein-reactive T-cells. *J Immunol* **151**: 5000-5010.

64. Wucherpfenning K, Strominger J. 1995. Molecular mimicry in T-cell-mediated autoimmunity: viral peptides active human T-cell clones specific for myelin basic protein. *Cell* **80**: 695-705.

65. Hemmer B, Vergelli M, Gran B, *et al.* 1998. Predicable TC antigen recognition based on peptide scans leads to the identification of agonist ligands with no squence homology, *J Immunol* **160**: 3631-3636.

66. Roudier C, Auger I, Roudier J. 1996. Molecular mimicry reflected through database screening: serendipty or survival strategy? *Immunology Today* **17**: 357-358.

67. Garcia K, Degano M, Stanfield R, *et al.* 1996. An $\alpha\beta$ T-cell receptor structure at 2.5A and its orientation in the TCR-MHC complex. *Science* **274**: 209-219.

68. Garboczi D, Ghosh P, Utz U, *et al.* 1996. Structure of the complex between human T-cell receptor, viral peptide and HLA-A2. *Nature* **352**: 67-70.

69. Seder R, Paul W. 1994. Acquision of lymphokine-producing phenotype by CD4+ T-cells. *Annu Rev Immunol* **12**: 635-673.

70. Khoury S, Hancock W, Weiner H. 1992. Oral tolerance to myelin basic protein and natural recovery from experimental autoimmune encephamyelitis are associated with down-regulation of inflammatory cytokines and differential upregulation of transforming growth factor beta, interleukin 4, and prostaglandin E expression in the brain. *J Exp Med* **176**: 1355-1364.

71. Merill L, Kono D, Clayton J. 1992. Inflammatory leukocytes and cytokines in the peptide-induced disease of experimental allergic encephamyelitisin SJL and B10. PL mice. *Proc Natl Acad USA* **89**: 574-578.

72. Miller S, Karpus W. 1994. The immunopathogenesis and regulation of T-cell-mediated demyelinating diseases. *Immunology Today* **15**: 356-361.

73. Rabinovitch A. 1994. Immunoregulatory and cytokine imbalances in the pathogenesis of IDDM: therapeutic intervention by immunostimulation? *Diabetes* **43**: 613.

74. Katz J, Benoist C, Mathis D. 1995. T helper cell subsets in insulin-dependent diabetes. *Science* **268**: 1185.

75. Rocken M, Racke M, Schevach E. 1996. IL-4 induced immune deviation as antigen-specific therapy for inflammatory autoimmune disease. *Immonol Today* **17**: 225.

76. Shindo M, Mullin G, Braun-Elwert L, *et al.* 1996. Cytokine mRNA expression in the liver of patients with primary biliary cirrhosis (PBC) and chronic hepatitis B (CHB). *Clin Exp Immunol* **105**: 254-259.

77. Tsai S, Lai M, Chen D. 1996. Analysis of rearranged T-cell receptor (TCR) Vα transcripts in livers of primary biliary cirrhosis: preferential Vα usage suggests antigen-driven selection. *Clin Exp Immunol* **103**: 99-104.

78. Berg P, Klein R, Rocken M. 1997. Cytokines in primary biliary cirrhosis. *Semin Liver Dis* **17**: 115-123.

79. Van de Water J, Ansari A, Prindiville T. 1995. Heterogeneity of autoreactive T-cell clones specific for the E2 component of the pyruvate dehydrogenase complex in primary biliary cirrhosis. *J Exp Med* **181**: 723-733.

80. Harada K, Van de Water J, Leung P, *et al.* 1997. *In situ* nuclein acid hybridization of cytokines in primary biliary cirrhosis: predominance of the Th1 subset. *Hepatology* **25**: 791-796.

81. Kemp M, Theander T, Kharazmi A. 1996. The contrasting roles of CD4+ T-cells in intracellular infections in humans: leishmaniasis as an example. *Immunology Today* **17**: 13-16.

82. Yamamura M, Uyemura K, Deans R, *et al.* 1991. Defining protective responses to pathogens: cytokine profiles in leprosy lesions. *Science* **254**: 277-279.

83. Rook G, Stanford J. 1998. Give us this day our daily germs. *Immunology today* **116**: 113-116.

84. Shirakawa T, Enomoto T, Shimazu S, *et al.* 1997, the inverse association between tuberculin responses and atopic disorder. *Science* **275**: 77-79.

85. Eerole E, Mottonen T, Hannonen P, *et al.* 1994. Intestinal flora in early rheumatoid arthritis. *Br J Rheumatol* **33**: 1030-1038.

86. Granfors K, Jalkanen S, von Essen R. 1989. *Yersinia* antigens in synovial-fluid cells from patients with reactive arthritis. *N Engl J Med* **320**: 216-221.

87. Shinebaum R, Neumann V, Cooke E, *et al.* 1987. Comparison of farcal flora in patients with rheumatoid arthritis and controls. *Br J Rheumatol* **26**: 329-333.

88. Olhagen B, Mansson I. 1974. *Clostridium perfringens* and rheumatoid arthritis. *J Infect Dis* **130**: 444-445.

89. Deighton C, Gray Z, Bint A, *et al.* 1992. Specificity of the Proteus antibody response in rheumatoid arthritis. *Ann Rheum Dis* **39**: 1206-1207.

90. Khalafpour S, Ebringer A, Abuljadayel I, *et al.* 1988. Antibodies to *Klebsiella* and *Proteus* microorganisms in ankylosing spondylitis and rheumatoid arthritis patients measured by ELISA. *Br J Rheum* **27** (Suppl 2): 86-89.

91. Bendelac A, Rivera M, Park S, *et al.* 1997. Mouse CD1-specific NK1 T-cells. *Annu Rev Immonol* **15**: 535.

92. MacDonald H. 1995. NK1.1+ T-cell receptor-αβ+ cells: new clues to their origin, specificity, and function. *J Exp Med* **182**: 633.

93. Vicari A, Zlotnik A. 1996. Mouse NK1.1+ cells: new family of T-cells. *Immunol Today* **17**: 71.

94. Lantz O, Bendelac A. 1994. An invariant T-cell receptor α chain is used by a unique subset of major histocompatibility complex class-I specific CD4+ and CD4-8- T-cells in mice and humans. *J Exp Med* **180**: 1097.

95. Makino Y, Kanno R, Ito T, *et al.* 1995. Predominant expression of invariant Vα14+ TCR α chain in NK1.1+ T-cell populations. *Int Immunol* **7**: 1157.

96. Arase H, Arase N, Ogasawara K, *et al.* 1992. An NK1.1+ CD4+8- single-positive thymocyte subpopulation that express a highly skewed T-cell antigen receptor Vα family. *Proc Natl Acad USA* **89**: 6506.

97. Zlotnik A, Godfrey D, Fischer M, *et al.* 1992. Cytokine production by mature and immature CD4-CD8- T-cells: αβ-T-cell receptor+ CD4-CD8- T-cells produce IL-4. *J Immunol* **149**: 1211.

98. Yoshimoto T, Paul W. 1994. CD4^{pos}, NK1.1^{pos} T-cells promptly produce interleukin 4 in response to *in vivo* challenge with anti-CD3. *J Exp Med* **179**: 1285.

99. Yoshimoto A, Bendelac A, Hu-Li J, *et al.* 1995. Defective IgE production by SJL mice is linked to the absence of CD4+, NK1.1+ T-cells that promptly produce interleukin 4. *Proc Natl Acad USA* **92**: 11931.

100. Yoshimoto T, Bendelac A, Watson C, *et al.* 1995. Role of NK1.1+ T-cells in a Th2 response and in immunoglobulin E production. *Science* **270**: 1845.

101. Arase H, Arase N, Saito T. 1996. Interferon γ production by natural killer (NK) cells and NK1.1+ T-cells upon NKR-P1 cross-linking. *J Exp Med* **183**: 2391.

102. Kawamura T, Takeda K, Mendiratta S, *et al.* 1998. Critical role of NK1.1+ T-cells in IL-12-induced immune responses *in vivo*. *J Immunol* **160**: 16-19.

103. Makino Y, Koseki H, Adachi Y, *et al.* 1994. Extrathymic differentiation of a T-cell bearing invariant V alpha 14J alpha 281 TCR. *Int Rev Immuol* **11**: 31-46.

104. Sumida T, Sakamoto A, Murata H, *et al.* 1995. Selective reduction of T-cells bearing invariant Vα24JαQ antigen receptor in patients with systemic sclerosis. *J Exp Med* **182**: 1163-1168.

105. Kawano T, Cui J, Koezuka Y, *et al.* 1997. CD1d-restricted and TCR-mediated activation of Vα14 NKT cells by glycosylceramides. *Science* **278**: 1626-1629.

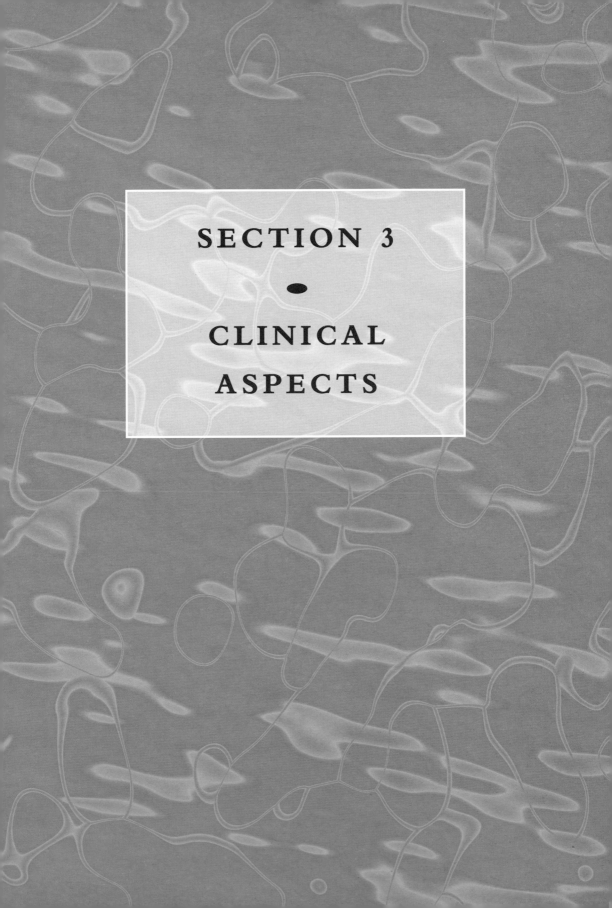

SECTION 3

•

CLINICAL
ASPECTS

PATHOLOGY OF VANISHING BILE DUCT SYNDROMES

Stefan G Hübscher

Department of Pathology, University of Birmingham,
Birmingham B15 2TT, U.K.

SUMMARY

Histological assessment has an important role in the diagnosis and management of patients with ductopenic syndromes in the liver. In primary biliary cirrhosis liver biopsy is still commonly used to confirm the clinical diagnosis. Whilst it could be argued that histological confirmation is not strictly necessary in cases of classical AMA positive PBC, liver biopsy still provides additional information which is not available by other means. This includes staging of fibrosis (most appropriate in the context of clinical trials), grading of necro-inflammatory activity (to identify a potentially treatable inflammatory component), identification of neoplastic or pre-neoplastic lesions and the exclusion of other intercurrent diseases. Finally, liver biopsy material provides a valuable resource for studies investigating mechanisms involved in bile duct damage in cases of PBC.

Primary biliary cirrhosis (PBC) is one of an increasingly large number of diseases which are recognised to be associated with a paucity of intrahepatic bile ducts. The purpose of this chapter is to review the pathological features of ductopenic syndromes in the liver, with particular reference to the pathology of primary biliary cirrhosis. The review will concentrate mainly on practical issues relating to the diagnosis of PBC and other duct losing diseases.

DEFINITION OF VANISHING BILE DUCT SYNDROME

The widely accepted definition for vanishing bile duct syndrome (VBDS) is bile duct loss in more than 50% of portal tracts[1]. The majority of vanishing bile duct syndromes (including PBC) affect small ducts of approximately interlobular size. However, larger bile duct branches may also be involved in some conditions (e.g. biliary atresia, sclerosing cholangitis, chronic liver allograft rejection).

In the normal liver, bile ducts accompany branches of the hepatic arterial system from which they receive a blood supply forming the peribiliary capillary plexus. The diagnosis of bile duct loss should therefore be based on the presence of unaccompanied hepatic arterial branches. However, up to 20-30% of small portal tracts in the normal liver may lack recognisable bile ducts[2-4].

The figure of 50% bile duct loss is arbitrary, but it is perhaps useful conceptually to think in terms of more than half of the liver's biliary drainage system being lost. There are problems in applying the definition of VBDS to the assessment of small needle biopsy specimens, in

which there may be few complete portal tracts with clearly defined hepatic arterial branches. There are also problems related to sampling variation which can be viewed at two levels. Firstly, in common with other histological abnormalities, bile duct loss in PBC and other ductopenic syndromes is often unevenly distributed within the liver. A small needle biopsy sample therefore may not be representative of what is going on in the remainder of the liver. Secondly, even if bile duct loss were present uniformly throughout the liver, a sufficient number of portal tracts would still be required to ensure adequate sampling. Using a mathematical model, it has been calculated that a minimum of 20 portal tracts are required in order for a figure of 50% bile duct loss to become statistically significant (i.e. fewer ducts than could be expected to be present as a consequence of normal variation)[5]. Since many needle biopsy specimens contain less than 20 portal tracts, accurate quantitation of bile duct loss in these small specimens may not be possible.

Another factor which impairs the assessment of bile duct numbers in many cases of chronic cholestatic liver disease is the presence of bile ductular proliferation. The mechanisms and pathological significance of bile ductular proliferation are discussed further below. In theory, it should be relatively easy to distinguish native interlobular bile ducts from neocholangioles on the basis of their morphology and location. Interlobular ducts are located centrally (usually in close promimity to an hepatic arteriole), are lined by cuboidal epithelium and have a clearly identifiable lumen. By contrast, proliferating ductules are mainly located towards the periphery of portal areas, have a flatter lining epithelium and usually lack a recognisable lumen. However, in cases where ductular proliferation is extensive, it can be very difficult to determine if the original bile duct has been lost.

Immunohistochemical staining for bile duct cytokeratins (or other bile duct specific markers) can be useful for identifying bile ducts in cases where they are effaced by a dense portal inflammatory infiltrate[6]. Conversely, the absence of cytokeratin-positive cells within portal areas confirms that duct loss is indeed present.

DISEASES ASSOCIATED WITH BILE DUCT LOSS

These can be divided into seven main categories[7,8]:

Developmental

Diseases associated with the disordered development of the embryonic biliary tree are the commonest cause of the VBDS in neonates and young children. They can be subdivided into two main forms, (extra-and intrahepatic biliary atresia) reflecting the main sites at which bile duct loss is thought to occur.

Extrahepatic biliary atresia is characterised by fibrous obliteration of the extrahepatic bile ducts. There is frequently also a paucity of intrahepatic bile ducts. It is not clear whether the latter occurs as a secondary phenomenon (analogous to secondary sclerosing cholangitis)[9] or whether it is a manifestation of a more widespread developmental abnormality involving intrahepatic as well as extrahepatic bile ducts[10]. Either way, histological distinction between extra-and intrahepatic atresia may not be possible in needle biopsy specimens.

Extrahepatic biliary atresia may also co-exist with other developmental abnormalities affecting the embryonic ductal plate, from which the definitive bile ducts are formed by a process of re-modelling[9]. Ductal plate malformations, resembling those seen in congenital hepatic fibrosis are sometimes present in cases of extrahepatic biliary atresia[11]. Conversely, cases of congenital hepatic fibrosis may be associated with a paucity of true (portal) bile ducts.'

Intrahepatic biliary atresia (also known as paucity of intrahepatic bile ducts) occurs in two main forms, syndromic and non-syndromic[12]. In the syndromic form (Alagille's syndrome or arteriohepatic dysplasia), hepatic abnormalities are associated with characteristic facies and abnormalities involving the cardiovascular, skeletal, renal and ocular systems. Most patients with Alagille's syndrome have relatively mild liver disease and progressive liver damage is uncommon. Non-syndromic paucity of interlobular bile ducts has a less favourable outcome, with most patients developing progressive liver damage resulting in cirrhosis. An association between non-syndromic paucity of bile ducts and idiopathic adult ductopenia has been postulated[13].

A number of metabolic diseases may also be associated with bile duct loss in neonates. These include alpha-1-antitrypsin deficiency, cystic fibrosis, Byler's disease and Zellweger syndrome.

Immune-mediated

These are the commonest causes of ductopenic syndromes in adults.

Primary biliary cirrhosis is characterised by non-suppurative destructive cholangitis principally involving small (interlobular) bile ducts. Focal inflammatory damage to medium sized (septal) ducts is sometimes also seen. Other pathological features of PBC are discussed in further detail below.

In **primary sclerosing cholangitis**, bile duct lesions affect ducts of all sizes[14]. Bile duct loss predominantly affects small (interlobular) ducts which usually disappear without trace. In some cases surviving interlobular ducts may show basement membrane thickening, revealed by PAS staining. Portal tract granulomas can also be seen in up to 10% of cases of PSC[15,16]. However, in contrast with PBC, portal granulomas do not appear to be involved with bile duct damage. The characteristic histological lesion of PSC is a fibrous obliterative cholangitis, which is generally most prominent in medium sized (septal) bile ducts. In the early stages of the disease, this is present as loose 'onion skin'-like periductal fibrosis. Later on the bile duct is completely replaced by a nodular fibrous scar. Inflammation, dilatation and ulceration are commonly present in large (hilar) bile ducts and account for the characteristic abnormalities identified by endoscopic retrograde cholangiopancreatography (ERCP)[17]. In a small proportion of patients, the disease appears to be confined to small/medium-sized bile ducts, without demonstrable radiological abnormalities being present in larger ducts ("small duct PSC")[18].

Overlap syndromes involving PBC, PSC and autoimmune hepatitis have been recognised recently. The term **'autoimmune cholangiopathy'** may be used in this context and is discussed further later.

Hepatic involvement is common in patients with **sarcoidosis**. Granulomas tend to be mainly located in portal and periportal regions. In a small proportion of cases there is granulomatous destruction of bile ducts resulting in a chronic cholestatic syndrome closely resembling PBC[19].

Bile ducts are important targets of immunological damage in **liver allograft rejection**[20]. Acute (cellular) rejection is characterised by inflammatory bile duct infiltration. In most cases this is reversible with the use of additional immunosuppression. In a small proportion of patients there is progressive destruction of bile ducts resulting in chronic (ductopenic) rejection in which there is severe intractable cholestasis requiring re-transplantation.

Bile duct damage is also a characteristic feature of **graft-versus-host** disease in the liver, usually occurring as a complication of bone marrow transplantation[21]. Early stages are characterised by inflammatory infiltration of bile ducts, generally less marked than is seen in liver allograft rejection. Progressive bile duct loss occurs in a small proportion of cases.

Vascular

Bile ducts receive a single arterial blood supply from branches of the hepatic arterial system. It is therefore not surprising that they are more susceptible to ischaemic injury than hepatocytes, which receive a dual blood supply from hepatic artery and portal vein branches.

Arterial causes of bile duct injury include hepatic artery thrombosis, traumatic injury, intra-arterial infusions (e.g. chemotherapeutic agents or ethanol embolisation for the treatment of hepatic neoplasms) and vasculitis (e.g. polyarteritis nodosa). It has also been postulated that bile duct loss in chronic liver allograft rejection may partly have an ischaemic basis, secondary to the obliterative foam cell arteriopathy which occurs in this condition[3,22].

Bile duct ischaemia produces a spectrum of lesions which closely resemble those seen in sclerosing cholangitis. In the native liver this rarely gives rise to diagnostic difficulties. However, in the assessment of patients following liver transplantation, it may be impossible to distinguish recurrent primary sclerosing cholangitis from ischaemic causes of bile duct injury in the liver allograft[23,24].

Portal venous obstruction rarely gives rise to problems involving the biliary tree. However, a PSC-like syndrome ('pseudosclerosing cholangitis') has been reported in association with portal vein thrombosis, possibly reflecting compression of bile ducts due to choledochal varices[25].

Infective

Bacterial infection of the biliary tree in ascending cholangitis may rarely be associated with inflammatory bile duct destruction[8].

A number of viruses have been implicated in the pathogenesis of VBDS. These include cytomegalovirus (CMV), reovirus 3 and hepatitis C virus (HCV). CMV has been postulated as a factor contributing to bile duct

loss in extrahepatic biliary atresia,[26] chronic liver allograft rejection[27,28] and AIDS associated sclerosing cholangitis[29]. Reovirus 3 has also been implicated in the pathogenesis of biliary atresia[30]. Portal lymphoid aggregates are a characteristic histological feature of chronic hepatitis C infection, and are frequently centred on small bile ducts. Whilst there is a suggestion that minor degrees of bile duct loss may occur in chronic HCV infection[31,32], it is very uncommon to see advanced duct loss associated with other features of chronic biliary disease.

Protozoal infection of the biliary tree (e.g. cryptosporidia or microsporidia) is sometimes seen in immunocompromised individuals and may result in a sclerosing cholangitis-like syndrome.[33]

Bile duct destruction has been described as a rare complication of a Echinococcus granulosus infection of the liver, due to rupture of hydatid cyst into the biliary tree.

Drugs

Cholestatic reactions are a common manifestation of drug induced liver injury[34]. An increasing number of drugs have been associated with VBDS. Some of the commoner ones are listed in table 1.

In some cases VBDS may be an early presenting feature of drug induced liver injury[35]. Liver biopsy assessment is particularly important in this context. Diagnosis of drug induced bile duct loss requires exclusion of other causes of ductopenia. However histological features which might favour a drug reaction include dispro-portionately severe cholestatis, or an inflammatory infiltrate which includes eosinophils and/or granulomas.

Neoplastic

Histiocytosis X is characterised by proliferation of dendritic cells (Langerhans cells). Although Langerhans

TABLE 1. DRUGS ASSOCIATED WITH LOSS OF INTRAHEPATIC BILE DUCTS	
Phenothiazines	Chlorpromazine Prochlorperazine
Penicillins	Ampicillin Flucloxacillin
Tricyclic antidepressants	Amitryptiline Imipramine
Antiepileptics	Carbamazepine Phenytoin
Other	Cimetidine Methyltestosterone Tolbutamide

cell proliferation in this condition is now thought to be an inflammatory/reactive process, possibly related to disordered immune regulation, rather than a true neoplasm, disseminated disease (of which hepatic involvement is one component) is usually rapidly progressive and fatal. Hepatic infiltration is characteristically seen in portal and periportal regions and is frequently associated with destructive lesions involving small bile ducts[36].

A syndrome of severe intrahepatic cholestasis associated with bile duct loss, has been reported to occur in a small proportion of patients with Hodgkin's lymphoma[37]. The mechanism of bile duct loss in these cases is uncertain. PSC-like changes have also been documented in association with hepatic involvement in systemic mastocytosis[38].

Unknown

The term 'idiopathic adult ductopenia' was first used by Ludwig et al to describe a small group of patients who had a chronic biliary disease associated with bile duct loss, for which no obvious cause could be found[39]. Whether this diagnosis of exclusion represents a specific disease process is uncertain. Some cases may represent small bile duct PSC. A relationship to the non-syndromic paucity of interlobular bile ducts has also been postulated[13]. Cases occurring in siblings have also been reported suggesting the possibility of a familial tendency[13].

PRIMARY BILIARY CIRRHOSIS – HISTOLOGICAL FEATURES

Early Disease

The early stages of PBC are characterised by inflammatory infiltration, mainly located in portal and periportal areas associated with bile duct damage leading eventually to bile duct loss[40]. Portal inflammatory cells comprise a mixed population including lymphocytes (the predominant cell type), histiocytes (associated with granuloma formation), plasma cells, eosinophils and neutrophils. Lymphocytes are mainly CD3 positive T-cells which are dispersed throughout portal areas. CD8+ T-cells are most abundant during the early stages of the disease and may be involved in cytotoxic bile duct injury. As the disease progresses a higher proportion of CD4+ T-cells is observed. Frequently T-cells are most prominent at the periphery of portal areas, where they may be associated with interface hepatitis. By contrast, B-cells are mainly located centrally. Evidence exists to implicate all of the cell types noted in portal infiltrates in the pathogenesis of bile duct damage in PBC.[41-45]

Bile duct injury in PBC is largely confined to interlobular ducts approximately 40 to 80µm in diameter. Inflammatory infiltration of biliary epithelium is associated with degenerative changes such as swelling, cytoplasmic vacuolation and fragmentation of the basement membrane (Figure 1). In some cases there may be frank disruption of bile duct epithelium (the so called 'florid duct lesion'). Granulomatous bile duct destruction is generally regarded as the most characteristic bile duct lesion in PBC (Figure 2). However, granulomatous cholangitis can also occur in other conditions such as sarcoidosis[19] and chronic hepatitis C infection[46]. Granulomatous cholangitis is also a feature of so called 'autoimmune cholangitis'. The precise relationship of this entity to PBC will be discussed later.

It is worth noting that bile duct lesions in PBC are patchy in distribution and may therefore not be sampled in small needle biopsy specimens. Although they are generally regarded as a feature of early disease, inflammatory bile duct lesions are commonly present in hepatectomy specimens obtained from patients undergoing liver transplantation (Figure 2). This observation indicates that bile duct damage in PBC is an ongoing process which takes place over a period of many years.

The reasons why small bile ducts are selectively damaged in PBC are still not clearly understood. Immunohistochemical studies have demonstrated a number of phenotypic changes in bile duct epithelial cells, which may render them more susceptible to immunological injury[47]. These are summarised in table 2 and are also discussed elsewhere. However, the functional significance of these phenotypic changes in the pathogenesis of bile duct damage remains uncertain, for two main reasons. Firstly, most of the changes noted are not specific for PBC and can also be seen in other liver diseases, including non-immunological diseases such as mechanical bile duct obstruction. Secondly, some changes (e.g. class

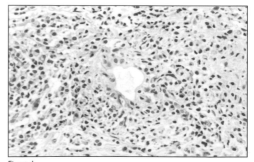

Figure 1.
Inflammatory bile duct lesion in PBC. Epithelium of an interlobular bile duct shows lymphocytic infiltration and cytoplasmic vacuolation.
Haematoxylin and eosin

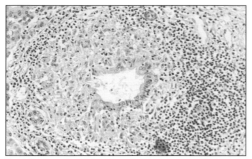

Figure 2.
Granulomatous bile duct lesion in PBC. Medium sized bile duct is surrounded by a granulomatous infiltrate associated with disruption of biliary epithelium. This "florid bile duct lesion" is generally regarded as the characteristic histological feature of early (stage 1) disease. However, the bile duct shown in this illustration was present in a cirrhotic hepatectomy specimen obtained at liver transplantation, indicating that active bile duct damage can be seen at all stages of the disease.
Haematoxylin and eosin

II MHC expression) appear to occur as a relatively late event and are thus unlikely to be involved in initiating bile duct damage[48].

Inflammatory bile duct lesions eventually give rise to bile duct loss. There is increasing evidence to implicate apoptosis as the final mode of biliary epithelial cell death in PBC. Apoptosis of BECs has been demonstrated by electron microscopy[49,50] and by DNA fragmentation studies[51,52]. Expression of Fas (CD95), which is important in mediating apoptosis, has also been demonstrated in biliary epithelial cells[51,53]. Once bile ducts have disappeared, distinction from other duct losing diseases is rarely possible on the basis of histological findings alone (Figure 3). Portal lymphoid aggregates are commonly seen in PBC and may still be present after bile ducts have disappeared. In some cases these lymphoid aggregates appear to be marking the site of former bile ducts ('tombstone aggregates'). (Figure 3)

Although most studies have concentrated on mechanisms of bile duct destruction in PBC, it is worth noting that damaged bile ducts may also show increased proliferative activity[54]. The final outcome of immune activation in PBC is thus likely to depend on the balance that exists between factors mediating bile duct damage and those stimulating biliary epithelial cell proliferation.

Parenchymal changes during the early stages of the disease are usually rather mild. Minor degrees of inflammatory infiltration are commonly seen, and may include occasional epithelioid granulomas. Zonal necrosis associated with an infiltrate of activated T-cells can also be seen in a small proportion of cases. This suggests that hepatocytes may also be targets for immunological damage in PBC[55]. Nodular regenerative hyperplasia (NRH) has also been recognised as a common abnormality in the early stages of PBC[56] and may be an important factor in the pathogenesis of portal hypertension which often occurs before a true cirrhosis supervenes.

TABLE 2. SUMMARY OF BILIARY EPITHELIAL CELL (BEC) ANTIGENS SHOWING INCREASED OR *DE NOVO* EXPRESSION IN PRIMARY BILIARY CIRRHOSIS		
BEC Antigen	**Ligand/Binding Antibody**	**Functional Significance/Comments**
MHC Antigens		
MHC Class I	CD8/TCR Complex	Immune recognition by CD8+ T cells. Involved in cytotoxic T cell mediated damage
MHC Class II	CD4/TCR Complex	Immune recognition by CD4+ T cells. Involved in afferent arm of immune response
Adhesion Molecules		
ICAM-1 (CD54)	LFA-1	Facilitates T cell binding
VCAM-1	VLA-4	Facilitates T cell binding
LFA-3 (CD58)	LFA-2 (CD2)	Facilitates T cell binding
Other Antigens		
PDC-E2	Anti-M2	Epitope recognised by PBC-specific antimitochondrial antibodies. Also involved in T cell responses
B7 (CD80)	CD28	Important costimulatory molecule for T cell activation. Conflicting evidence regarding BECs capacity to express B7
Heat-shock protein (HSP 27-kD, 90kD)	?	May be involved in 'non-specific' pathways of BEC damage

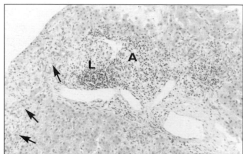

Figure 3.
Bile duct loss in PBC. Portal tract contains an arterial branch (A), without an accompanying bile duct. A lymphoid aggregate (L) possibly marks the site where the bile duct once was. There is also fibrous portal expansion associated with marginal ductular proliferation (arrows), indicating progressive liver damage. In the absence of diagnostic bile duct lesions, histological distinction from other duct losing diseases is not possible at this stage.
Haematoxylin and eosin

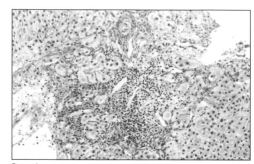

Figure 4.
Periportal inflammation and fibrosis in PBC. Portal tract contains a moderately dense infiltrate of lymphoid cells. There is inflammatory spillover into the periportal region (interface hepatitis) associated with deposition of collagen fibres between hepatocytes.
Haematoxylin van Gieson

Progressive liver injury

As the disease progresses there is development of fibrosis leading eventually to a true cirrhosis. Fibrosis can be divided into three main phases. First, there is fibrous portal expansion (periportal fibrosis). This is followed by the formation of linkages between vascular structures (mainly portal-portal, some portal-central). Normal vascular relationships are still retained at this stage. Finally, there is development of a true cirrhosis with nodular regeneration and loss of the normal liver architecture. There is marked variation in the rate of progression of fibrosis, both between different individuals with the disease and in different areas of the same liver. This variation gives rise to problems with the histological staging of PBC in needle biopsy specimens and these are discussed further later.

Two main factors are involved in the pathogenesis of periportal fibrosis in PBC. The first is spillover of inflammatory cells from portal areas into periportal regions (interface hepatitis). This is associated with damage to periportal hepatocytes and, in some cases, death of these cells mainly by apoptosis. Periportal inflammatory infiltration is also associated with deposition of new collagen fibres (Figure 4). These are initially present as delicate strands between individual

hepatocytes, but later on may coalesce to form broader fibrous septa. Although interface hepatitis (or 'piecemeal necrosis') is generally regarded as a characteristic feature of chronic viral or autoimmune hepatitis, it is also commonly seen in chronic cholestatic liver diseases such as PBC. In cases where interface hepatitis is a prominent feature, the possibility of an overlap syndrome with autoimmune hepatitis might be considered.

The other main factor driving the development of periportal fibrosis is bile ductular proliferation (also known as 'ductular reaction' or 'ductular hyperplasia')[57,58] (Figure 3). Bile ductular proliferation is a common response seen in many forms of liver injury. However, it is particularly prominent in ductopenic syndromes, where it may have a protective role enabling resorption of bile and recirculation within the liver (cholehepatic cycling) when the normal pathway of enerohepatic circulation is blocked as a consequence of bile duct loss.

Three main sources of bile ductular proliferation have been postulated (see table 3). Of these, ductular metaplasia of periportal hepatocytes is thought to be the most important mechanism in chronic cholestatic liver diseases such as PBC. Immunohistochemical studies have shown that periportal hepatocytes in chronic biliary disease express antigens that are confined to bile ducts in the normal liver. These include bile duct cytokeratins (cytokeratin 7 and 19), blood

TABLE 3. SOURCES OF PROLIFERATING BILE DUCTILES IN DIFFERENT TYPES OF LIVER DISEASE		
Histological type	**Source of Ductules**	**Associated diseases**
1. Typical Ductular Prolifereration	Pre-existing bile ductules	Extrahepatic biliary obstruction
2. Atypical Ductular Proliferation	Periportal hepatocytes (ductular metaplasia)	Chronic cholestatic diseases
3. Oval Cell Proliferation	Oval cells	Experimental hepatocarcinogenesis

group antigens, TPA, neuroendocrine markers (e.g. chromogranin), bile duct integrins (VLA 2, 3 and 6) and other bile duct specific antibodies (e.g. human epithelial antigen 125) (Figure 5). Three dimensional reconstruction studies have demonstrated that periportal hepatocytes showing feature of biliary metaplasia are in continuity with ductular structures at the periphery of portal areas[59]. Cells with an intermediate morphology can sometimes be seen in a transitional zone.

There is recent evidence to suggest that oval cell proliferation may also be involved in the ductular reaction which occurs in human liver disease, including chronic cholestatic diseases such as PBC. Immunohistochemical studies using the oval cell marker OV6 have shown OV6 expression in proliferating ductules from cases of PBC and PSC[60,61]. In addition individual small OV6 positive oval cells were also present in periportal areas suggesting the possibility of a progenitor cell population in these areas.

Bile ductular proliferation is commonly associated with an inflammatory infiltrate rich in neutrophils (cholangiolitis) (Figure 6). These cells may represent a non-specific inflammatory response to bile or be recruited more specifically as a consequence of cytokines released from bile ductules themselves (e.g. interleukin 8). Whatever their source, the presence of a dense neutrophilic infiltrate accompanying bile ductules may be another factor involved in damage to periportal hepatocytes in PBC.

There are two main mechanisms whereby bile ductular proliferation is associated with the development of periportal fibrosis[57]. The first is direct production of basement membrane related proteins (e.g. collagen type 4 or laminin) by bile ductules themselves (ductular fibrosis). Secondly, bile ductules are capable of releasing

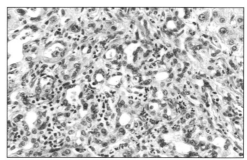

Figure 6.
Bile ductular proliferation in this case of PBC is associated with a dense infiltrate of neutrophils and with deposition of collagen fibres between bile ductules.
Haematoxylin van Gieson

cytokines (e.g. TGF beta) which can stimulate portal fibroblasts or myofibroblasts to produce fibrous tissue. Either way, a delicate framework of new collagen fibres can be demonstrated around neocholangioles in diseases where marginal ductular reaction occurs. (Figure 6)

Further evidence for the role of bile ductular proliferation as a driving force for the development of periportal fibrosis comes from observations made in bile duct losing diseases in which ductular proliferation is not seen. Two good examples of this phenomenon are chronic liver allograft rejection and Alagille's syndrome, in which advanced bile duct loss is seen in normal sized portal tracts which have no ductular proliferation or fibrosis. (Figure 7)

Other (secondary) changes

A number of other abnormalities are seen in the liver parenchyma, principally in periportal regions. These are thought to be related to toxic injury caused by the accumulation of bile salts or bile itself. Changes seen

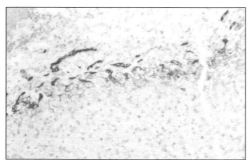

Figure 5.
Ductular metaplasia of periseptal hepatocytes in chronic cholestatic liver disease. This section of cirrhotic PBC liver has been stained with an antibody to HEA-125, which recognises a biliary-specific glycoprotein in the normal liver. HEA-125 immunoreactivity is present both in proliferating bile ductules at the periphery of a fibrous septum and in adjacent periseptal hepatocytes (with a membranous pattern).
Immunoalkaline phosphatase

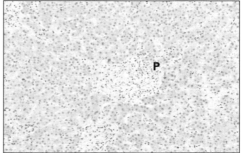

Figure 7.
Bile duct loss in chronic liver allograft rejection. This specimen was obtained at re-transplantation 6 months after the original transplant operation Portal tract (P) has a characteristic "burnt out" appearance with scanty inflammatory cells, and no recognisable bile duct. In contrast to most other duct losing diseases there is no ductular proliferation or periportal fibrosis.
Haematoxylin and eosin

include hepatocyte ballooning and feathery degeneration ("cholate stasis"), formation of Mallory's hyaline and deposition of copper associated protein. Eventually bile pigment deposition may be visible histologically. Lipid laden macrophages (xanthoma cells) and hepatocytes (pseudoxanthoma cells) are also commonly seen in periportal regions.

In addition to degenerative changes in periportal hepatocytes, 'halo zones' of loose fibrosis are commonly present at the periphery of portal areas and/or fibrous septa in chronic cholestatic liver diseases. (Figure 8).

Hepatocellular carcinoma

Hepatocellular carcinoma (HCC) has been recognised as a relatively rare complication of PBC. The apparently low incidence compared with other forms of chronic liver disease probably reflects two main factors. Firstly, PBC is largely confined to women who have a lower risk of developing HCC than men. Secondly, true cirrhosis occurs as a relatively late event in most cases of PBC. If one 'corrects' for these factors (e.g. by looking at male PBC patients with advanced liver

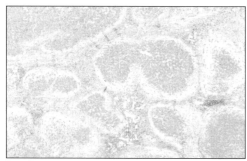

Figure 8.
Established cirrhosis in PBC. This specimen obtained at liver transplantation has a characteristic biliary pattern of cirrhosis with small nodules, often irregular in shape, surrounded by "halo zones" of loose fibrosis.
Haematoxylin and eosin

disease), the incidence of HCC in PBC is comparable to other forms of cirrhosis.[62]

HISTOLOGICAL GRADING AND STAGING OF PRIMARY BILIARY CIRRHOSIS

The concepts of histological 'grading' and 'staging' have been used for many years in the pathological assessment of neoplastic diseases. More recently, a similar approach has been advocated in the histological evaluation of chronic liver disease[63-65]. The histological 'grade' is regarded as a measure of ongoing inflammatory activity, which is potentially treatable, whereas the fibrosis 'stage' is a marker of progressive liver injury, which is less likely to be reversible. It still accepted that these two processes are interrelated, in that increasing grades of necroinflammatory activity are more likely to be associated with the development of progressive fibrosis. However, in the assessment of a liver biopsy from an individual patient, the two patterns of liver injury may have different therapeutic implications, and they are thus best regarded as separate pathological processes.

Several staging systems have been described in the histological assessments of patients with PBC. Four of the more commonly used ones are summarised in table 4[66-69]. All four systems agree that early (stage 1) disease is characterised by bile duct damage and/or portal inflammation and that late (stage 4) disease is defined by the presence an established cirrhosis. However, some confusion exists regarding the criteria used to define the intermediate stages (stage 2 and 3). Bile ductular proliferation, interface hepatitis (periportal hepatitis) and fibrosis are all used to varying degrees. In line with current concepts of staging liver disease, it might be more appropriate to adopt a simplified staging system, which is based purely on the degree of fibrosis present. An example of such a system is also included in table 4.

	Rubin et al (1965)	Scheuer (1967)	Popper and Schaffer (1970)	Ludwig (1978)	Simplified System
TABLE 4. SUMMARY OF FOUR STAGING SYSTEMS WHICH HAVE BEEN USED IN THE HISTOLOGICAL ASSESSMENT OF PRIMARY BILIARY CIRRHOSIS. A SIMPLIFIED SYSTEM, BASED PURELY ON THE EXTENT OF FIBROSIS, IS ALSO INCLUDED FOR COMPARISON.					
Stage 1	Bile duct damage	Florid duct lesion	Cholangitis	Portal Hepatitis	No fibrosis
Stage 2	Ductular proliferation	Ductular proliferation	Ductular proliferation & destruction	Periportal hepatitis	Periportal fibrosis
Stage 3	Ductular proliferation	Scarring	Precirrhotic stage	Bridging necrosis and or fibrosis	Bridging fibrosis
Stage 4	Cirrhosis	Cirrhosis	Cirrhosis	Cirrhosis	Cirrhosis

Histological staging is particularly relevant in the context of clinical trials, where traditional descriptive reports can be replaced by numerical scores which are more amenable to statistical manipulation. However, there are problems with applying histological scores to needle biopsies from individual patients. These mainly relate to sampling variation. Disease progression in PBC is patchy in distribution. Examination of whole livers obtained at orthotopic liver transplantation (OLT) has shown a marked variation in histological stage in different parts of the same liver. In a study by Garrido et al only ten (20%) of 50 hepatectomy specimens obtained at OLT had the same stage throughout the liver[70]. Of the remaining 40 cases 23 (46%) varied by one stage, 14 (28%) by 2 stages and 3 (6%) by 3 stages (Figure 9). A similar (though less marked) variation in histological stage has also been noted in a study of paired needle biopsies from patients with primary sclerosing cholangitis[71].

Problems also exist with observer variation, particularly if assessments are made on an infrequent basis by pathologists with relatively little experience in liver biopsy interpretation. In the context of clinical trials, this problem can be overcome by having a central review of specimens by a small panel of experienced liver pathologists, who have agreed on the precise criteria to be used to define different histological scores. Better interobserver agreement is generally obtained for fibrosis stage than for necroinflammatory grade[72,73].

OVERLAP SYNDROMES IN AUTOIMMUNE LIVER DISEASE

The concept of overlap syndromes in autoimmune liver disease has been recognised fairly recently[74]. These syndromes may involve primary biliary cirrhosis (PBC), primary sclerosing cholangitis (PSC) and autoimmune hepatitis (AIH) in any combination. In most cases, these overlapping features present simultaneously. However, there are a small number of well documented cases in which patients presented initially with features of one disease (e.g. autoimmune hepatitis), for which successful treatment was given, and then presented again after an interval of several years with typical features of another disease (e.g. primary biliary cirrhosis)[75,76]. Although the concept of overlap syndromes is widely accepted, problems exist regarding diagnostic criteria, confusing terminology and the clinical significance in terms of therapeutic implications.

The main criteria used to diagnose PBC, PSC and AIH are summarised in a simplified form in table 5. The diagnosis of 'overlap syndrome' may be based on overlapping features involving any of the 5 main

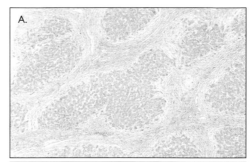

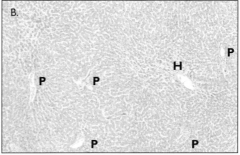

Figure 9.
Sampling variation in the severity of fibrosis in PBC. These two slides are both taken from a single block of liver obtained at transplantation. In one area there is an established cirrhosis (A). Another area shows preservation of normal vascular relationships with no obvious fibrosis (B). P=portal tract, H=hepatic vein
Haematoxylin and eosin

diagnostic criteria listed in table 5, or on combinations thereof. However, to simplify matters 2 main forms of overlap syndrome can be recognised. These are summarised in table 6. Patient 1 has serological, biochemical and histological features which would be compatible both a diagnosis of autoimmune hepatitis and with a diagnosis of PBC. This could be regarded as an example of a 'true' overlap syndrome. By contrast, patient 2 has a 'cross-over' syndrome in which the serological profile is typical of autoimmune hepatitis (with negative antimitochondrial antibodies), but the biochemical and histological features suggest PBC as the most likely diagnosis. The term 'autoimmune cholangitis' has been used to describe this combination of findings[74,77].

One of the main problems relating to the diagnosis of overlap syndrome concerns the criteria used to make the diagnosis. For example, in a hypothetical patient who is AMA positive, with a raised serum alkaline phosphatase and histological findings compatible with PBC, what additional features are required to make a diagnosis of 'overlap syndrome'? Should it be based on the presence of hepatitic biochemistry (if so, what level of transaminitis is required?), positive autoantibodies (if so which antibodies and at what titre?) or on the presence of inflammatory changes in a liver biopsy (if so

TABLE 5. SUMMARY OF MAIN CRITERIA USED TO DIAGNOSE THREE AUTOIMMUNE LIVER DISEASES WHICH MAY BE ASSOCIATED WITH AN OVERLAP SYNDROME.

THE DIAGNOSIS OF OVERLAP SYNDROME CAN BE BASED ON OVERLAPPING FEATURES INVOLVING ANY OF THE FIVE DIAGNOSTIC FEATURES LISTED BELOW, OR COMBINATIONS THEREOF.

	Autoimmune Hepatitus	Primary Biliary Cirrhosis	Primary Sclerosing Cholangitis
1. Serology	ANA, SMA (type 1)	AMA, anti-M2	ANCA
2. Biochemistry	Hepatitic	Cholestatic	Cholestatic
3. Immunoglobulins	Raised IgG	Raised IgM	–
4. Radiology (ERCP)	Normal	Normal	Beading, strictures
5. Histology	Hepatitic	Biliary	Biliary
Bile duct loss	No	Yes	Yes
Biliary fibrosis/cirrhosis	No	Yes	Yes

TABLE 6. EXAMPLES OF TWO MAIN FORMS OF OVERLAP SYNDROME WHICH HAVE BEEN RECOGNISED IN AUTOIMMUNE LIVER DISEASE.

PATIENT 1 HAS A "TRUE" OVERLAP SYNDROME IN WHICH SEROLOGICAL, BIOCHEMICAL AND HISTOLOGICAL FEATURES OF AUTOIMMUNE HEPATITIS (AIH) AND PRIMARY BILIARY CIRRHOSIS (PBC) ARE SIMULTANEOUSLY PRESENT. BY CONTRAST, PATIENT 2 HAS THE SEROLOGICAL PROFILE OF AIH, WITH BIOCHEMICAL AND HISTOLOGICAL FEATURES TYPICAL OF PBC ("AUTOIMMUNE CHOLANGITIS")

1. **'True' Overlap Syndrome (AIH/PBC)** (autoimmune hepatitis / primary biliary cirrhosis)

Autoantibodies	ANA+, SMA+, AMA+
Biochemistry	AST raised, Alk Phos raised
Histology	Mixed hepatitic and biliary features

2. **'Cross-over' Overlap Syndrome** ("autoimmune cholangitis")

Autoantibodies	ANA+, SMA+, AMA-
Biochemistry	AST normal, Alk Phos raised
Histology	PBC like features

what grade of interface hepatitis is required?). Can a diagnosis of overlap syndrome be based on overlapping features involving one of these three main components or should all three be involved? Unfortunately, no clear answers exist for any of these important questions. In the absence of clearly defined guidelines, it could be argued that the hypothetical patient outlined above should simply be regarded as having primary biliary cirrhosis, irrespective of any other abnormalities noted, as this is likely to be the main pathway determining progressive liver injury.

Problems relating to confusing terminology apply particularly to the term 'autoimmune cholangitis', as defined above. It is now widely accepted that this is best regarded as AMA negative PBC[78-80]. However, differences exist between patients with 'autoimmune cholangitis' and classical cases of AMA positive PBC. Other suggestions for the nature of autoimmune cholangitis include a subtype of autoimmune hepatitis with prominent biliary features[77] and a distinctive syndrome which is neither PBC nor AIH[81]. It has also been

suggested that the term 'autoimmune cholangitis' could be used to describe all (presumed) autoimmune liver diseases in which there is prominent bile duct damage. Using this approach, classical PBC and PSC could both be regarded as subtypes of autoimmune cholangitis (AMA positive and fibrosing autoimmune cholangitis respectively).

In terms of clinical management, the main purpose of identifying overlap syndromes concerns therapeutic implications. There is some evidence to suggest that the hepatitic component of an overlap syndrome may respond to immunosuppressive therapy, but biliary features will still persist.

REFERENCES

1. Leevy CM, Sherlock S, Tygstrup N, Zetterman R (eds) International Hepatology Informatics Group. Diseases of the liver and biliary tract. Standardisation of nomenclature, diagnostic criteria and prognosis. New York Raven Press, 1994.

2. Nakanuma Y, Ohta G. Histometric and serial section observations of the intrahepatic bile ducts in primary biliary cirrhosis. Gastroenterology 1979; 76: 1326-1332.

3. Oguma S, Belle S, Starzl TE, Demetris AJ. A histometric analysis of chronically rejected human liver allografts: insights into mechanisms of bile duct loss: direct immunological and ischaemic factors. *Hepatology* 1989; **9**: 204-209.

4. Hübscher SG, Buckels JAC, Elias E, McMaster P, Neuberger J. Vanishing bile duct syndrome following liver transplantation – is it reversible? *Transplantation* 1991; **51**: 1004-1010.

5. Tadrous PJ, Goldin RD, How many portal tracts are necessary to make a diagnosis of significant bile duct loss (SBDL)? An exercise in evidence based pathology. *Journal of Pathology* 1997; **181**: A11.

6. Harrison RF, Patsiaoura K, Hübscher SG. Cytokeratin immunostaining for detection of biliary epithelium: its use in counting bile ducts in cases of liver allograft rejection. *J Clin Pathol* 1994; **47**: 303-308.

7. Sherlock S. The syndrome of disappearing intrahepatic bile ducts. *Lancet* 1987; **2**: 493-496.

8. Woolf GM, Vierling JM. Disappearing intrahepatic bile ducts: the syndromes and their mechanisms. *Semin Liver Dis* 1993; **13**: 261-275.

9. Desmet VJ. Congenital disease of intrahepatic bile ducts: variations on the theme 'ductal plate malformation'. *Hepatology* 1992; **16**: 1069-1083.

10. Calder CJ, Davison S, Kelly DA, Hübscher SG. Ductopenia in end stage paediatric liver disease. *J Pathol* 1994; **173**: 157A.

11. Raweily EA, Gibson AA, Burt AD. Abnormalities of intrahepatic bile ducts in extrahepatic biliary atresia. *Histopathology* 1990; **17**: 521-527.

12. Kahn E. Paucity of interlobular bile ducts. Arteriohepatic dysplasia and nonsyndromic duct paucity. In: Abramowsky CR, Bernstein J, Rosenberg HS (eds). Perspectives in Pediatric Pathology. Transplantation Pathology – Hepatic Morphogenesis. Vol 14. Basel: Karger; 1991: pp. 168-215.

13. Bruguera M, Llach J, Rodes J. Nonsyndromic paucity of intrahepatic bile ducts in infancy and idiopathic ductopenia in adulthood: the same syndrome? *Hepatology* 1992; **15**: 830-834.

14. Harrison RF, Hübscher SG. The spectrum of bile duct lesions in end-stage primary sclerosing cholangitis. *Histopathology* 1991; **19**: 321-327.

15. Chapman RW, Arborgh BMA, Rhodes JM, Summerfield JA, Dick R, Scheuer PJ. Primary sclerosing cholangitis: A review of its clinical features, cholangiography and hepatic histology. *Gut* 1980; **21**: 870-877.

16. Ludwig J, Colina F, Poterucha JJ. Granulomas in primary sclerosing cholangitis. *Liver* 1995; **15**: 307-312.

17. Ludwig J, MacCarty RL, LaRusso NF, Krom RA, Wiesner RH. Intrahepatic cholangiectasis and large-duct obliteration in primary sclerosing cholangitis. *Hepatology* 1986; **6**: 560-568.

18. Ludwig J. Small duct primary sclerosing cholangitis. *Semin Liver Dis.* 1991; **11**: 11-17.

19. Ishak KG. Sarcoidosis of the liver and bile ducts. *Mayo Clinic Proceedings* 1998; **73**: 467-472.

20. Hübscher SG. Histological findings in liver allograft rejection – new insights into the pathogenesis of hepatocellular damage in liver allografts. *Histopathology* 1991; **18**: 377-383.

21. Sloane JP, Norton J. The pathology of bone marrow transplantation. *Histopathology* 1993; **22**: 201-209.

22. Wiesner RH, Ludwig J, van Hoek B, Krom RA. Current concepts in cell-mediated hepatic allograft rejection leading to ductopenia and liver failure. *Hepatology* 1991; **14**: 721-729.

23. Harrison RF, Davies MH, Neuberger JM, Hübscher SG. Fibrous and obliterative cholangitis in liver allografts: evidence of recurrent primary slcerosing cholangitis? *Hepatology* 1994; **20**: 356-361.

24. Sebagh M, Farges O, Dubel L, Samuel D, Bismuth H, Reynes M. Sclerosing cholangitis following human orthotopic liver transplantation. *Americal Journal of Surgical Pathology* 1995; 19: 81-90.

25. Dilawari JB, Chawala YK. Pseudosclerosing cholangitis in extrahepatic portal venous obstruction. *Gut* 1992; **33**: 272-276.

26. Tarr PI, Haas JE, Christie DL. Biliary atresia, cytomegalovirus and age at referral. *Pediatrics* 1996; **97**: 828-831.

27. Lautenschlager I, Hockerstedt K, Loginov R, Salmela K, Taskinen E, Ahonen J. Persistent cytomegalovirus in liver allografts with chronic rejection. *Hepatology* 1997; **25**: 190-194.

28. Martelius T, Krogerus L, Hockerstedt K, Bruggeman C, Lautenschlager I. Cytomegalovirus infection is associated with increased inflammation and severe bile duct damage in rat liver allografts. *Hepatology* 1998; **27**: 996-1002.

29. Forbes A, Blanshard C, Gazzard B. Natural history of AIDS related sclerosing cholangitis: a study of 20 cases. *Gut* 1993; **34**: 116-121.

30. Morecki R, Glaser JH, Cho S, Balistreri WF, Horwitz MS. Biliary atresia and reovirus type 3 infection. *New England journal of Medicine* 1982; **307**: 481-484.

31. Bach N, Thung SN, Schaffner F. The histological features of chronic hepatitis C and autoimmune chronic hepatitis: A comparative analysis. *Hepatology* 1992; **15**: 572-576.

32. Goldin RD, Patel NK, Thomas HC. Hepatitis C and bile duct loss. *J Clin Pathol* 1996; **49**: 836-838.

33. Lucas SB. Other viral and infectious diseases and HIV-related liver disease. In: MacSween RNM, Anthony PP, Scheuer PJ, Burt AD, Portmann BC (eds). Pathology of the liver. 3rd Edition Edinburgh: Churchill Livingstone; 1994: pp 269-316.

34. Degott C, Feldmann G, Larrey D et al. Drug-induced prolonged cholestasis in adults: a histological semiquantitative study demonstrating progressive ductopenia. *Hepatology* 1992; **15**: 244-251.

35. Davies MH, Harrison RF, Elias E, Hübscher SG. Antibiotic-associated acute vanishing bile duct syndrome: a pattern associated with severe, prolonged intrahepatic cholestasis. *Journal of Hepatology* 1994; **20**: 112-116.

36. Thompson HH, Pit HA, Lewin KJ, Longmire WP. Sclerosing cholangitis and histiocytosis X. *Gut* 1984; **25**: 526-530.

37. Hübscher SG, Lumley MA, Elias E. Vanishing bile duct syndrome: a possible mechanism of intrahepatic cholestasis in Hodgkin's lymphoma. *Hepatology* 1993; **17**: 70-77.

38. Baron TH, Koehler RE, Rodgers WH, Fallon MB, Ferguson SM. Mast cell cholangiopathy: Another cause of sclerosing cholangitis. *Gastroenterology* 1995; **109**: 1677-1681.

39. Lugwig J, Wiesner RH, LaRusso NF. Idiopathic adulthood ductopenia. A cause of chronic cholestatic liver disease and biliary cirrhosis. *Journal of Hepatology* 1988; **7**: 193-199.

40. Portmann B, MacSween RNM. Diseases of the intrehepatic bile ducts. In: MacSween RNM, Anthony PP, Scheuer PJ, Burt AD Portmann BC (eds). Pathology of the Liver. 3rd Edition. Edinburgh: Churchill Livingstone; 1994: pp. 477-512.

41. Van Den Oord JJV, Fevery J, De Groote J, Desmet VJ. Immunohistochemical characterization of inflammatory infiltrates in primary biliary cirrhosis. *Liver* 1984; **4**: 264-274.

42. Krams SM, Van de Water J, Coppel RL, Esquivel C, Roberts J, Ansari A et al. Analysis of hepatic T lymphocyte and immunoglobulin deposits in patients with primary biliary cirrhosis. *Hepatology* 1990; **12**: 306-113.

43. Nakanuma Y. Distribution of B lymphocytes in nonsuppurative cholangitis in primary biliary cirrhosis. *Hepatology* 1993; **18**: 570-575.

44. Teraskai S, Nakanuma Y, Yanazaki M, Unoura M. Eosinophilic infiltration of the liver in primary biliary cirrhosis: A morphological study. *Hepatology* 1993; **17**: 206-112.

45. Martinez OM, Villanueva JC, Gershwin ME, Sheri MK. Cytokine patterns and cytotoxic mediators in primary biliary cirrhosis. *Hepatology* 1995; **21**: 113-119.

46. Hoso M, Nakanuma Y, Kawano M, Oda K, Tsuneyama K, van de Water J et al. Granulomatous cholangitis in chronic hepatitis C: a new diagnostic problem in liver pathology. *Pathology International* 1996; **46**: 301-305.

47. Nakanuma Y, Tsuneyama K, Gershwin ME et al. Pathology and immunopathology of primary biliary cirrhosis with emphasis on bile duct lesions: recent progress. *Semin Liver Dis* 1995; **15**: 313-328.

48. Tsuneyama K, Van de Water J, Leung PSC, Cha S, Nakanuma Y, Kaplan M et al. Abnormal expression of the E2 component of the pyruvate dehydrogenase complex on the luminal surface of biliary epithelium occurs before major histocompatibility complex class II and BB1/B7 expression. *Hepatology* 1995; **21**: 1031-1037.

49. Bernuau D, Feldmann G, Degott C, Gisselbrecht C. Ultrastructural lesions of bile ducts in primary biliary cirrhosis. A comparison with the lesions observed in graft versus host disease. *Human Pathology* 1981; **12**: 782-793.

50. Nakanuma Y, Ohta G, Kono N, Kobayashi K, Kato Y. Electron microscopic observation of destruction of biliary epithelium in primary biliary cirrhosis. *Liver* 1983; **3**: 238-248.

51. Kuroki T, Seki S, Kawakita N, Nakatani K, Hisa T, Kitada T *et al.* Expression of antigens related to apoptosis and cell proliferation in chronic nonsuppurative descrtuctive cholangitis in primary biliary cirrhosis. *Virchows Archiv* 1996; **429**: 119-129.

52. Koga H, Sakisaka S, Ohishi M, Sata M, Tanikawa K. Nuclear DNA fragmentation and expression of Bcl-2 in primary biliary cirrhosis. *Hepatology* 1997; **25**: 1077-1084.

53. Harada K, Ozaki S, Gershwin ME, Nakanuma Y. Enhanced apoptosis related to bile duct loss in primary biliary cirrhosis. *Hepatology* 1997; **26**: 1399-1405.

54. Nakanuma Y, Harada K. Florid duct lesion in primary biliary cirrhosis shows highly proliferative activity. *Hepatology* 1993; **19**: 216-220.

55. Nakanuma Y. Necroinflammatory changes in hepatic lobules in primary biliary cirrhosis with less well defined cholestatic changes. *Human Pathology* 1993; **24**: 378-383.

56. Nakanuma Y, Ohta G. Nodular regenerative hyperplasia of the liver in primary biliary cirrhosis of early histological stages. *Am J Gastroentrol* 1987; **82**: 8-10.

57. Burt AD, MacSween RNM. Bile duct proliferation – its true significance. *Histopathology* 1993; **23**: 599-602.

58. Desmet V, Roskams T, Van Eyken P. Ductular reaction in the liver. *Path Res Pract* 1995; **191**: 513-524.

59. Nagore N, Howe S, Boxer L, Scheuer PJ. Liver cell rosettes: structural differences in cholestasis and hepatitis. *Liver* 1989; **9**: 43-51.

60. Crosby HA, Hübscher SG, Fabris L, Joplin R, Sell S, Kelly D *et al.* Immunolocalization of putative human liver progenitor cells in livers from patients with end-stage primary biliary cirrhosis and sclerosing cholangitis using the monoclonal antibody OV-6. *Am J Pathol* 1998; **152**: 771-779.

61. Roskams T, De Vos R, Van Eyken P, Myazaki H, Van Damme B, Desmet V. Hepatic OV-6 expression in human liver disease and rat experiments: evidence for hepatic progenitor cells in man. *J Hepatol* 1998; **29**: 455-463.

62. Jones DE, Metcalf JV, Collier JD, Bassendine MF, James OF. Hepatocellular carcinoma in primary biliary cirrhosis and its impact on outcomes. *Hepatology* 1997; **26**: 1138-1142.

63. Scheuer PJ. Classification of chronic viral hepatitis: a need for reassessment. *J Hepatol* 1991; **13**: 372-374.

64. Desmet VJ, Gerber M, Hoofnagle JG, Manns M, Scheuer PJ. Classification of chronic hepatitis: diagnosis, grading and staging. *Hepatology* 1994; **19**: 1513-1520.

65. Ishak K, Baptista A, Bianchi L, Callea F, De Groote J, Gudat F *et al.* Histological grading and staging of chronic hepatitis. *J Hepatol* 1995; **22**: 296-699.

66. Rubin E, Schaffner F, Popper H. Primary biliary cirrhosis. Chronic non-suppurative destructive cholangitis. *Am J Pathol* 1965; **46**: 387-407.

67. Scheuer PJ. Primary biliary cirrhosis. *Proc Roy Soc Med* 1967; **60**: 1257-1260.

68. Popper H, Schaffner F. Non-suppurative destructive chronic cholangitis and chronic hepatitis. In: Popper H, Schaffner F, eds. Progress in liver diseases, vol III. New York: Grune & Stratton, 1970; pp 336-354.

69. Ludwig J, Dickson ER, McDonald GS. Staging of chronic non-suppurative cholangitis (syndrome of primary biliary cirrhosis). *Virchows Arch (A)* 1978; **379**: 103-112.

70. Garrido MC, Hübscher SG. Accuracy of staging in primary biliary cirrhosis. *J Clin Pathol* 1996; **49**: 556-559.

71. Olsson R, Hagerstrand I, Broome U, Danielsson A, Jarnerot G, Loof L *et al.* Sampling variability of percutaneous liver biopsy in primary sclerosing cholangitis. *J Clin Pathol* 1995; **48**: 933-935.

72. Goldin RD, Goldin JG, Burt AD, Dhillon AP, Hübscher SG, Wyatt J *et al.* Intraobserver and interobserver variation in the histopathological assessment of chronic viral hepatitis. *J Hepatology* 1996; **25**: 649-654.

73. Bedossa P, Bioulac-Sage P, Callard P, Chevallier M, Degott C, Deugnier Y *et al.* Intraobserver and interobserver variations in liver biopsy interpretation in patients with chronic hepatitis C. *Hepatology* 1994; **20**: 15-20.

74. Brunner G, Klinge O. A cholangitis with antinunclear antibodies (immunocholangitis) resembling chronic destructive non-suppurative cholangitis. *Dtsch Med Wochenschr* 1987; **112**: 1454-1458.

75. Horsmanns Y, Piret A, Brenard R, Rahier J, Geuvel AP. Autoimmune chronic active hepatitis responsive to immunosuppressive therapy evolving into a typical primary biliary cirrhosis syndrome: a case report *J Hepatol* 1994; **21**: 194-198.

76. Colombato LA, Alvarez F, Cote J, Huet PM. Autoimmune cholangiopathy: The result of consecutive primary biliary cirrhosis and autoimmune hepatitis? *Gastroenterology* 1994; **107**: 1839-1843.

77. Ben-Ari Z, Dhillon AP, Sherlock S. Autoimmune cholangiopathy: part of the spectrum of autoimmune chronic active hepatitis. *Hepatology* 1993; **18**: 10-15.

78. Taylor SL, Dean PJ, Riely CA. Primary autoimmune cholangitis. An alternative to antimitochondrial antibody-negative primary biliary cirrhosis. *Am J Surg Pathol* 1994; **18**: 91-99.

79. Goodman ZD, McNally PR, Davis Dr, Ishak KG. Autoimmune cholangitis: a variant of primary biliary cirrhosis. Clinicopathologic and serologic correlations in 200 cases. *Dig Dis Sci* 1995; **40**: 1232-1242.

80. Heathcote J. Autoimmune cholangitis. *Gut* 1997; **40**: 440-442.

81. Michieletti P, Wanless IR, Katz A *et al.* Antimitochondrial antibody negative primary biliary cirrhosis: a distinct syndrome of autoimmune cholangitis. *Gut* 1994; **35**: 260-265.

DEFINITION AND EPIDEMIOLOGY OF PRIMARY BILIARY CIRRHOSIS

Oliver FW James

Centre for Liver Research, Department of Medicine,
University of Newcastle Upon Tyne, NE2 4HH.

SUMMARY

Definitions: PBC can be considered as either definite or probable.

Definite PBC is characterised by the triad of cholestatic liver tests, positive antimitochondrial antibodies and diagnostic or compatible liver histology.

Probable PBC defines three groups of patients: those with cholestatic liver tests and positive anti-mitochondrial antibodies but no histology available; those with anti-mitochondrial antibodies and compatible/diagnostic histology but whose liver tests are normal, and those with cholestatic liver tests, liver histology compatible with or diagnostic of PBC but negative anti-mitochondrial antibodies.

Epidemiology: Developments in the definition of PBC and advances in epidemiological techniques have meant that appreciation of the epidemiology of PBC has radically altered over the last decade. There is great geographical variation in the reported incidence and prevalence of PBC: in Northern Europe, the prevalence of PBC exceeds 100/million whereas in Africa and the Indian subcontinent, the prevalence is much lower. Studies in the North-East of England have shown that the reported prevalence of PBC is rising from 149/million in 1987 to 251/million in 1994. It remains unclear whether this increase represents better diagnosis or an true increase in prevalence.

DEFINITION OF PRIMARY BILIARY CIRRHOSIS (PBC)

The International Hepatology Informatics Group define PBC as "cirrhosis of unknown aetiology associated with destruction of small intrahepatic bile ducts". Clinical (symptomatic, laboratory, morphological, and aetiological) criteria are then described[1]. Although this description is correct it is of little everyday use to practising clinicians. I will suggest more pragmatic, and I hope useful definitions of PBC (Table 1).

Definite PBC

Few would argue with the traditional diagnostic triad for PBC of abnormal (usually cholestatic) liver function tests, positive antimitochondrial antibody (AMA) – usually titre 1 in 40 or greater, and compatible or diagnostic liver histology. This triad has been used to define PBC in most descriptive studies and clinical trials for many years. Note that it contains no clinical criteria for the diagnosis.

Probable PBC

Such is the specificity of finding a positive AMA (if by indirect immunofluorescence then titre 1 in 40 or greater) in the serum of a patient with cholestatic liver function tests that such patients may be regarded as having a high probability of PBC.[2] In a recent study our own group found that only 3% of over 1000 patients who had abnormal liver function tests and positive AMA and subsequently underwent liver biopsy showed liver histology not compatible with or diagnostic of PBC (unpublished observations).

TABLE 1: CLASSIFICATIONS OF PRIMARY BILIARY CIRRHOSIS				
Definition		Cholestatic liver tests	AMA	Compatible/diagnostic liver histology
Definite		+	+	+
Probable	I	+	+	not done
	II*	+	−ve	+
	III	normal	+	+
*also known as autoimmune cholangiopathy				

The second group who I contend should be regarded as having "probable PBC" are individuals with positive AMA (titre 1 in 40 or greater) and compatible or diagnostic liver histology, but with normal liver function tests. We have recently shown that at least 80% of such patients will ultimately develop abnormal liver function tests to complete a "definite" diagnosis, and in over 75% classic symptoms of liver disease will also develop over a prolonged follow-up period.[3]

The third group of the "probable PBC" triad contains patients with abnormal cholestatic liver function tests and liver histology compatible with or diagnostic of PBC but who have negative antimitochondrial antibodies. This entity also called "autoimmune cholangiopathy" has been shown in several studies to be, to all intents and purposes, identical with classical PBC.[4-6] Whether such patients ultimately form a distinct sub-group from the generality of PBC patients remains to be determined. At present it is helpful to consider such patients at least under the "PBC diagnostic umbrella".

PBC symptoms

It should be noted that none of the above definitions have mentioned symptoms or any other clinical features of the disease. In considering symptoms of PBC a distinction should be drawn between symptoms of the liver disease and such symptoms as dry eyes and dry mouth (Sjogrens Syndrome), or Raynaud's phenomenon which are characteristic of disorders often associated with PBC but not directly symptomatic of the liver disease itself.

The most characteristic symptoms of PBC are pruritus, persistent mental and physical fatigue, and persistent ill-defined upper abdominal discomfort. Later signs of the complications of more advance liver disease and cirrhosis – jaundice, ascites, bleeding varices, and encephalopathy – are common to all forms of late stage liver disease, indeed none of the above is pathognmonic of PBC. While this is the case, a high suspicion of PBC may be entered in a middle-aged or older women presenting with symptoms of persisting pruritus and fatigue. If a patient has none of the above symptoms, even in the presence of such "associated" symptoms as dry eyes or dry mouth, then they should be regarded as asymptomatic of PBC for the purposes of classification needed, for example, in design of clinical trials.

It is intended that the above rather pragmatic definitions should be clinically useful, even if in each of the three "probable" PBC categories there is a very small proportion of error. The error of excluding patients who only fulfil two of the three diagnostic criteria on investigation, particularly those who have cholestatic liver function tests and positive AMA but who have not had a liver biopsy, from a diagnosis of PBC is far greater than the possible error of including all such individuals, and possibly with them around 5% patients who do not truly have the disease.

EPIDEMIOLOGY

Although case series of patients with PBC had been described in the 1950s the epidemiology of PBC was not studied until Hamlyn and Sherlock's review of PBC deaths using death certification in England and Wales in 1974.[7] Just as the science of molecular biology has led to an explosion of knowledge and understanding in biomedical sciences over the past 20 years, so the science of epidemiology has also developed very rapidly in this time. Descriptive epidemiology is an important research tool with which to explore possible temporal and geographic variations in the occurrence of a disease and thus to generate and test hypotheses about its cause.[8]

Real interest in the epidemiology of PBC was first generated by the fascinating study of Triger of the distribution of PBC cases in the City of Sheffield from a 3 year period 1977-1979.[9] In this study Triger found that the distribution of the cases did not follow population density within the City. Of the 34 cases identified, 30 lived in homes supplied with water provided by a single reservoir. Since five reservoirs provided water for the City in proportions roughly equal to the population, the prevalence of PBC within the area supplied by the Rivelin reservoir was about ten times that of the other four reservoirs. Despite careful investigation at that time no difference in composition or content of the water was found between reservoirs. There were no other socio-economic, familial or geographical associations with these findings.

Between 1980 and 1990 there was an explosion of information concerning the epidemiology of PBC from the United Kingdom, Scandinavia, elsewhere in Europe, and from Canada. Subsequently studies have also been reported from Australia, Russia and, most recently, Wales. Before examining these findings in some detail it is important to understand the principles which should govern good modern descriptive epidemiology of a disease. These will be briefly described in turn (Table 2).

Case definition

In any study of descriptive epidemiology case definition is extremely important, hence it is appropriate that this account of PBC epidemiology should begin with a discussion of the definition of the disease. Few early

TABLE 2: FEATURES OF EPIDEMIOLOGICAL STUDIES	
Definition of	Disease Time period of study Geographical area of study Date of disease onset
Case finding methods	Use multiple approaches
Avoid potential sources of bias	e.g. tertiary referral

accounts of the epidemiology of PBC gave a clear definition. Those which did almost all used the "definite" definition (all three of abnormal liver function tests, positive AMA, diagnostic/compatible histology) – hence, as I have argued above, probably excluding a number of patients with the disease from consideration. Explicit case definition is important for interpretation of comparative studies between different regions.[10]

Define time and place

In order to examine prevalence and incidence of a disease precise definition of the time of study and of the exact region of study is vital. Thus, if these parameters are not defined the tendency will be to draw in patients from outside a strictly defined geographical area – perhaps due to tertiary referral bias – or to include individuals who either died before the beginning of the study period (although they lived within the study area), or in whom a diagnosis was made after the end of the study period. Almost none of the earlier studies of PBC epidemiology were rigorous in respect of both careful definition of time and study region, and hence population.

Thoroughness of case finding methods

Clearly the number of cases reported in a descriptive case finding epidemiological study will depend upon the thoroughness of case finding methods used. Use of multiple case finding methods will ensure the greatest completeness of data collection. In an ideal study the whole population in the defined area, over the defined time, would be screened for a disease. In the case of PBC this is not practicable. Use of multiple case finding methods is particularly important as we will see, in PBC where a high proportion of patients are asymptomatic at a time when a diagnosis may be made. For understandable reasons, almost all earlier epidemiological studies of PBC have used incomplete case finding methods – many relying only upon collecting patients known to physicians, within a region, to have PBC and/or hospital case record analysis.

Definition of date of disease onset

Definition of the date of onset of a disease is not a problem in a disease which is always accompanied by definite symptoms or signs – for example, rubella, or psoriasis. The definition is much more difficult in a disease with a phase that is frequently asymptomatic and which may extend for many years.[11,12] The matter is made more complex by debate over case definition – should a patient be regarded as having PBC only when all three diagnostic criteria are fulfilled – "definite PBC" – or, as I would strongly contend, when two out of three of the diagnostic criteria have been fulfilled – "probable PBC"? It will be seen that the potential for sources of error over date of diagnosis in respect of epidemiological studies of PBC is very great. For example, if some form of case finding is carried out in the course of the epidemiological survey of a region then a number of "incident" cases may be ascribed to the period of the case finding. In fact closer examination would show that many of these patients had PBC, as defined above, up to many years earlier than in the case finding exercise. Thus, if, for example, 80 patients are found by a case finding exercise in 1998 within a certain area is the incidence of the disease 80 within this area for 1998 or can and should these 80 cases be attributed to earlier years if it is possible to ascribe at least a "probable" diagnosis to them at some earlier stage?

In our recent studies my colleagues in Newcastle and I have made a pragmatic decision to define date of diagnosis as "the earliest date at which the patient was found to have fulfilled any two of the three diagnostic criteria". This is, therefore, frequently a retrospective diagnosis made following examination of patient case records.[13]

Other sources of variation

Apart from the above potential systemic errors in examination of descriptive epidemiology of PBC two other variables should be considered. The first is access to health care – in this case particularly to physicians interested in liver disease. Comparison of the epidemiology of PBC in, for example, Rochester, Minnesota – home of one of the worlds foremost centres for PBC research – compared with, say, Khartoum, Sudan, would be misleading since physicians in Khartoum have many higher health priorities than PBC and have probably little knowledge of or interest in the disease. Similarly, the level of appropriate diagnostic activity – in this case number of liver biopsies, frequency with which autoantibody profiles (AMAs), and liver function tests are carried out – is also very important. Again, a meaningful comparison between Rochester and Khartoum might be

TABLE 3: EPDEMIOLOGICAL STUDIES OF PRIMARY BILIARY CIRRHOSIS

Area of reference	Year of Publication	Case Finding Methods	Case Criteria	Number of Patients	Incidence (per million)	Point Prevalence (per million)
Sheffield, England[9]	1980	1,3	a+b or a+c	34	5.8	54
Dundee, Scotland[14]	1980	5	a+c	21	10.6	40.2
Northeast England[15]	1983	1,3,4	a+b+c	117	10.0	37–144
Malmo, Sweden[16]	1984	1,3,4	a+b+c	33	4–24	92
EASL[17]	1984	1	none (but most had a+b or a+c)	569	4.0	5–75
Erebro, Sweden[18]	1985	3	a+b+c	43	14.0	128
Glasgow, Scotland[19]	1987	3	a+c	373	11–15	70–93
Umea, Sweden[20]	1990	1,2 (3: incomplete data)	c	111	13.0	151
Northeast England[21]	1990	1,2,3	a+b+c or a+c	347	11–18	129
Ontario, Canada[22]	1990	1	a+c	206	3.0	22
Victoria, Australia[23]	1995	1 (2+3: incomplete data)	a+b+c (definite) a+b (probable)	71	– 84.0	19
Estonia, Russia[24]	1995	1,2 (probable)	at least 2/3 of a,b,c	69	2.0	27
Newcastle, England[13]	1997 (1994 FIGS)	1,2,3,4,5	a+b+c (definite) 2/3 of a,b,c (probable)	99 160	14–32 15–41	240 392
Swansea, Wales[25]	1998	1,2	a+b	65	20.0	200

1.Survey of physicians; 2.Hospital admission/acivity data; 3. Laboratory data on AMA positive individuals; 4.Death notifications: 5.Liver histology data.
a.AMA positive; b.cholestatic liver function tests; c.compatible liver histology

extraordinarily difficult because the frequency with which members of the population received these important investigations for the diagnosis of PBC would probably be vastly different.

Table 3 describes a number of the major studies of PBC epidemiology together with the case finding methods used and case criteria. No study apart from our own[13] has attempted to deal with all the possible sources of error outlined above.

World-wide trends

In general, notwithstanding the variation in quality of data described in Table 3, and using information from case series described elsewhere the following observations concerning world-wide distribution of PBC may be made.[10] The disease appears to be commonest in Northern Europe with prevalence, or likely prevalence, over 100/10[6] in Sweden, Norway, England, Wales and Scotland. Case series, preliminary epidemiological data, and descriptive studies also suggest that PBC is relatively common throughout Europe, for example in Spain, France, Italy and Greece. In North America only data from Canada is available suggesting that PBC is moderately common at between 20 and 30/10[6] during the 1980s.[22,26] It should be noted, however, that both of these studies were essentially surveys only of PBC cases known to interested physicians. In Australasia a case finding study suggested that prevalence of PBC was quite low in the State of Victoria (19/10[6] of the total population). However, if Australian born women over age 64 were considered alone then prevalence reached 122/10[6] [23]. Elsewhere in Asia case series suggest that the disease is moderately common in Japan but extraordinarily rare in the Indian Subcontinent. Indeed no case of PBC has ever been described in Sri Lanka (OFWJ, personal observation). In Africa PBC is extraordinarily rare, having only been described in a series of 8 cases all of white or Indian racial origin[27].

THE NEWCASTLE PROJECT

There has been an interest in PBC epidemiology in North-East England for almost 20 years. From 1987 a careful study of PBC epidemiology has been carried out. This study has tried to minimise the possible sources of error in descriptive epidemiology outlined above. My colleagues and I would suggest that by describing our methodology here, standards may be set so that future studies elsewhere can be carried out in a similar fashion and hence far greater comparability between regions can be achieved. Hence more meaningful hypotheses concerning possible environmental factors involved in PBC aetiology or progression may be examined.

Case definition

We have defined "definite" PBC as fulfilling all three diagnostic criteria described above, "probable PBC" as fulfilling any two of the criteria. We have and will provide figures for both "definite" and for "probable" cases in our reports. As I have indicated above, my own strong view is that the total "probable" prevalence and incidence is far closer to reality than merely the "diagnostic" figures.

Definition of disease onset

In our studies we have defined disease onset as the earliest date at which the patient was found to have fulfilled any two of the three diagnostic criteria. This avoids the need for different criteria for date of diagnosis in asymptomatic versus symptomatic patients.

Case finding methods

These are described fully in reference 13. They were briefly as follows:

1. Request to all physicians in the study area for notification of all their possible cases of PBC.

2. Search of hospital admission data on regional information systems for all hospitals in the region for admission episodes for PBC (using appropriate ICD codes).

3. Examination of all hospital immunology data for patients with AMA reported positive ≥1 in 40.

4. All listings from the Office of National Statistics (ONS) of deaths within the region where PBC was recorded on the death certificate with appropriate ICD code.

Definition of population area and time

The study area was defined using postal (zip) codes within county boundaries. The population for the area was recorded from the ONS and adjusted for each year of the study from ONS data.

Definition of time of study

Only cases prevalent or incident within the study period resident within the defined study area are included in our studies.

Data collection

This has been carried out as follows:

1. Hospital case records from all cases detected by the above case finding methods are exhaustively sought except in the few cases who have never attended hospital. These are sought after requesting permission from their general practitioner and invited to attend our liver clinic for assessment.

2. All cases no longer under hospital care are invited to attend the liver clinic.

3. All cases flagged by the ONS as having died, not previously known to the study group have had case records sought.

Symptom status

Symptoms of PBC have been defined as described earlier. Patients without PBC symptoms at the time of presumed diagnosis are regarded as being asymptomatic at presumed diagnosis. The appearance of any of the "PBC symptoms" has led to definition as "symptomatic".

FINDINGS

These have been fully described for the City of Newcastle upon Tyne – part of our study area[13]. The results for the whole study area – population about 2.05 million have been submitted for publication[28]. Briefly, these suggest that the overall prevalence for PBC in the Region was $251/10^6$ in 1994, the prevalence among women over age 40 being $940/10^6$. The apparent overall prevalence had risen from $149/10^6$ in 1987 or $541/10^6$ among women over 40. From an earlier, less complete study in the Region[21] apparent prevalence in 1976 (extremely incomplete data) was $16/10^6$.

Overall incidence showed a trend to increasing, mean annual incidence 1991-1994 was $31/10^6$ within the Region.

Symptom status

Of the 770 "definite" or "probable" cases, 469 (60.9%) were asymptomatic at presumed diagnosis. In June 1994 when 514 cases were prevalent, 62% had experienced PBC symptoms as their most recent clinical assessment. Thus it is possible to assume that at any one time at least 40% of PBC patients in a region have experienced no symptoms of their liver disease.

Case identification

Review of case records suggested that PBC was suspected by the original hospital consultant in 57% patients at a time when the probable diagnosis could have been made. The diagnosis was neither made nor apparently considered in the remainder. This points up the gross underestimate which will be made if only cases "known to physicians" are included in epidemiological studies of PBC.

Case distribution

We are currently examining the distribution of cases within the Region. The address (postal code) of each case is recorded on the database from two aspects. First, in the five health districts within the Region to establish whether variations in access to appropriate expertise – using numbers of gastroenterologists as a proxy for expertise – and diagnostic activity (as assessed by numbers of liver biopsies and autoantibody screens carried out each year by district per 100,000 population), are likely to account for variations in the incidence and prevalence of the disease found within the region of interest. Second, to examine the possibility that there may be clusters of patients within certain close geographic areas within the region of interest suggesting the possibility of sources of environmental agents involved in the pathogenesis or progression of the disease.

Case control study

We have also completed a pilot case control study of possible risk factors for PBC within the Region[29]. One hundred and five unselected PBC patients incident between 1993 and 1995 within the region were studied and information was obtained from 105 age and sex matched controls from the same primary health care registers by means of a postal questionnaire. The two groups were well matched in all demographic details. Cases did not differ significantly from controls in regard to family history of any liver disease, history of urinary tract infection, D & C procedures, hysterectomy, median number of births, history of TB, measles, mumps, rubella, or a variety of other infective diseases. Interestingly, cases were more likely to have a history of psoriasis (cases 10% controls 1% OR 9.0), less likely to have a history of eczema (cases 0 controls 10%).

CONCLUSIONS

There is a general perception that PBC is becoming much commoner. It is still unclear whether this is due to increased recognition of the disease and increasing diagnostic activity – autoantibody screening, routine use of liver biochemistries – or whether this apparent marked increase in incidence and prevalence in many countries is due to a true increase of the disease. Future studies using similar methodology to that described above, together with a continuation of the present studies in Northern England should provide answers to these important questions.

If figures from North East England and Swansea are extrapolated to the United Kingdom there are probably 10-15,000 patients with PBC in the United Kingdom.

REFERENCES

1. International Hepatology Informatics Group in "Diseases of the liver and biliary tract" 1994, pp65-66. Raven Press, New York

2. Sherlock S and Dooley J in "Diseases of the Liver and Biliary System" 9th edn 1993 pp236-248, Blackwell, Oxford

3. Metcalf JV, Mitchison HC, Palmer JM, Jones De, Bassendine MF, James OFW. Natural history of early primary biliary cirrhosis. *Lancet* 1996;**348**:1399-1402

4. Michieletti P, Wanless IR, Katz A, Scheuer PJ, Yeaman SJ, Bassendine MF, Palmer JM, Heathcote EJ. Antimitochondrial antibody negative primary biliary cirrhosis: a distinction syndrome of autoimmune cholangitis. *Gut* 1994;**35**:260-265.

5. Lacerda MA, Ludwig J, Dickson ER, Jorgensen RA, Lindor KD. Antimitochondrial antibody-negative primary biliary cirrhosis. *Am J Gastroenterol* 1995;**90**:247-2149.

6. Invernizzi P, Crosignani A, Battezzati PM, Covini G, De Valle G, Larghi A, Zuin M, Podda M. Comparison of the clinical features and clinical course of antimitochondrial antibody-positive and –negative primary biliary cirrhosis. *Hepatology* 1997;**25**:1090-1095

7. Hamlyn AN, Sherlock S. The epidemiology of primary biliary cirrhosis: a survey of mortality in England and Wales. *Gut* 1974;**15**:473-479

8. Metcalf JV, Howel D, Bhopal RS, James OFW. Primary biliary cirrhosis – epidemiology helping the clinician. *Br Med J* 1996;**312**:1181-1182

9. Triger DR. Primary biliary cirrhosis: an epidemiological study. *Br Med J* 1980;**281**:772-775

10. Metcalf JV, James OFW. The Geoepidemiology of primary biliary cirrhosis. *Seminars in Liver Disease* 1997;**17**(1):13-22

11. Mitchison HC, Lucey MR, Kelly PJ, Neuberger JM, Williams R, James OFW. Symptom development and prognosis in primary biliary cirrhosis: a study in two centres. *Gastroenterology* 1990;**99**:778-84.

12. Balasubramanian K, Grambasch PM, Wiesner RH, Lindor KD, Dickson ER. Diminished survival in asymptomatic primary biliary cirrhosis: a prospective study. *Gastroenterology* 1990;**90**:1567-71

13. Metcalf JV, Bhopal RS, Gray J, Howel D, James OFW. Incidence and prevalence of primary biliary cirrhosis in the City of Newcastle upon Tyne, England. *Int J Epidemiol* 1997;**26**:830-836

14. Hislop W. Primary biliary cirrhosis: an epidemiological study,. *Br Med J* 1980;**281**:772

15. Hamlyn AN, Macklon AF, James O. Primary biliary cirrhosis: geographical clustering and symptomatic onset seasonality. *Gut* 1983; **24**:940-945

16. Eriksson S, Lindgren S. The prevalence and clinical spectrum of primary biliary cirrhosis in a defined population. *Scand J Gastroenterol* 1984;**19**:971-976

17. Triger DR, berg PA, Rodes J. Epidemiology or primary biliary cirrhosis. *Liver* 1984;**4**:195-200

18. Lofgren J, Jarnerot G, Danielsson D, Hemdal I. Incidence and prevalence of primary biliary cirrhosis in a defined population in Sweden. *Scand J Gastroenterol* 1985;**20**:647-650

19. Goudie B, MacFarland G, Boyle P et al. Epidemiology of antimitochondrial antibody seropositivity and primary biliary cirrhosis in the west of Scotland. *Gut* 1987;**28**:A1346

20. Danielsson A, Boqvist L, Uddenfeldt P. Epidemiology of primary biliary cirrhosis in a defined rural population in the northern part of Sweden. *Hepatology* 1990;**11**:458-464

21. Myszor M, James OF. The epidemiology of primary biliary cirrhosis in northern England: an increasingly common disease? *Quar J Med* 1990;**75**:377-385

22. Witt-Sullivan H, Heathcote, J, Cauch K et al. The demography of primary biliary cirrhosis (PBC) in Ontario, Canada. *Hepatology* 1990;**12**:98-105

23. Watson R, Goss B, Angus P. Low prevalence of primary biliary cirrhosis (PBC) in Victoria, Australia. *Gut* 1995;**36**:927-930

24. Remmel T, Remmel H, Uibo R, Saluprere V. Primary biliary cirrhosis in Estonia, with special reference to incidence, prevalence, clinical features, and outcome. *Scand J Gastroenterol* 1995;**30**:367-371.

25. Kingham JGC, Parker DR. The association between primary biliary cirrhosis and coeliac disease, a study of relative prevelances. *Gut* 1998;**42**:120-122

26. Villeneuve J, Fenyves D, Infante-Rivard C. Descriptive epidemiology of primary biliary cirrhosis in the province of Quebec, Canada. *J Gastroenterol* 1991;**5**:174-178

27. Robson S, Hift R, Kirsch R. Primary biliary cirrhosis: a retrospective survey at Groote Schuur Hospital, Capetown. *So Afr med J* 1990;**78**:19-21.

28. James OFW, Bhopal R, Howel D, Gray J, Metcalf JV. Epidemiology of PBC in Northern England: is the disease truly increasing? (Submitted to Gastroenterology August 1998)

29. Fischbacker CM, Metcalf JV, Howel D, Bhopal R, Jones DE, James OFW. A pilot case control study of possible risk factors for primary biliary cirrhosis. *Hepatology* 1988;**28**:540A

I greatly acknowledge the very hard work of Dr Jane Metcalf in carrying out the studies described above from Newcastle and of my colleagues in the University of Newcastle Department of Epidemiology and Public Health who have been responsible for the design of these studies and for (partially) educating me in descriptive epidemiology.

AETIOPATHOGENESIS OF PRIMARY BILIARY CIRRHOSIS

Roger Chapman

Dept of Gastroenterology, Oxford Radcliffe Hospital,
Headley Way, Headington, Oxford OX3 9DU.

SUMMARY

Current evidence suggests that primary biliary cirrhosis is an immune mediated disease triggered in susceptible individuals by an environmental agent which remains unknown. Enterobacteria, atypical mycobacteria and retroviruses have all been suggested as infectious agents triggering the disease. However, there is little data to support these hypotheses at the present time.

Introduction

Primary biliary cirrhosis (PBC) is a chronic cholestatic liver disease characterized by the immunological destruction of interlobular and septal bile ducts leading to cholestasis, fibrosis, and biliary cirrhosis. PBC is considered to be one of the group of autoimmune liver diseases in which the biliary epithelial cells lining the interlobular and septal bile ducts from the target for key cell related immune mediated damage. The identification of the major auto-antigens (part of the pyruvate dehydrogenase complex) has meant that the immunopathogenesis of the disease has been extensively studied and this has been discussed in earlier chapters. Although the aetiological factors remain unknown, it is widely accepted that PBC arises in a susceptible individual, usually female, as a result of one or more environmental trigger factors. In common with other diseases which are thought to be immune mediated, PBC occurs predominantly in females with a male/female ratio of 1:9.

Environmental Factors

Recent epidemiological studies have highlighted marked variations in the prevalence of PBC in certain geographical regions, with genetically similar populations. The prevalence of PBC in a recent study from Newcastle in the United Kingdom, has suggested a disease point prevalence of approximately 1 per thousand of urban women.[1,2] In addition, marked geographical variations of prevalence have been noticed in adjacent and apparently genetically similar populations such as in Scandinavia where the prevalence is low and high in different areas of Sweden[3,4] (Table 1).

Moreover, a remarkably low prevalence of PBC has been noted in Victoria, Australia, and Ontario, Canada where in both cases the population is largely Caucasian of Western European origin[5,6]. There have been few studies in the Third World, but the prevalence is believed to be very low. It is still unclear as to whether these variations are artifactual due to variations in methods used for case finding[7], but if these temporal and geographical variations in the prevalence of PBC

TABLE 1: GEOGRAPHICAL VARIATIONS IN THE PREVALENCE OF PBC

Country	Year	Cases	Prevalence per million of population	Methods (*)
Newcastle, England	1989	347	128.5	PS; AMA, HR
Newcastle, England	1995	303	96	PS; AMA, HR
Umea, Sweden	1990	86	151	PS; AMA, HR
Malmo, Sweden	1984	92	92	HR
Ontario, Canada	1990	206	22	PS
Victoria, Australia	1995	84	19	PS; AMA,HR
Delhi, India	1991	?	<5.0	HR

(*) PS = Postal survey of physicians. AMA = Follow-up of positive antimitochondrial antibody tests. HR = Retrospective review of hospital records.

prove to be correct, then this has important implications in the investigation of aetiopathogenesis of the condition suggesting there is a locally variable environmental factor.

Circumstantial evidence that an environmental agent may induce PBC was provided from a three-year study of PBC in Sheffield, UK. The prevalence of PBC was ten times greater in that area of the city supplied by one water reservoir compared with five other areas of Sheffield supplied by different reservoirs[8]. Chemical and bacteriological investigation failed to find any infectious or chemical factors unique to this reservoir, but the Sheffield observations have been repeated within the same city recently with similar findings (Gleeson D, Personal Communication 1998).

Infectious Agents

It has been suggested that antimitochondrial antibody and ultimately PBC are induced by exposure to enterobacterial antigens. Immunoblotting studies have shown that PBC specific antibodies recognise enterobacterial proteins which correspond to mitochondrial target proteins has a molecular weight of between 50-70RDa[9]. Studies by Stemerowicz et al. have shown that all Gram-negative bacteria contain these proteins[10]. The structure and metabolism of mitochondria and aerobic bacteria are similar and it has been suggested that mitochondria derive phylogenetically from bacteria as the result of integration of bacteria into amoeboid cells[11]. According to this endosymbiotic hypothesis, the inner mitochondrial membrane represents the outer bacterial membrane and this interpretation is compatible with the reactivity of PBC specific antimitochondrial antibody. Rabbits who are immunized with enterobacteria R mutants produce antimitochondrial antibody although enterobacteria wild forms which are not R mutants do not develop antimitochondrial antibody[10]. Hopf has suggested that this is because the R (rough) mutants have a defect in

TABLE 2: SERUM & PLASMA PROTEINS ENCODED AT CLASS III REGION ON CHROMOSOME 6

Classical complement pathway components – C4A, C4B, and C2
Alternative complement pathway components – Bf (factor B or properdin factor)
Tumor necrosis factor α and β
Heat shock protein -hsp 70
Steroid cytochrome P450 21 - hydroxylase enzymes (Cyp 21 A and Cyp 21 B)

the liposaccharide molecule which alters the membrane characteristics of the bacteria leading to the expression of other superficial antigens which are more lipophilic and less water soluble than other forms[11]. These workers have also suggested that stool samples from patients of PBC contain R forms of E. coli which represent up to 50% of all aerobic Gram-negative bacteria in the samples which are much less commonly found in patients with other diseases and healthy controls[12]. These findings were extended by the demonstration by the Royal Free Group that patients with PBC commonly suffer asymptomatic urinary tract infections with Gram-negative bacteria[13] and that these have a high proportion of R forms[14]. This has not been confirmed and although PBC sera contain antibodies capable of binding both mammalian and bacterial PBC E2 proteins, there is poor cross reactivity indicating that separate antibodies against these prokaryotic and eukaryotic antigens are present in PBC serum[15]. On the current evidence it is difficult to conclude that enterobacteriaceae are the trigger factors for PBC.

It is, perhaps not surprising, since granulomata occurring either as aggregates of histirocytes or of non-caseating lesions adjacent to damaged bile ducts are commonly found in PBC and since granulomata may be induced by Mycobacteria, that a search has been made for Mycobacteria as an effective cause of PBC. In a study from Spain, all primary biliary cirrhotic sera from nineteen patients and none of thirty-five controls (twenty-five patients with other liver diseases and ten healthy subjects) reacted with an extract from Mycobacterium gordonae[16]. No reaction was found in PBC patients or controls with extracts from nine other atypical Mycobacteria tested. These results were not confirmed by a study from the UK in which western blotting was used to test membrane extracts of Mycobacterium gordonae and seven other atypical Mycobacterium species with the serum of patients with PBC[17]. No reaction was seen with any of the Mycobacterium although antibodies to a 65RDa Mycobacteria protein was found in most patients with PBC as well as in normal controls and patients with other chronic liver diseases[17]. Although it is an attractive hypothesis, it remains unproven as to whether Mycobacterium play any role in the pathogenesis of PBC.

A preliminary report from the United States found the presence of false positive antibodies to human immunodeficiency virus, HIV I, in a proportion of PBC patients[18] which led to a search for retroviral antibodies in PBC and other idiopathic biliary disorders. There is a close association between PBC and Sjogren's syndrome which occurs in about 70% of patients with PBC. Similar reports of false positive HIV I antibodies have been found Sjogren's syndrome[19] and in addition, the human intra-cisternal A-type protein (HIAP) ahs been detected from the salivary glands of Sjogren's syndrome patients[20]. Using Western blotting, Mason et al.[21], found HIV I p24 gag seroreactivity in 35% of patients with PBC compared with 29% of patients with SLE and 39% of patients with either primary sclerosing cholangitis or biliary atresia compared with only 4% of control patients with non-biliary diseases and normal controls[21]. The serum did not react with other epitopes of the HIV virus. Western blot activity was also found more than two HIAP proteins which was found in 51% of patients with PBC but was also found in a high proportion of patients with other autoimmune diseases and biliary diseases. This non-specific antibody activity could represent the result of the autoimmune response to cross reactive cellular proteins, or response to infection with an uncharacterized retroviral element. The finding that these antibodies are non-specific, and are found in other immune mediated biliary disease such as primary sclerosing cholangitis do not provide strong evidence for a retroviral aetiology. The authors, however, demonstrated that the presence of retroviral (HIAP) antigens did correlate closely with autoantibody production and it may be that retroviral infection is important in this process.

Genetic Susceptibility

Evidence from family studies has shown that inherited factors play an important role in determining disease susceptibility[22]. Two studies have shown that the prevalence of PBC in first degree relatives is between 4–6%, significantly higher than the highest reported whole population prevalence[23,24]. Unfortunately, there are no reports of twin studies in PBC apart from one case report which showed discordant disease in a monozygotic pair confirming the suggestion that environmental factors are important[25].

Unlike the two other autoimmune diseases, autoimmune hepatitis and primary sclerosing cholangitis, PBC is not associated with an over representation of the HLA A1 B8 DR3 DR52a haplotype, nor are there secondary associations with HLA DR4 OR DR2 as reported in these conditions. A number of genotyping studies from different populations have demonstrated a positive association between HLA class II antigen DR8 and PBC.

Early studies of HLA antigen frequency in PBC provided contradictory and inconclusive results. However, in 1987 Gores et al.[26] in a study of one hundred and fourteen patients from the Mayo Clinic described an increase in the frequency of DR8 in patients with PBC.

Thirty per cent of patients were DR positive compared with 4.7% of one hundred and seventy one controls[26]. Since the initial report, a number of other studies have been reported in different population groups. A first publication from Japan reported a very high association with HLA DR8, 79% in patients compared with 23% in the control group[27], although a subsequent report from Japan revealed the association to be less strong[28]. Whilst it is true that in the majority of PBC populations that have been tested DR8 is increased in frequency, in Caucasians, the association only accounts for a minority of patients with PBC. This may reflect the fact that the susceptibility allele lies some distance from the HLA DR genes. Possibilities include susceptibility genes within the HLA class III region or within the closely linked DQ and DP loci. Seki et al. from Japan reported that 84% of PBC patients in their study were DPBI*0501 positive compared with 55% of controls[29]. The authors suggested that DPBI*0501 may be the primary susceptibility allele in PBC[29]. These results, however, have not been confirmed in a study from Kings College Hospital by Underhill et al.[30].

The term HLA class III is confusing since the products of this region are not all surface glycoproteins or human leucocyte antigens. The genes from this region encode an important collection of immunologically active serum and plasma proteins (Table 1). The class III complement genes have been studied in PBC. The first report from England by Briggs et al. described a significant increase of C4B2 in patients with PBC[31] (45% of PBC patients compared with 17% in the control group). In addition, C4A4 was increased to 21% compared with 6% in the control groups[31]. A second study from Germany confirmed an increase in C4B2[32]. In addition, a significant increase in C4A-Q0 alleles was detected. Tumour necrosis factor beta is encoded in the class region of chromosome 6; however, studies in PBC have shown no significant differences in the occurrence of tumour necrosis factor alleles in PBC patients compared with controls[33]. Other genes which may contribute to the susceptibility of autoimmune liver disease, for example, the contribution of TAP genes upstream promoter sequences and T-cell receptor and complement genes elsewhere in the human genome have not been well studied. Gregory et al. have examined TAP1 and TAP 11 antigen processing genes n PBC and showed an increase frequency of TAP 1Beta 42% DR positive versus 16% DR negative patients[34] but this was also found HDR positive controls indicating a linkage disequilibrium between these loci. Although the effect of HLA types on disease progression has not been extensively studied Gregory *et al.*[35] in 1993 suggested that DR positivity may identify a clinical sub-group with a worse prognosis. This remains to be confirmed by other workers. In the light of the strong association with DR8 which has been found in Japan, it has been suggested that a leucine at position 35 of the antigen binding group of the class II molecules may be important for determining the susceptibility of Japanese patients with PBC[29]. This is analogous to the leucine in position 38 felt to be important for susceptibility for PSC.

A weak association has been shown with the promoter polymorphism of the pro-inflammatory cytokine tumour necrosis factor alpha[36]. The functional significance of this polymorphism remains unclear, although it is interesting it has been postulated that the presence of this polymorphism together with the presence of DR8 causes a more rapid progression to cirrhosis[36].

REFERENCES

1. Myszor M, James OF. The epidemiology of primary biliary cirrhosis in north-east England: an increasingly common disease? *Q. J. Med.* 1990; **75**: 377-385.

2. Metcalf JV, Bhopal RS, Scott LMD, Gray J, Howel D, James OF. Temporal and geographical variations in the prevalence of primary biliary cirrhosis (PBC) in a stable population. *Hepatology* 1995; **22**: 384A.

3. Lofgren J, Jarnerot G, Danielsson A, Hemdal I. Incidence and prevalence of primary biliary cirrhosis in a defined population in Sweden. *Scand. J. Gastroenterol.* 1985; **20**: 647-650.

4. Danielsson A, Boqvist L, Uddenfeldt P. Epidemiology of primary biliary cirrhosis in a defined rural population in the northern part of Sweden. *Hepatology* 1990; **11**: 458-464.

5. Watson R, Angus PW, Dewar M, Goss B, Sewell RB, Smallwood RA. Low prevalence of primary biliary cirrhosis in Victoria, Australia. *Gut* 1995; **36**: 927-930.

6. Witt-Sullivan H, Heathcote EJ, Couch K. The demography of primary biliary cirrhosis in Ontario, Canada. *Hepatology* 1990; **12**: 98-105.

7. Metcalf JV, Howel D, James OF, Bhopal R. Primary biliary cirrhosis: epidemiology helping the clinician. *British Medical Journal* 1996; **312**: 1181-1182.

8. Triger DR. Primary biliary cirrhosis: is there an environmental contribution? *J. Gastroenterol. Hepatol.* 1991; **6**: 568-569.

9. Lindenborn-Fotinos J, Baum H, Berg PA. Mitochondrial antigens in primary biliary cirrhosis; further characterization of the M2 antigen by immunoblotting, revealing, species and non-species determinants. *Hepatology* 1985; **5**: 763-9.

10. Stemerowicz R, Hopf U, Möller B, Wittenbrink C, Rodloff A, Reinhardt R, Frendenberg M, Galanos C. Are mitochondrial antigens in primary biliary cirrhosis induced by R (rough)-mutants of Enterobacteriaceae? *Lancet* 1988; **2**: 1166-70.

11. Hopf U, Stemerowicz R. Can enterobacterial antigens induce a primary biliary cirrhosis? In: Immunology and Liver, Meyer Zum, Büschenfelde K-H, Hoofnagle J, Manns M, Eds, Klewer, London, 1993, pp447-458.

12. Hopf U, Möller B, Sternerowicz R, Rodloff A, Lobeck H, Freudenberg M, Galanos C, Huhn D. Escherichia Coli rough (R) mutants in the gut and lipid A in the liver from patients with primary biliary cirrhosis (PBC). *Lancet* 1989; **2**: 1419-22.

13. Burroughs AK, Rosenstein IJ, Epstein O, Hamilton-Miller JMT, Brumfitt W, Sherlock S. Bacteriuria and primary biliary cirrhosis. *Gut* 1984; **25**: 133-7.

14. Butler P, Falle F, Hamilton-Miller JMT, Brumfitt W, Baum H, Burroughs AK. M2 mitochondrial antibodies and urinary rough mutant bacteria in patients with primary biliary cirrhosis and in patients with recurrent bacteriuria. *J. Hepatol.* 1992; **17**: 483-488.

15. Fussey SPM, Lindsay JG, Fuller C, Perham RN, Dale S, James OJ, Bassendine MF, Yeaman SJ. Autoantibodies in primary biliary cirrhosis: analysis of reactivity against eukaryotic and prokaryotic 2-oxo-acid dehydrogenase complexes. *Hepatology* 1991; **13**: 467-74.

16. Bilagut L, Vila J, Vinas O, Pares A, Gines A, Jimenez de Anta M, Rodes J. Cross reactivity of anti-mycobacterium gordonae antibodies with the major mitochondrial autoantigens in primary biliary cirrhosis. *J. Hepatol.* 1994; **21**: 673-677.

17. O'Donohue J, McFarland B, Bromford A, Yates M, Williams R. Antibodies to atypical mycobacteriae in primary biliary cirrhosis. *J. Hepatol.* 1994; **21**: 887-889.

18. Munoz SJ, Ballas SK, Norberg R, Maddrey WC. Antibodies to human immunodeficiency virus (HIV) in primary biliary cirrhosis. *Gastroenterology* 1988; **94**: A574 (abstr).

19. Talal N, Dauphinee M, Dang H, Alexander S, Hard D, Garry R. Detection of serum antibodies to retroviral proteins in patients with Sjögren's syndrome. *Arthritis Rheum.* 1990; **33**: 741-81.

20. Talal N, Garry R, Alexander S et al. A conserved idiotype and antibodies to retroviral proteins in systemic lupus erythematosus. *J. Clin. Invest.* 1990; **85**: 1866-71.

21. Mason AL, Xu L, Guo L, Munoz S, Jaspan JB, Bryer-Asl M, Cao Y, Sander D, Van de Water J, Gershwin ME, Garry RF. Detection of retroviral antibodies in primary biliary cirrhosis and other idiopathic biliary disorders. Lancet 1998; **351**: 1620-1624.

22. Bach N, Schaffner F. Familial primary biliary cirrhosis. *J. Hepatol.* 1994; **20**: 698-701.

23. Brind AM, Bray GP, Portmann BC, Williams R. Prevalence and pattern of familial disease in primary biliary cirrhosis. *Gut* 1995; **36**: 615-617.

24. Metcalf JV, Bhopal RS, Gray J, James OJ. Incidence and prevalence of primary biliary cirrhosis in the city of Newcastle upon Tyne, England. *Int. J. Epidemiol.* 1997; **26**: 830-836.

25. Kaplan MM, Robson AR, Lee YM. Discordant occurrence of primary biliary cirrhosis in monozygote twins. *N. Engl. J. Med.* 1994; **331**: 932.

26. Gores GJ, Moore SB, Fisher LD, Powell FC, Dickson ER. Primary biliary cirrhosis association with class II major histocompatibility complex antigens. *Hepatology* 1987; **7**: 889-92.

27. Aguilar HI, Nuako K, Kro RAF, Wiesner RH. Do primary sclerosing cholangitis (PSC) patients who express HLA-DR4 hapolype have a more rapidly progressive disease? *Hepatology* (abs) 1994; **20**: 154A.

28. Maeda T, Onoshi S, Saibara T, Iwasaki S, Yamamoto J. HLA DR8 and primary biliary cirrhosis. *Gastroenterology* 1992; **103**: 1118-19.

29. Seki T, Kiyosawa K, Ota M, Furata S. Association of primary biliary cirrhosis with human leucocyte antigen DPB1*0501 in Japanese patients. *Hepatology* 1993; **18**: 33-78.

30. Underhill JA, Donaldson PT, Doherty DG, Manake K. HLA DPB polymorphis in primary sclerosing cholangitis and primary biliary cirrhosis. *Hepatology* 1995; **21**: 959-62.

31. Briggs DC, Donaldson PT, Hayes P, Welsh KI, Williams R. A major histocompatibility complex class III allotype C4 B2 associated with primary biliary cirrhosis. *Tissue Antigens* 1987; **29**: 141-5.

32. Manns MP, Bremm A, Schneider PM, Notghi A, Gerken G, Prager-Eerbele M, Bellinghausen B, Meyer zum Buschenfelde KH, Ritner C. HLA DRw8 and complement C4 deficiency as risk factors in primary biliary cirrhosis. *Gastroenterology* 1991; **101**: 1367-73.

33. Messer G, Spengler U, Jung MC, Hoaold G, Eisenburg J, Scholz S, Albert ED, Pape GR, Riethmuller G, Weiss EH. Allelic variation in the TNF beta gene does not explain the low TNF beta response in patients with primary biliary cirrhosis. *Scnd. J. Immunol.* 1991; **34**: 735-740.

34. Gregory WL, Daly AK, Dunn AN, Cavanagh G, Idle JR, James OF, Bassendine MF. *Quarterly Journal of Medicine* 1994; **87**: 237-44.

35. Gregory WL, Mehal W, Dun AN, Cavanagh G, Chapman RW, Fleing KA, Daly AK, Idle JR, James OF, Bassendine MF. *Quarterly Journal of Medicine* 1993; **86**: 393-9.

36. Watt FC, Grove J, Daly AK, Jones DE, Bassendine M, James OJ. Tumour necrosis factor 308 polymorphism and disease progression in primary biliary cirrhosis. *Gastroenterology* 1997; **112**: A1414.

CLINICAL PATTERNS AND NATURAL HISTORY OF PRIMARY BILIARY CIRRHOSIS

Stephen M Riordan, Roger Williams

Institute of Hepatology, University College London
Medical School and Hospitals, London, England.

SUMMARY

- A wide range of clinical patterns of primary biliary cirrhosis (PBC) are recognised, including a classical presentation with jaundice and syndromes in which pruritus, fatigue, portal hypertension and abdominal pain predominate; up to 60% of patients in recent series have no liver-related symptoms at diagnosis.

- The prevalences of abnormal physical signs and advanced histological stage of disease at diagnosis are significantly lower in the asymptomatic group, although stage III or IV PBC is still evident in up to 57%.

- Less than 15% of PBC patients in most series are male; the prevalences of pruritus, hyperpigmentation and associated Sjögren's syndrome are lower in men than in women, but clinical features are otherwise indistinguishable.

- There is an inherited component to PBC, with a familial prevalence of up to 5.4%.

- An overlap syndrome with autoimmune hepatitis occurs in 8% of patients with PBC, in which the clinical features of autoimmune hepatitis predominate.

- Antimitochondrial antibody (AMA)-negative patients account for 5-10% of cases of PBC; high titres of antinuclear and smooth muscle antibodies and reduced levels of IgM are found in this group.

- The natural history of PBC is extraordinarily variable; however, symptomatic PBC is a progressive disorder in the majority of patients.

- Most patients diagnosed while asymptomatic and without biochemical evidence of cholestasis will also have progressive disease, with over 80% developing cholestasis a median 5.6 years after detection of AMA.

- Up to 33% of patients with biochemical evidence of cholestasis but asymptomatic at diagnosis remain asymptomatic after a median 12 years of follow up; survival in this persistently asymptomatic group is significantly longer than in symptomatic patients; the survival rate in those initially asymptomatic patients who develop symptoms during follow-up becomes indistinguishable from that of patients symptomatic at the outset.

- Elderly PBC patients who remain persistently asymptomatic may follow a particularly indolent clinical course.

- There is no difference in overall survival related to gender, although an increased proportion of male deaths is attributable to the development of hepatocellular carcinoma.

- Available data suggests that there is no significant difference in the natural histories of AMA-positive and -negative PBC.

- PBC may first present during pregnancy; in patients with known PBC, the disease worsens, especially during the third trimester, in approximately one third; conversely, resolution of jaundice and other biochemical abnormalities has occasionally been reported.

Introduction

Primary biliary cirrhosis (PBC) was first described nearly 150 years ago as a condition of middle-aged women presenting with jaundice, pruritus and generalised xanthomas and considered to be an uncommon and inexorably progressive disorder[1]. Although the substantial female preponderance remains, with males comprising less than 15% of cases

in most series, the recognised clinical profile of patients with this disorder has otherwise expanded substantially with a growing number of clinical associations. The more widespread availability of biochemical and immunological screening tests has led not only to the recognition of cases at an earlier stage in the disease process but also to an appreciation that the "classical" clinical, biochemical and even immunological features of the disorder need not necessarily be present. This chapter reviews the modes of presentation and natural history of PBC in the variety of these clinical settings, including those with and without symptoms at presentation and subsequently, as well as those with and without positive anti-mitochondrial antibody (AMA) titres. Possible differences in the clinical manifestations and course of the disease in males and females will be considered, along with the features of familial involvement, of PBC in pregnancy and in the elderly and of a syndrome overlapping with autoimmune hepatitis.

Modes of Presentation

Patients with PBC may develop a wide range of symptoms and signs and several patterns of presentation are recognised (Table 1)[2,5]. In addition, as already referred to, an increasing number of patients are identified in the absence of any disease-related symptoms.

Classical Pattern of Disease

The classical presentation of PBC at an advanced stage with the combination of jaundice, steatorrhoea and generalised xanthomas is decidedly less common nowadays, as is well shown in Table 1. In the 1950s, some 80% of patients were noted to be icteric at the time of diagnosis[6] whereas in more recent series jaundice was the presenting complaint in only 3.8 to 12.0% of patients[2,5]. Serum bilirubin levels are generally observed to increase slowly over time in PBC. More abrupt rises may occur in pregnancy, with the use of exogenous oestrogen preparations for contraception or hormone replacement, with choledocholithiasis, in the setting of sepsis or, rarely, due to associated hyperthyroidism or treatment with azathioprine[7-9]. In the absence of these complicating factors, the progression of jaundice is consequent on increasing destruction of interlobular bile ducts, and, thus, is a reflection of advancing disease. In this classical setting of disease, the onset of clinical jaundice usually precedes that of other manifestations of hepatic decompensation, such as ascites, coagulopathy and hepatic encephalopathy[7].

The destruction of interlobular bile ducts also leads to decreased hepatic secretion of conjugated bile salts into the small intestinal lumen. Steatorrhoea with faecal fat excretion up to 68g/day has been reported[10-12]. Kaplan et al.[13] investigated the prevalence of fat-soluble vitamin deficiency in 52 consecutive patients, including 21 (40.4%) with stage I or II disease and 31 (59.6%) with more advanced disease (stage III or IV histology), of whom 11 were clinically jaundiced. Only one patient was receiving a low fat diet for steatorrhoea. Serum vitamin A and 25-hydroxyvitamin D levels were reduced and prothrombin times prolonged in 17/52 (32.6%), 10/52 (19.2%) and 7/52 (13.5%), respectively. The prothrombin time improved with vitamin K supplementation in the majority of patients, indicating that coagulopathy was predominantly due to vitamin K deficiency rather than hepatocellular dysfunction. Vitamin E deficiency was present in only 4/52 (7.7%) patients. Despite the high prevalence of fat-soluble vitamin deficiencies, only one (1.9%) patient had clinical manifestations, namely night blindness. Variables most predictive of fat-soluble vitamin deficiency were an advanced histologic stage, jaundice and hypoalbuminaemia. The potentially exacerbating effect on luminal bile salt deficiency of resins such as cholestyramine, used for treatment of pruritus, must also be borne in mind.

Xanthomas are evident during the life-time course of PBC in 16 to 27% of patients[3,14] but represent the first symptom or sign in less than 1% of patients[3]. Xanthomas may paradoxically regress as the disease reaches end-stage. The presence or absence of xanthomas does not reliably correlate with the height of the raised serum cholesterol level, which in the early

TABLE 1: PREDOMINANT PRESENTING FEATURES IN PRIMARY BILIARY CIRRHOSIS (PBC)				
	Sherlock & Scheuer, 1973[2]	Christensen et al, 1980[3]	Crowe et al, 1985[4]	Nyberg & Loof, 1989[5]
Jaundice	33.0%	12.0%	10.6%	3.8%
Pruritus	57.0%	47.0%	35.3%	26.3%
Fatigue	0.0%	7.6%	4.7%	11.3%
Gastrointestinal bleeding/ascites	4.0%	7.6%	12.9%	0.0%
Abdomininal pain	0.0%	6.8%	4.7%	7.5%
Hepatomegaly	3.0%	0.8%	0.0%	1.3%
No disease-related symptoms or signs	4.0%	16.4%	31.8%	48.8%

stages is due to a marked increase in high density lipoprotein (HDL) cholesterol, a shift from HDL$_2$ to HDL$_3$ and only a modest increase in the low density lipoprotein (LDL) fraction. Conversely, patients with advanced PBC usually have a predominant elevation of LDL, with a reduced HDL component[15,16]. Levels of lipoprotein AI, which is associated with protection against atherosclerosis, are generally increased, except in advanced disease, and may contribute to the lack of an increased incidence of atherosclerosis reported in this disorder[17]. Nonetheless, in our experience, coronary artery disease is not an uncommon finding in older PBC patients with advanced disease coming to liver transplantation assessment.

I. Predominant Pruritus

Among patients with its classical disease pattern, pruritus is the predominant presenting symptom in up to 57% in series reported over the past 25 years[2-5]. Indeed, it is not unusual for the initial referral to come from a dermatology clinic. Diurnal and seasonal variations in the severity of pruritus are common, with exacerbations at night and during winter, possibly due to increasing dryness of the skin. The intensity of pruritus is not correlated with other clinical features or laboratory indices of cholestasis and is not a reflection of the intrinsic severity of the lesion. On the contrary, it often resolves, or at least improves, for periods particularly during the later stages of the disease. Pruritus may first become evident or worsen during the third trimester of pregnancy, failing to resolve post-partum as would be expected with idiopathic cholestasis of pregnancy. The use of exogenous oestrogens can also trigger pruritus in PBC. As a consequence of chronic scratching, hyperpigmentation of the skin, most evident on the trunk and arms and due to an increased deposition of melanin, becomes increasingly marked[18].

II. Predominant Fatigue

Persistent fatigue is the predominant presenting complaint in up to 11.3% of patients[2-5]. As with pruritus, the presence of fatigue bears no significant relation to objective markers of disease severity[19]. Nonetheless, this symptom may be associated with considerable psychological distress, as evidenced by increased prevalences of sleep disturbance and depression[19]. The degree to which fatigue may interfere with normal daily activities has been estimated to be comparable to that reported by patients with disorders such as end-stage renal failure[19,20].

III. Predominant Portal Hypertension

Even though portal hypertension is a common complication of PBC, in less than 15% of patients is the presentation with variceal haemorrhage or ascites[2-5]. These features do not necessarily imply the presence of cirrhosis, as pre-sinusoidal portal hypertension may occur in early stage PBC, possibly due to the presence of nodular regenerative hyperplasia[21,22]. The latter scenario according to a number of reports pertains to 24 to 50% of PBC patients with oesophageal varices[4,23-25]. An increased incidence of portal vein thrombosis has also been reported in PBC compared to other aetiologies of cirrhosis[26] and abnormalities on thrombelastography reflecting an underlying hypercoagulable state have recently been described in almost one third of patients[27].

IV. Predominant Abdominal Pain

Right upper quadrant or epigastric pain may be particularly marked in some patients and is the presenting feature in up to 7.5%[2-5]. The aetiology often remains obscure and this symptom commonly resolves spontaneously. Although gallstones have been reported in approximately 30% of PBC patients[28], these generally remain asymptomatic. Hepatocellular carcinoma (HCC) is a complication of late-stage disease only, the overall incidence including both males and females (see later) being low at 5.9%[29].

"ASYMPTOMATIC" PRESENTATION

Up to 60% of patients in recently reported series have no liver-related symptoms at the time of diagnosis[30], compared to only 4% some 25 years ago[2]. The diagnosis of PBC in this group is usually established after the chance finding of an abnormal physical sign, such as hepatomegaly, or, more often, an elevated serum alkaline phosphatase level during the course of an unrelated illness. Alternatively, patients may be diagnosed after biochemical and immunological screening is carried out either as part of a routine health check or following the documentation of one of the extrahepatic disorders known to be associated with PBC, listed in Table 2 and discussed in detail elsewhere in this volume. The most common of these associated conditions include Sjögren's syndrome, arthropathy (predominantly non-erosive), Raynaud's phenomenon and osteoporosis. Coeliac disease and lichen planus are increasingly recognised, such that patients with "asymptomatic" PBC are referred from a wide range of other clinics. Mahl et al[31] compared clinical features at diagnosis in "asymptomatic" PBC patients and a symptomatic group. Although the prevalence of abnormal physical signs was significantly lower in the latter group, hepatomegaly was still detectable in 50%. Serum bilirubin and cholesterol levels were significantly lower and serum albumin higher in the asymptomatic group (Table 3). The general

TABLE 2: DISORDERS ASSOCIATED WITH PRIMARY BILIARY CIRRHOSIS (PBC)
Common
Sjögren's syndrome
Arthropathy (predominantly non-erosive)
Raynaud's phenomenon
Osteoporosis
Scleroderma
CREST syndrome
Coeliac disease
Lichen planus
Other
Pulmonary fibrosis
Autoimmune thyroid dysfunction
Systemic lupus erythematosis
Glomerulonephritis
Transverse myelitis
Myasthenia gravis
Autoimmune thrombocytopoenia
Acquired IgG deficiency
Periostitis
Carcinoma of the breast
Dermatomyositis
Polymyositis
Pancreatic insufficiency
Collagenous colitis
Anti-phospholipid syndrome
Uterine fibroids
Renal tubular acidosis

experience is that a higher proportion of patients asymptomatic at diagnosis are at an earlier histological stage of disease, although stage III or IV disease is still found at the time of presentation in 34 to 57% of patients with "asymptomatic" PBC[5,31,32] (Table 4).

PBC IN MALES

Whether men with PBC have the same pattern of disease as women has been the subject of several studies. Rubel et al[33] compared clinical and histological

features of PBC in 30 men with 30 age-matched women and found no difference between the two groups. However, the small number of enrolled female patients may not have adequately represented the wide spectrum of clinical manifestations and presentations of this disorder, as discussed above.

Subsequently, Lucey et al[14] compared clinical parameters at the time of diagnosis in 39 men and 191 women presenting to King's College Hospital, London over a 15 year period. The mean age and alkaline phosphatase levels at diagnosis were similar in each group. The distributions of early and advanced disease, as shown by both the serum bilirubin level and histological staging, were also comparable. Comparison of symptoms and signs at diagnosis showed that pruritus was present in significantly fewer men than women (Table 5). Stratification of female patients into pre- and post-menopausal groups demonstrated that differences in prevalence of pruritus between men and women were more marked in the pre-menopausal group, raising the possibility that the higher prevalence of pruritus in the latter group was related to differences in circulating levels of sex hormones. Hyperpigmentation was also recorded significantly less often in males, almost certainly related to the lower prevalence of pruritus and, hence, chronic scratching in this group. There were no gender-related differences in the frequencies of gastrointestinal haemorrhage, ascites, hepatomegaly, splenomegaly or xanthomas. Twenty-three % of men and 12% of women had no liver-related symptoms at the time of diagnosis. Symptoms of associated Sjögren's syndrome were significantly less common in men than in women, compatible with the known association of autoimmunity with female sex.

FAMILIAL PBC

There is some evidence for an inherited component to PBC, based on well documented instances of multiple

TABLE 3: COMPARISON OF PHYSICAL SIGNS AND LABORATORY DATA AT DIAGNOSIS IN SYMPTOMATIC AND ASYMPTOMATIC PATIENTS WITH PBC[31]			
	Symptomatic (n=243)	Asymptomatic (n=36)	P
Physical Signs			
Jaundice	59%	6%	0.001
Hyperpigmentation	42%	13%	0.002
Hepatomegaly	74%	50%	0.003
Splenomegaly	47%	12%	0.0001
Ascites	7%	3%	NS
Oedema	17%	14%	NS
Laboratory Data			
Median bilirubin (range)	48 μmol/L (3.2-493)	8 μmol/L (3.2-50)	0.0001
Median albumin (range)	34 g/L (14-54)	39 g/L (29-47)	0.0001
Median cholesterol (range)	8.8 mmol/L (2.2-54.5)	6.5 mmol/L (4.0-11.8)	0.0001

		At Diagnosis		P
		Asymptomatic (%)	Symptomatic (%)	
USA[31]	Stage I/II	42	21	<0.0005
	Stage III/IV	57	79	<0.0005
England[32]	Stage I/II	51	18	<0.0005
	Stage III/IV	49	82	<0.0005
Sweden[5]	Stage I/II	66	21	<0.0005
	Stage III/IV	34	79	<0.0005

cases of PBC occurring within single families, even though reported associations with standard genetic markers such as major histocompatibility alleles are weak[34]. Three studies have systematically investigated prevalence in family members of affected patients. Bach et al[35] found the prevalence of familial cases to be 5.5% (22/405) in a New York series, while Myszor et al[32] reported a familial prevalence of 2.4% (8/347) in a series from North-east England. Brind et al[36] recently determined the prevalence and pattern of familial PBC in a large series of 736 patients from a single United Kingdom centre over a 25 year period. PBC was found in eight mother and daughter pairs, yielding a familial prevalence of 1.1%. All mothers and two (25%)

daughters were cirrhotic at presentation. Of the eight affected daughters, three were asymptomatic at diagnosis, which followed the detection of abnormal liver function tests, whereas all the mothers were symptomatic at presentation. The daughters had each been diagnosed at an earlier age (median: 36 years; range: 24-54) than their mothers (median: 52 years: range: 50-81). Indeed, in all but three the diagnosis of PBC had been made in the daughter before the mother. It is likely that increased awareness of the disease and the more widespread availability of screening nowadays contributed to the greater proportion of daughters than their mothers being diagnosed while asymptomatic, at a younger age and with earlier stage disease.

	Men (n=39)	Women (n=191)
Liver-related Symptoms (%)		
Pruritus	**45**	68[1]
Jaundice	44	53
Gastrointestinal haemorrhage	23	15
None	23	12
Physical Signs (%)		
Hyperpigmentation	**35**	55[2]
Hepatomegaly	89	95
Splenomegaly	51	56
Ascites	14	10
Xanthoma	8	18
Associated Disorders (%)		
Sjögren's syndrome	**15**	33[2]
Scleroderma	8	13
Raynaud's phenomenon	3	13
Fibrosing alveolitis	3	2
Thyroid dysfunction	5	8
Rheumatoid arthritis	0	3
Laboratory Data		
Median bilirubin (range) (µmol/L)	44 (3-192)	33 (4-390)
Median alkaline phosphatase (range) (IU/L)	645 (102-1900)	640 (51-2100)
Histological stage (%)		
I or II	41	42
III or IV	59	58

[1] P<0.01; [2] P<0.5

OVERLAP SYNDROME WITH AUTOIMMUNE HEPATITIS

Nearly 30% of previously reported instances of a positive AMA titre in patients with otherwise classical autoimmune hepatitis were subsequently shown to be false positives, the immunofluorescence pattern being confused with that of the liver-kidney microsomal type I antibody[37]. However, 8% of adult patients with autoimmune hepatitis do appear to have a true overlap syndrome with PBC. In these cases, histological features of autoimmune hepatitis are combined with the bile duct damage, ductular proliferation and granuloma formation in the portal tract characteristic of PBC. Analysis of liver enzyme profiles in serum shows cholestatic liver enzyme abnormalities in addition to the elevated serum transaminases typical of autoimmune hepatitis. Patients may be of either sex of any age, although more commonly they are women aged 40 years or younger. The clinical features are predominantly those of autoimmune hepatitis and typical symptoms of PBC such as pruritus are usually absent[38]. In contradistinction to a true overlap syndrome in which features of both disorders are present simultaneously, AMA-positive PBC has very rarely been reported to evolve into autoimmune hepatitis, with loss of serum AMA and development of ANA, high serum transaminases and prominent interface hepatitis on liver biopsy[39].

A first case of AMA-positive autoimmune hepatitis in a child has recently been reported[40]. However, the clinical picture was that of autoimmune hepatitis alone, with no clinical, biochemical or histological features to suggest a biliary component. There remain no reports of a true autoimmune hepatitis/PBC overlap syndrome in the paediatric setting.

AMA-NEGATIVE PBC

It has long been recognised that 5 to 10% of patients with clinical, histological and biochemical features typical of PBC are AMA-negative when tested by standard indirect immunofluorescence[41,42]. Approximately 80% of these cases remain AMA-negative when serum is re-tested using more sensitive immunoblotting techniques[43]. Such AMA-negative patients, who otherwise meet diagnostic criteria for PBC, have a high prevalence of other serium autoantibodies, notably anti-nuclear (ANA) and anti-smooth muscle (SMA) antibodies. This has led to the use of terms such as immune cholangitis[44], autoimmune cholangiopathy[45] and autoimmune cholangitis[43]. Such terminology has in turn led to some confusion with primary sclerosing cholangitis, in which a comparable pattern of serum

autoantibody abnormalities can be found but which has distinct histological and cholangiographic manifestations, and for this reason a recent editorial[46] reinforces use of the term AMA-negative PBC, rather than those including cholangiopathy or cholangitis.

Several studies have been performed to compare clinical, biochemical, serological and histological characteristics of AMA-negative and -positive cases[30,43,47]. A North American study of 17 AMA-negative patients and an equal number of AMA-positive patients matched for serum bilirubin concentration found that serum IgM concentrations were significantly lower in AMA-negative patients. Each of this latter group had serum positive for ANA, usually in high titre (>1:160), whereas only 3/17 (17.6%) AMA-positive patients were ANA positive. Similarly, more of the AMA-negative group were positive for SMA than were AMA-positive patients (7/17, 41.2% vs 1/17, 5.9%). Aside from these serological parameters, the AMA-positive and -negative patients were indistinguishable, with comparable symptoms, liver histology and prevalence of other autoimmune disorders[43]. Similar findings have been reported from the Mayo Clinic[47].

Ivernizzi et al[30] have recently reported an historical cohort study from an Italian centre in which presenting clinical, biochemical, serological and histological features of 273 AMA-positive and 24 AMA-negative patients were compared. As with the American experiences, no significant differences were noted with respect to sex, age or prevalences of symptomatic disease, advanced histological stage or complications of cirrhosis, while the reduced serum IgM levels and increased prevalences of positive ANA and SMA titres in the AMA-negative group were confirmed (Table 6).

Other pathological studies have yielded no convincing evidence that the lack of AMA positivity in serum should be taken to reflect a disorder distinct from AMA-positive PBC. Kaserer et al[48] found no immuno-histochemical differences in the inflammatory infiltrate associated with bile duct damage in AMA-positive and -negative patients. Similarly, Tsuneyama et al[49] reported abnormal expression of the E2 component of the pyruvate dehydrogenase complex on the apical surface of biliary epithelial cells in both AMA-positive and -negative patients, suggesting a common pathogenetic mechanism in the two groups. Although, Gordon et al[50] have demonstrated antibodies against carbonic anhydrase, an enzyme found in biliary epithelial cells, in AMA-negative but not -positive patients, others have to date been unable to confirm these findings[46].

	AMA-Positive (n=273)	AMA-Negative (n=24)

TABLE 6: PATIENT CHARACTERISTICS AND BIOCHEMICAL, SEROLOGICAL AND HISTOLOGICAL FEATURES AT PRESENTATION ACCORDING TO AMA POSITIVITY OR NEGATIVITY[30]

	AMA-Positive (n=273)	AMA-Negative (n=24)
Women (%)	244 (89)	21 (88)
Age (years)	54 ± 11	52 ± 11
Asymptomatic (%)	166 (61)	17 (71)
Histological stage III or IV (%)	111 (41)	7 (29)
Complications of cirrhosis (%)	22 (8)	3 (13)
Bilirubin (mg/dL)	2.2 ± 3.5	2.2 ± 2.9
Cholesterol (mg/dL)	260 ± 114	267 ± 75
IgM (mg/dL)	**591 ± 553**	**409 ± 242**[1]
Positive ANA (%)	**84 (31)**	**17 (71)**[2]
Positive SMA (%)	**26 (9)**	**9 (37)**[2]

± values are means ± SD; [1] P=0.0002; [2] P=0.05

NATURAL HISTORY, INCLUDING SYMPTOMATIC AND ASYMPTOMATIC VARIANTS

The natural history of PBC in individual patients is extraordinarily variable. Nonetheless, the multicentre, prospective study of 236 patients reported by Christensen et al[3] demonstrated that symptomatic PBC is a progressive disorder in the majority of cases. Patients who had been symptomatic for a median of 2.1 years at study entry, including 14% with histological stage I disease, 40% with stage II, 19% with stage III and 27% with stage IV, were followed for a median 18 months. Using life-table analysis, the proportion of patients with pruritis rose from 75% at presentation to an estimated 95% at five years, with corresponding figures for jaundice of 9% and 82%. The proportion of patients with cirrhosis rose from 27% to 82% in four years, in keeping with experience from the Mayo Clinic, in which only 20% of pre-cirrhotic PBC patients showed no histological progression over this time[51].

Other studies have addressed the natural history in asymptomatic patients, including those without biochemical evidence of cholestasis at the outset. Metcalf et al[52] have investigated such a group and, as in symptomatic patients, found a progressive course in the majority. A cohort of 29 patients without symptoms or cholestasis were found by indirect immunofluorescence to have an AMA titre of at last 1:40 and followed for a median

period of nearly 18 years. Liver histology at the outset had been compatible with PBC in 24/29 (82.8%) and completely normal in only 2/29 (6.9%). During follow-up, biochemical evidence of cholestasis ensued in 24/29 (82.8%) patients. The median time from the first positive AMA test to the development of cholestasis was 5.6 years.

In patients with cholestasis, several authors over the past 20 years have investigated the proportion of initially asymptomatic patients who will subsequently become symptomatic (Table 7). In the United Kingdom, Long et al[53] found that 50% of such patients developed symptoms of liver disease during a mean follow-up period of 4.5 years, while 36% of those enrolled in another dual-centre study became symptomatic during a median follow-up period of 5.8 years[54]. Similarly high rates of progression to symptomatic disease have been reported from Sweden[5], the Mayo Clinic[55] and Yale[31] over longer mean/median follow-up periods ranging from 7.6 to 12.1 years.

The survival rate of initially asymptomatic patients in comparison to their symptomatic counterparts has also been addressed. A cohort of 243 initially symptomatic and 36 asymptomatic PBC patients from Yale, most of each group with alkaline phosphatase levels at least twice normal, was followed for a median time from diagnosis of 6.4 years (range: 0.04-24.2 years) and 12.1 years (range 1.1-19.2 years), respectively[31]. Despite similar

TABLE 7: THE PROPORTION OF ASYMPTOMATIC PBC PATIENTS WITH BIOCHEMICAL EVIDENCE OF CHOLESTASIS WHO DEVELOP DISEASE-RELATED SYMPTOMS

Authors	Location	n	% Developing Symptoms	Mean/Median Follow-up (yr)
Long et al, 1977[53]	Royal Free, England	20	50	4.5
Mitchison et al, 1980[54]	Newcastle/King's College, England	95	36	5.8
Nyberg & Loof, 1989[5]	Sweden	56	37	9.5
Balasubramaniam et al, 1990[55]	Mayo Clinic, USA	37	89	7.6
Mahl et al, 1994[31]	Yale, USA	36	66	12.1

ages at diagnosis, survival in the asymptomatic group (median 16 years) was significantly longer than in symptomatic patients (median 7.5 years). However, the survival of patients asymptomatic at diagnosis is not normal, falling significantly below that of gender- and age-matched control groups after 6-12 years of follow up in various series (Figure 1)[5,31,55]. As already discussed, a substantial proportion of patients asymptomatic at diagnosis ultimately become symptomatic and once this occurs, their survival rate becomes indistinguishable from that of patients who had been symptomatic from the outset[31,54] (Figure 2). Nonetheless, up to 33% of patients asymptomatic at diagnosis may remain so during a median follow up period of over 12 years and survival in this group is significantly higher than that in patients who develop symptoms[31]. Unfortunately, no factors have yet been identified which can be used to predict which asymptomatic patients will remain symptom free and who will not and, therefore, to identify those who may benefit from early treatment.

The possible influence of gender on the natural history of PBC has also been addressed in several studies. Christensen et al[3] reported no significant gender-related differences in the course of PBC in 25 men and 236 women, predominantly symptomatic at enrollment and followed for a median 18 months. Lucey et al[14] similarly found no significant difference in survival in 39 men and 191 women, the majority with stage III or IV disease at the outset and with similar proportions of symptomatic to asymptomatic patients in each group, who were followed for a median 37 and 42 months, respectively. However, an increased prevalence of complicating HCC was noted in men (10.3% vs 1.6%), all in patients with established cirrhosis. It is presumably because HCC only develops during the end-stage of the clinical course that overall survival is not significantly reduced in men. Jones et al[29] similarly found an increased

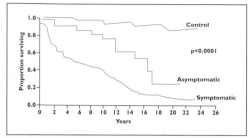

Figure 2.

Kaplan-Meier life table analysis of 36 initially asymptomatic and 243 symptomatic patients with PBC. Sixty-seven percent of the initially asymptomatic group became symptomatic during follow-up. Survival is significantly longer in the initially asymptomatic group (p<0.0001), although not comparable to an age- and gender-matched control group after 11 years of follow up (modified from reference 31).

prevalence of HCC complicating advance PBC in men than in women (20% vs 4%), with a significantly increased proportion of male than female deaths attributable to this cause (46% vs 8%).

Available data, obtained in AMA-positive and -negative patients predominantly asymptomatic but cholestatic at diagnosis and followed up for a mean 75 and 53 months, respectively, suggests that there is no significant difference in the clinical course, including survival, of these two groups[30]. However, more prolonged follow up is required to confirm these observations. The natural history of the AMA-positive PBC/autoimmune hepatitis overlap syndrome also remains to be clarified.

The influence of pregnancy on the natural history of PBC is variable. Jaundice and pruritis worsen, especially in the third trimester, in approximately one third of cases[56]. Rabinovitz et al[57] have reported a previously asymptomatic patient in whom PBC was diagnosed during the third trimester of pregnancy following the onset of jaundice who continued to deteriorate post-partum. Conversely, jaundice may improve[58] or liver biochemistry even revert entirely to normal during pregnancy[56].

Each of three survival models reported from Yale[59], the Mayo Clinic[60] and Europe[61] have identified advancing age as one of several independent adverse prognostic indicators in PBC, even when deaths from liver disease alone are considered. Nonetheless, there is increasing evidence that elderly PBC patients, whether male or female, who remain persistently asymptomatic may follow a particularly indolent clinical course[62].

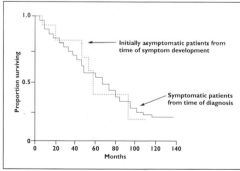

Figure 1.

Cumulative proportional survival of symptomatic patients from the time of diagnosis (____) and asymptomatic patients from the time of subsequent symptom appearance (____). No significant difference in survival is evident[54].

REFERENCES

1. Addison T, Gull W. On a certain affection of the skin, vitiligoidea-α plana, β tuberosa. Guy's Hosp Rep 1851; **7**: 265-276.

2. Sherlock S, Scheuer PJ. The presentation and diagnosis of 100 patients with primary biliary cirrhosis. N Engl J Med 1973; **289**: 674-678.

3. Christensen E, Crowe, Doniach D, *et al.* Clinical pattern and course of disease in primary biliary cirrhosis based on an analysis of 236 patients. *Gastroenterology* 1980; **78**: 236-246.

4. Crowe J, Christensen E, Doniach D, Popper H, Tygstrup N, Williams R. Early features of primary biliary cirrhosis: an analysis of 85 patients. *Am J Gastroenterol* 1985; **80**: 466-468.

5. Nyberg A, Loof L. Primary biliary cirrhosis: clinical features and outcome with special reference to asymptomatic disease. *Scand J Gastroenterol* 1989; **24**: 57-64.

6. Ahrens EH, Rayne MA, Kunkel HG, *et al.* Primary biliary cirrhosis. *Medicine* 1950; **29**: 299-364.

7. Heathcote J. The clinical expression of primary biliary cirrhosis. *Sem Liver Dis* 1996; **17**: 23-33.

8. Thompson NP, Leader S, Jamieson CP, Burnham WR, Burroughs AK. Reversible jaundice in primary biliary cirrhosis due to hyperthyroidism. *Gastroenterology* 1994; **106**: 1342-1343.

9. Yela C, Manzano L, Castellano G, Garfia C, Solis JA. Primary biliary cirrhosis treated with azathioprine and liver transplantation. *J Hepatol* 1997; **27**: 599.

10. Herlong HF, Recker RR, Maddrey WC. Bone disease in primary biliary cirrhosis: histologic features and response to 25-hydroxyvitamin D. *Gastroenterology* 1982; **83**: 103-108.

11. Matloff DS, Kaplan MM, Neer RM, Goldberg MJ, Bitman W, Wolfe HJ. Osteoporosis in primary biliary cirrhosis: effects of 25-hydroxyvitamin D₃ treatment. *Gastroenterology* 1982; **83**: 97-102.

12. Hodgson SF, Dickson ER, Wahner HW, Johnson KA, Mann KG, Riggs BL. Bone loss and reduced osteoblast function in primary biliary cirrhosis. *Ann Intern Med* 1985; **103**: 855-860.

13. Kaplan MM, Elta GH, Furie B, Sadowski JA, Russell RM. Fat-soluble vitamin nutriture in primary biliary cirrhosis. *Gastroenterology* 1988; **95**: 787-792.

14. Lucey MR, Neuberger JM, Williams R. Primary biliary cirrhosis in men. *Gut* 1986; **27**: 1373-1376.

15. Aly A, Carlson K, Johansson C, Kirstein P, Rossner S, Wallentin L. Lipoprotein abnormalities in patients with early primary biliary cirrhosis. *Eur J Clin Invest* 1984; **14**: 155-162.

16. Jahn CE, Schaefer EJ, Taam LA, *et al.* Lipoprotein abnormalities in primary biliary cirrhosis. *Gastroenterology* 1985; **89**: 1266-1278.

17. O'Kane MJ, Lynch PL, Callender ME, Trimble ER. Abnormalities of serum apo A1 containing lipoprotein particles in patients with primary biliary cirrhosis. *Atherosclerosis* 1997; **131**: 203-210.

18. Reynolds TB. The butterfly sign in patients with chronic jaundice and pruritus. *Ann Intern Med* 1973; **78**: 545-546.

19. Cauch-Dudek K, Abbey S, Stewart DE, Heathcote EJ. Fatigue and quality of life in primary biliary cirrhosis. *Hepatology* 1995; **22**: 108A.

20. Huet PM, Deslauriers J. Impact of fatigue on quality of life in patients with primary biliary cirrhosis. *Gastroenterology* 1996; **110**: A1215.

21. Nakanuma Y, Ohta G. Nodular hyperplasia of the liver in primary biliary cirrhosis of early histological stages. *Am J Gastroenterol* 1987; **82**: 8-10.

22. Scheuer PJ. Pathologic features and evolution of primary biliary cirrhosis and primary sclerosing cholangitis. *Mayo Clin Proc* 1988; **73**: 179-183.

23. Zeegan R, Standfield Ag, Dawson AM, *et al.* Bleeding oesophageal varices as the presenting feature in primary biliary cirrhosis. *Lancet* 1969; **2**: 9-13.

24. Kew MC, Varma RR, Don Santos HA, *et al.* Portal hypertension in primary biliary cirrhosis. *Gut* 1971; **12**: 830-834.

25. Navasa M, Pares A, Bruguera M, Caballeria J, Bosch J, Rodes J. Portal hypertension in primary biliary cirrhosis. *J Hepatol* 1987; **5**: 292-298.

26. Shannon P, Wanless IR. The site of vascular obstruction in early stage primary biliary cirrhosis with portal vein (PV) thrombosis. *Hepatology* 1995; **22**: 253A.

27. Ben-Ari Z, Panogou M, Patch D, *et al.* Hypercoagulability in patients with primary biliary cirrhosis and primary sclerosing cholangitis evaluated by thrombelastrography. *J Hepatol* 1997; **26**: 554-559.

28. Summerfield JA, Ellias E, Hungerford GD, Nikapota VL, Dick R, Sherlock S. The biliary system in primary biliary cirrhosis: a study by endoscopic retrograde cholangiopancreatography. *Gastroenterology* 1976; **70**: 240-243.

29. Jones De, Metcalf JV, Collier JD, Bassendine MF, James OF. Hepatocellular carcinoma in primary biliary cirrhosis and its impact on outcomes. *Hepatology* 1997; **26**: 1138-1142.

30. Ivernizzi P, Crosignani A, Battezzatti PM, *et al.* Comparison of the clinical features and clinical course of antimitochondrial antibody-positive and -negative primary biliary cirrhosis. *Hepatology* 1997; **25**: 1090-1095.

31. Mahl TC, Schockcor W, Boyer JL. Primary biliary cirrhosis: survival of a large cohort of symptomatic and asymptomatic patients followed for 24 years. *J Hepatol* 1994; **20**: 707-713.

32. Myszor M, James OFW. The epidemiology of primary biliary cirrhosis in north-east England: an increasingly common disease? *Quart J Med* 1990; **276**: 377-385.

33. Rubel LR, Rabin L, Seeff LF, Licht H, Cuccherini BA. Does primary biliary cirrhosis in men differ from primary biliary cirrhosis in women? *Hepatology* 1984; **4**: 671-677.

34. Mehal WZ, Gregory WL, Lo D, *et al.* Defining the immunogenetic susceptibility to primary biliary cirrhosis. *Hepatology* 1994; **20**: 1213-1219.

35. Bach N, Schaffner F. Prevalence of primary biliary cirrhosis in family members of affected patients. *Gastroenterology* 1991; **102**: A776.

36. Bring AM, Bray GP, Portman BC, Williams R. Prevalence and pattern of familial disease in primary biliary cirrhosis. *Gut* 1995; **36**: 615-617.

37. Czaja AJ, Manns MP, Homburger HA. Frequency and significance of antibodies to liver/kidney microsome type 1 in adults with chronic active hepatitis. *Gastroenterology* 1992; **103**: 1290-1295.

38. Czaja AJ. The variant forms of autoimmune hepatitis. *Ann Intern Med* 1996; **125**: 588-598.

39. Colombato LA, Alvarez F, Cote J, Huet PM. Autoimmune cholangiopathy: the result of consecutive primary biliary cirrhosis and autoimmune hepatitis? *Gastroenterology* 1994; **107**: 1839-1843.

40. Gregorio GV, Portmann B, Mowat AP, Vergani D, Mieli-Vergani G. A 12-year-old girl with antimitochondrial antibody-positive autoimmune hepatitis. *J Hepatol* 1997; **27**: 751-754.

41. Kaplan MM. Primary biliary cirrhosis. *N Engl J Med* 1987; **316**: 521-528.

42. Gershwin ME, Mackay IR. Primary biliary cirrhosis: paradigm or paradox for autoimmunity. *Gastroenterology* 1991; **100**: 822-833.

43. Michieletti P, Wanless IR, Katz A, *et al.* Antimitochrondrial antibody-negative primary biliary cirrhosis: a distinct syndrome of autoimmune cholangitis. *Gut* 1994; **35**: 260-265.

44. Brunner G, Glinge O. A cholangitis with antinuclear antibodies (immunocholangitis) resembling chronic destructive non-suppurative cholangitis. *Dtsch Med Wochenschr* 1987; **112**: 1454-1458.

45. Ben-Ari Z, Dhillon AP, Sherlock S. Autoimmune cholangiopathy: part of the spectrum of autoimmune chronic active hepatitis. *Hepatology* 1993; **18**: 10-15.

46. Heathcote J. Autoimmune cholangitis. *Gut* 1997; **40**: 440-442.

47. Lacerda MA, Ludwig J, Dickson ER, *et al.* Antimitochondrial antibody-negative primary biliary cirrhosis. *Am J Gastroenterol* 1995; **90**: 247-249.

48. Kaserer K, Exner M, Mosberger I, Penner E, Wrba F. Characterization of the inflammatory infiltrate in autoimmune cholangitis. *Virchows Arch* 1998; **432**: 217-222.

49. Tsuneyama K, Van de Water J, Van Thiel D, *et al.* Abnormal expression of PDC-E1 on the apical surface of biliary epithelial cells in patients with antimitochondrial antibody-negative primary biliary cirrhosis. *Hepatology* 1995; **22**: 1140-1146.

50. Gordon SC, Quattrociocchi-Longe TM, Khan BA, *et al.* Antibodies to carbonic anhydrase in patients with immune cholangitis. *Gastroenterology* 1995; **108**: 1802-1809.

51. Locke GR, Therneau TM, Ludwig J, Dickson ER, Lindor KD. Time course of histological progression in primary biliary cirrhosis. *Hepatology* 1996; **23**: 52-56.

52. Metcalf JV, Mitchison HC, Palmer JM, Jones DE, Bassendine MF, James OFW. Natural history of early primary biliary cirrhosis. *Lancet* 1996; **348**: 1399-1402.

53. Long RG, Scheuer PJ, Sherlock S. Presentation and course of asymptomatic primary biliary cirrhosis. *Gastroenterology* 1977; **72**: 1204-1207.

54. Mitchison HC, Lucey MR, Kelly PJ, Neuberger JM, Williams R, James OFW. Symptom development and prognosis in primary biliary cirrhosis: a study in two centres. Gastroenterology 1990; **99**: 778-784.

55. Balasubramaniam K, Grambsch PM, Wiesner RH, Lindor KD, Dickson ER. Diminished survival in primary biliary cirrhosis. *Gastroenterology* 1990; **98**: 1567-1571.

56. Poupon R, Poupon RE. Primary biliary cirrhosis. In Zakim D, Boyer TD (Eds). Hepatology. A Textbook of Liver Disease, Third edition. Philadelphia, WB Saunders, 1996: 1329-1365.

57. Rabinovitz M, Appasamy R, Finkelstein S. Primary biliary cirrhosis diagnosed during pregnancy. *Dig Dis Sci* 1995; **40**: 571-574.

58. Nir A, Sorokin Y, Abramovici H, Theodor E. Pregnancy and primary biliary cirrhosis. *Int J Gynecol Obstet* 1989; **28**: 279-282.

59. Roll J, Boyer JL, Barry D, Klatskin G. The prognostic importance of clinical and histologic features in asymptomatic and symptomatic primary biliary cirrhosis. *N Engl J Med* 1983; **308**: 1-7.

60. Dickson ER, Grambsch PM, Fleming TR, *et al.* Prognosis in primary biliary cirrhosis: model for decision making. *Hepatology* 1989; **10**: 1-7.

61. Christensen E, Neuberger J, Crowe J, *et al.* Beneficial effect of azathioprine and prediction of prognosis in primary biliary cirrhosis: final result of an international trial. *Gastroenterology* 1985; **89**: 1084-1091.

62. James OFW. Parenchymal liver disease in the elderly. *Gut* 1997; **41**: 430-432.

PRURITUS AND LETHARGY IN THE PRIMARY BILIARY CIRRHOSIS PATIENT

Mark G Swain

Liver Unit, Gastroenterology Research Group
University of Calgary, Calgary, Canada.

SUMMARY

Two symptoms commonly associated with PBC are pruritus and lethargy.

Pruritus occurs in up to 65% of patients with PBC and is often severe. The cause of itching is uncertain. Whilst itching in PBC used to be attributed to elevated levels of bile acids, evidence for this hypothesis is less than convincing. More recently attention has focused on the importance of endogenous opioids which may act either centrally or peripherally. Treatment is symptomatic and Cholestyramine or Colestipol remain the first line treatment. Second line therapies include Rifampicin and opioid receptor antagonists. Anti-histamines and UDCA have a variable effect. Transplantation is effective but rarely required.

Lethargy occurs in up to 90% of patients and is a cause of significant morbidity. The fatigue is central is origin and is associated with mood and behaviour disorders. The pathogenesis remains unknown but some evidence suggests there may be a central defect in CRH release. Treatment is, at present, symptomatic.

PRURITUS IN PRIMARY BILIARY CIRRHOSIS

Clinical Presentation

Pruritus is a common complaint in patients with primary biliary cirrhosis (PBC), occurring in approximately 65% of patients and representing the second most common complaint in PBC patients behind fatigue[1]. Pruritus can be divided into two components, itch and scratching. Itch is an "unpleasant sensation provoking the desire to scratch", and may or may not be followed by the act of scratching[2]. Itch is considered an appropriate response if scratching results in the removal of deleterious agent from the skin. However, in PBC pruritus is not relieved by scratching[3,4]. The pruritus can be localized or generalized and often appears initially on the soles of the feet or palms of the hands. Typically pruritus in PBC patients is worse at night and during winter months. Pruritus in PBC patients does not correlate with disease stage. Moreover, the pruritus is often exacerbated during pregnancy, premenstrually and during hormonal replacement therapy. The persistence of pruritus in a postpartum woman may be the first indication of the diagnosis of PBC in some patients. After pruritus occurs in a PBC patient it is uncommon for it to disappear, although interestingly in some patients with end stage PBC pruritus has been reported to fade away despite the persistence of severe cholestasis. Since pruritus is a subjective sensation it is difficult to study and this has hampered progress in understanding and treating this condition in PBC patients. In its most severe form pruritus in PBC

patients is unresponsive to all medical interventions and can only be relieved by liver transplantation.

PRURITUS IN PBC: CLINICAL

- occurs in up to 65% of patients
- generalized or localized
- unrelieved by scratching
- not related to stage of disease
- may be indication for liver transplantation

Pathogenesis

The pathogenesis of pruritus in PBC patients remains unknown. Because itch is by definition subjective in nature, it must relate to nervous activity. Activation of cutaneous afferent nerves can induce a number of sensations, including itch. Traditionally pruritus in cholestasis has been proposed as being due to an interaction of cutaneous nerve endings with substances retained in plasma as part of the cholestatic syndrome. Classically pruritogens act in the superficial part of the skin and activate thin afferent nerves which project to the subepidermal region of the skin. The afferent nerves most strongly implicated in the transmission of itch are unmyelinated C-fibres (Figure 1)[2]. Once activated the C-fibres transmit their impulses through the dorsal roots to the dorsal horn of the spinal cord. After synaptic activation of spinal second order neurons impulses are transmitted to the anterolateral spinothalamic tract and subsequently to the thalamus

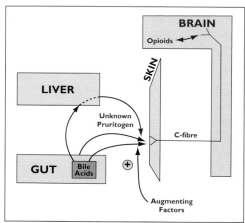

Figure 1.

Pathogenesis of Pruritus of Cholestasis: Peripheral theories for the genesis of the pruritus of cholestasis include retained bile acids acting directly on cutaneous C-fibres, or an unknown pruritogen either released from the gut or released from the liver as a result of a bile acid effect, acting to stimulate cutaneous C-fibres. Augmenting factors may be present in plasma which may enhance the pruritogenic effects of bile acids or an unknown pruritogen at the level of the skin. These augmenting factors may include histamine and/or endogenous opioids. C-fibres transmit nerve impulses from the skin to the spinal cord and ultimately to the cerebral cortex where itch is perceived. Endogenous pioids released within the brain may modulate the perception of itch or may induce itch *de novo*.

and then to the cerebral cortex (Figure 1). Therefore, the central nervous system plays an important role in the *perception* of itch. However, itch can also be generated *de novo* within the central nervous system as indicated by the generation of itch in patients with cerebral tumours and multiple sclerosis. Furthermore, the opiate morphine can induce itch via central opioid receptors after its injection epidurally or intrathecally, indicating that itch can also be induced centrally pharmacologically[5].

Possible Peripheral Causes of Pruritus

i) **Bile Acids**: Bile acids retained as part of the cholestatic syndrome have received the greatest attention as potential pruritogens. This theory was based on an early finding which correlated skin surface bile acid levels and pruritus in cholestatic patients. Furthermore, bile acids cause pruritus when administered to normal volunteers[6]. In addition the bile salt binding resin cholestyramine is effective in controlling pruritus in the majority of cholestatic patients with pruritus. However, more recent studies could not correlate skin bile acid levels with pruritus in cholestatic patients[7]. Moreover, elevated plasma bile acid levels are observed in many cholestatic patients who do not itch. A modification of the bile acid theory suggests that retained bile acids induce the release of an unknown pruritogenic substance from the liver (Figure 1)[8].

BILE ACIDS
For
• elevated plasma and tissue levels of bile acids in cholestatic patients
• bile acid sequestrants relieve cholestatic itch
• bile acids are pruritogenic
Against
• plasma and tissue levels of bile acids correlate poorly with itch
• bile acid sequestrants relieve itch in diseases not associated with elevated bile acid levels

ii) **Histamine**: Histamine was first recognised as pruritogen in the 1920's. Recently, plasma histamine levels have been shown to be elevated in cholestatic patients[9]. Furthermore, antihistamines are widely used to treat pruritus in cholestatic patients, although their effectiveness is unimpressive and their perceived clinical effects have been attributed by some to their sedative properties. Histamine, when injected intradermally, induces a wheal and flare response in association with the development of itch and these are prevented by antihistamines. Pruritic cholestatic patients do not demonstrate evidence of a cutaneous wheal and flare response in conjunction with their itch.

HISTAMINE
For
• elevated plasma histamine levels in cholestasis
• antihistamines widely used to treat cholestatic itch
Against
• antihistamines have poor clinical efficacy
• lack of cutaneous wheal and flare response in cholestatic patients who itch

iii) **Endogenous Opioids**: Itching is commonly observed after the peripheral administration of the opiate morphine[5]. This effect has been attributed to morphine-induced release of histamine from mast cells. However, very low doses of morphine and the opioid met-enkephalin, which do not induce histamine release or itch when injected alone, markedly enhance histamine-induced itch[10]. Therefore, endogenous opioids may potentiate peripherally generated itch. This has direct implications for patients with PBC as met-enkephalin accumulates in plasma in PBC patients[11] and opioid receptor blockade relieves itch in some PBC patients[12]. However, plasma levels of met-enkephalin do not appear to correlate with the presence of itch in PBC.

ENDOGENOUS OPIOIDS (PERIPHERAL)

For

- endogenous opioids accumulate in plasma in cholestasis
- opioids potentiate itch produced by other pruritogens
- itch in some PBC patients blocked by opioid receptor blockade

Against

- pruritus does not correlate well with plasma met-enkephalin levels

Possible Central Causes of Pruritus

Opiates also induce pruritus when injected centrally, suggesting that endogenous opioids released within the brain may also induce itch. Opiate induced central itch is often first perceived on the face and is relieved by the opioid receptor blocker naloxone. These observations suggested that the spinal cord or spinal roots are sites of itch genesis.

The central release of endogenous opioids has been implicated in the genesis of pruritus in PBC patients. Specifically, administration of opioid receptor blockers to pruritic PBC patients resulted in the development of an opiate withdrawal-like syndrome in addition to a relief of itching[12-14], highly suggestive of enhanced central opioidergic tone in these patients. Furthermore, rats with experimental cholestasis exhibit naloxone-reversible analgesia coupled with a down-regulation of central opioid receptors[15, 16]. These findings further support the possibility of enhanced central opioidergic tone in cholestasis. Unfortunately, opioid receptor blockade does not relieve itching in all pruritic cholestatic patients. Moreover, opioid receptor antagonists have been reported to relieve itch in patients with urticaria and atopic dermatitis, suggesting a modulatory role of endogenous opioids in a number of pruritic conditions[17].

ENDOGENOUS OPIOIDS (CENTRAL)

For

- opiate withdrawal-like syndrome in pruritic PBC patients given opioid receptor antagonists
- evidence for enhanced central opioidergic tone in cholestatic rats

Against

- opioid receptor antagonists don't relieve pruritus in all cholestatic patients
- opioid receptor blockade relieves itch in some non-cholestatic pruritic conditions

Treatment

Given a lack of a unifying theory to explain the genesis of cholestasis associated pruritus treatment of this condition is therefore empiric in nature. Traditionally treatment has been divided into first-line, second-line, and "last ditch" approaches.

i) First Line Therapies

a) **Bile Acid Sequestrants**: The most widely used anti-pruritic agent in PBC patients is the anion exchange resin cholestyramine, and more recently colestipol. This agent was first utilized because of its bile acid sequestering properties, but it is also choleretic. The mechanism underlying its antipruritic action in PBC is unknown. Cholestyramine can be given in 4gm doses up to a total dose of 16gm/day. Improved efficacy is achieved if the first doses are given before and after breakfast. Amelioration of pruritus occurs in up to 90% of patients, although patients often find it unpleasant to ingest and it is constipating.

b) **Antihistamines**: Antihistamines are also widely used to treat pruritic PBC patients, their use likely deriving from the extensive utilization of antihistamines to treat itch associated with allergic skin diseases. Hydroxyzine can be used in doses of 25-50mg every 6-8 hours; however, a single nocturnal dose is most useful in those whose itch is significantly worse at bedtime. The presumed benefit of antihistamines in treating cholestatic pruritus appears to be derived from their sedating properties.

c) **Ursodeoxycholic Acid (UDCA)**: UDCA has recently gained widespread acceptance as an effective agent in delaying the progression of PBC. Early studies suggested that UDCA may be of benefit with respect to pruritus in PBC patients; however, other studies have failed to confirm this. Given the current role for UDCA in treating PBC itself at a dose of 13-15mg/kg/day, potential beneficial effects of UDCA with respect to pruritus in a given patient will be determined on an individual basis. In some patients UDCA can exacerbate itch.

ii) Second Line Therapies

a) **Rifampicin**: In a number of well controlled studies the antibiotic rifampicin has been shown to be effective in treating cholestasis associated pruritus at a does of up to 10mg/kg/day in divided doses. Furthermore, the long term use of rifampicin to treat cholestatic pruritic patients has been shown to be safe[18]. The mechanism of action of rifampicin as an antipruritic agent is unknown but may be secondary to its hepatic enzyme inducing properties. Due to possible hepatotoxicity liver enzymes should be checked regularly.

b) **Opioid Receptor Antagonists**: Opioid receptor blockade is effective in relieving itch in 50-60% of pruritic PBC patients[13,14] and should be considered in patients who don't respond to rifampicin as a second line medication. The opioid receptor antagonist naloxone can be effective at a dose of 0.2μg/kg/min but needs to be given as an intravenous infusion, limiting its usefulness. However, the orally available opioid receptor antagonist naltrexone can be used at a dose of 50 mg/day[14]. Patients need to be observed for opiate withdrawal-like effects and as higher doses of naltrexone can be hepatotoxic, liver enzymes should be regularly monitored.

iii) Other Therapies

Many other therapies have been tried in an attempt to ameliorate itching in pruritic cholestatic patients refractory to the previously mentioned treatments. Therapies which may be considered include:

- propofol (up to 15mg.day)
- corticosteroids (10-20mg/day)
- phenobarbital (2-4mg/kg/day)
- methotrexate (7.5-15mg/week)
- plasmapheresis
- external biliary diversion
- transplantation

Summary

- pruritus in PBC is generalized or localized, not relieved by scratching, worse at night and in winter, and not related to disease stage.
- pathogenesis unclear but origin may be peripheral, central or combination of both.
- cholestyramine will ameliorate pruritus in up to 90% of patients.

LETHARGY IN PRIMARY BILIARY CIRRHOSIS

Clinical Presentation

The symptom of fatigue is commonly encountered in patients with PBC, occurring in up to 86% of patients[1,19]. In fact, fatigue is the most common complaint in PBC patients[1]. However, given the subjective nature of fatigue and the lack of therapies to treat fatigue this symptom is often overlooked or ignored by doctors caring for PBC patients. A number of terms have been used to describe fatigue in PBC patients including lethargy, malaise, lassitude and exhaustion but they are all part of the spectrum of complaints which I will term fatigue.

Fatigue has a significant impact on the quality of life of PBC patients. Specifically, fatigue constitutes the worst symptom in approximately 50% of patients with PBC and causes severely disabling effects on activities of daily life in up to 25% of patients[19-21]. Moreover, fatigue scores as determined by questionnaire in approximately one quarter of PBC patients are similar to those documented in patients with multiple sclerosis and lupus. The complaint of fatigue in PBC patients does not appear to correlate with disease stage and fatigue can be the presenting symptom even in patients with very early hepatic lesions. Furthermore, fatigue in PBC does not correlate with liver biochemistry or Mayo risk score and does not respond to ursodeoxycholic acid therapy.

Fatigue can derive from peripheral (ie. muscle, nerve) or *central* (ie. brain, spinal cord) causes. A recent study has suggested that fatigue in PBC patients is of central, not peripheral origin[22]. Specifically, peripheral fatigue was assessed in PBC patients by electromyography and central fatigue by a series of questionnaires. PBC patients had normal electromyography studies but demonstrated high fatigue scores on the questionnaires, suggesting a central cause of fatigue possibly related to defective central neurotransmission. This suggestion is supported by other investigators who have found a close link in PBC patients between fatigue and disorders of mood (ie. depression, obsessive compulsive disorder), which are also felt to be due to altered central neurotransmission[19-22]. This type of association is also observed in patients with the chronic fatigue syndrome. Specifically, in patients with PBC obsessive-compulsive scores were the best predictors of fatigue scores in patients less than 45 years of age and depression scores were the best predictors of fatigue scores in patients over 45 years of age[22].

FATIGUE IN PBC
<ul><li>occurs in up to 86% of patients</li><li>cause of significant morbidity</li><li>central in origin</li><li>does not correlate with disease stage</li><li>close association with mood/behavioural disorders</li></ul>

Pathogenesis

The etiology of fatigue in PBC patients is poorly understood, however, as indicated earlier the complaint of fatigue in these patients appears to be due to a central, as yet undefined, defect. Moreover, altered central neurotransmission has been implicated in the generation of fatigue in a number of disease states. Therefore, attempts to define the cause(s) of fatigue in PBC patients will need to involve assessments of central neural pathways.

Corticotropin-releasing hormone (CRH) is a neuropeptide located throughout the central nervous system. CRH was first characterized as the main central regulator of the hypothalamic-pituitary-adrenal (HPA) axis via hypothalamic projections to the median eminence. Activation of the HPA axis by CRH results ultimately in the release of glucocorticoids from the adrenal cortex. Glucocorticoids thus released are essential for the control of inflammatory processes within the body (Figure 2). However, CRH containing nerve fibres also project from the hypothalamus to brain stem autonomic nuclei and to other brain areas. CRH nerve projections to autonomic nuclei in the brainstem control, in part, spinal sympathetic outflow which is of central importance in maintaining internal homeostasis (Figure 2). Furthermore, CRH containing nerve fibres have been localized within a number of brain areas, including the limbic system, thereby providing a basis for CRH playing a direct role in behavioural responses. *Specifically, the central release of CRH has been implicated in behavioural arousal and defective central CRH release, in turn, in the genesis of fatigue* (Figure 2)[23].

The acute release of CRH in the brain can be induced by a number of stimuli. Both psychological and physical stress cause central CRH release and this release plays an important role in the response of the individual to these stressors (Figure 2). Furthermore, a number of other stimuli induce CRH release including:

i) **Neurotransmitters**: A number of neurotransmitters have been shown to be capable of inducing central CRH release (Figure 2); however, serotonin and norepinephrine have received the greatest attention. Furthermore, defects in both of these neurotransmitter systems have been implicated in the genesis of mood disorders (e.g. depression) which are closely associated with the complain of fatigue in PBC patients. The serotonin receptor subtype $5HT_{1A}$ has been closely linked with central CRH release as well as with depression. Interestingly, we have recently identified central fatigue in cholestatic rats which is relieved by the repeated administration of a $5HT_{1A}$ agonist, suggesting a role for serotonin and this receptor subtype in cholestasis associated fatigue[24].

ii) **Cytokines**: Cytokines are soluble protein mediators released during inflammatory and immune responses. A number of cytokines, including IL-1, IL-6 and TNFα can induce central CRH release (Figure 3). However, the central release of IL-1β has been most strongly implicated in the genesis of fatigue/lethargy in experimental animals[25]. We have recently demonstrated that cholestatic rats exhibit enhanced central sensitivity to IL-1β-induced depression of locomotor activity suggesting a role for altered central cytokine sensitivity in the genesis of cholestasis associated fatigue[26]. Furthermore, IL-1β induced lethargy in experimental animals has been shown to involve a number of secondary mediators in addition to CRH (Figure 3) potentially implicating alterations in these other secondary mediators in IL-1β-induced fatigue in cholestasis.

The central synthesis and release of CRH appears to be *inhibited* by **chronic** inflammatory or psychological stress (Figure 2)[23]. As PBC is a disease characterized by both chronic inflammatory and psychological stress an

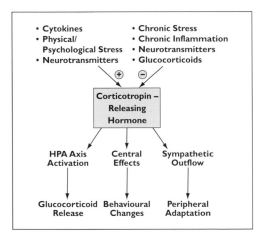

Figure 2.
Corticotropin-releasing hormone (CRH) and Fatigue: Acute stimuli inducing CRH release within the brain include cytokines (e.g. IL-1β), physical or psychological stress and neurotransmitters (e.g. serotonin and norepinephrine). CRH thus released plays a critical role in the regulation of activation of the hypothalamic-pituitary-adrenal (HPA) axis as well as in the control of sympathetic outflow. In addition, central CRH release results in behavioural activation and defective central CRH release has been implicated in the genesis of fatigue. Chronic inflammation or stress, neurotransmitters (e.g. GABA, substance P), and glucocorticoids have been shown to decrease central CRH levels and release.

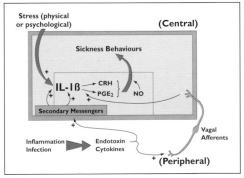

Figure 3.
Central Interleukin-1 and Sickness Behaviours: The central release of Il-1β has been implicated in the genesis of sickness behaviours including lethargy and fatigue. Inflammation and cytokines as well as physical and psychological stress induce the synthesis and release of Il-1β within the brain. Il-1β via secondary messengers such as CRH, prostaglandin E₂ PGE₂) and nitric oxide (NO) then induce sickness behaviours.

impairment in the central CRH system might be expected to occur in these patients. We have some evidence which supports this hypothesis. PBC patients exhibit enhanced pituitary ACTH release in response to exogenous CRH administration, suggesting an upregulation of pituitary CRH receptors secondary to chronic understimulation by endogenous CRH[27]. Furthermore, we have documented decreased hypothalamic CRH levels, mRNA expression and release coupled with defective CRH mediated behaviours in rats with experimental cholestasis[28,29]. These findings support the hypothesis that PBC is associated with defective central CRH release which may potentially be implicated in the genesis of fatigue.

PATHOGENESIS OF FATIGUE

- defective central CRH release appears to play a central role in the genesis of fatigue in PBC.
- alterations in central serotonin receptor sensitivity and sensitivity to IL-1β effects also potentially implicated.

Treatment

Since the etiology of fatigue in PBC is poorly understood, no specific therapies are currently available. However, a systematic approach can benefit a significant number of patients.

Rule Out Other Causes of Fatigue

i) **History**: A thorough history should be obtained which includes specific inquiry about "normal" causes of fatigue:

- symptoms of hypothyroidism
- sleeping patterns, behaviours
- exercise
- caffeine and alcohol ingestion
- life stresses
- medication review – benzodiazepines, β blockers, etc

ii) **Laboratory Tests**:

- CBC, electrolytes, BUN, Cr, glucose, TSH, Ca^{2+}, Mg^{2+}
- if muscle weakness documented then do CK

Rule Out Depression

If the patients history is suggestive of a depressive disorder consider psychiatric assessment or neuro-psychiatric testing.

Treatment of Fatigue

- appropriate diet, sleep, exercise
- limit caffeine, alcohol
- if possible, discontinue any possibly contributing medication(s)
- try graded exercise program
- if depressed, try antidepressant

Treatment of Fatigue: Future Directions

- centrally active CRH agonists
- 5HT$_{1A}$ receptor agonists
- anticytokines

REFERENCES

1. Witt-Sullivan H, Heathcote J, Cauch K, Blendis L, Ghent C, Katz A, Milner R, Pappas SC, Rankin J, Wanless IR. The demography of primary biliary cirrhosis in Ontario, Canada. *Hepatology* 1990; **12**: 98-105.

2. Ekblom A. Some neurophysiological aspects of itch. *Sem. Dermatol* 1995; **14**: 262-270.

3. Bergasa NV. The pruritus of cholestasis. *Sem. Dermatol* 1995; **14**: 302-312.

4. Gillespie DA, Vickers CR. Pruritus of cholestasis: Therapeutic options. J Gastroenterol. *Hepatol* 1993; **8**: 168-173.

5. Ballantyne JC, Loach AB, Carr DB. Itching after epidural and spinal opiates. *Pain* 1988; **33**: 149-160.

6. Kirby J, Heaton KW, Burton JL. Pruritic effect of bile salts. *BMJ* 1974; **4**: 693-695.

7. Freedman MR, Holzback RT, Ferguson DR. Pruritus in chlestasis: No direct causative role for bile acid retention. *AM J Med* 1981; **70**: 1011-1016.

8. Ghent CN. Pruritus of cholestasis is related to effects of bile salts on the liver, not the skin. *AM J Gastro* 1987; **82**: 117-118.

9. Gittlen SC, Schulman ES, Maddrey WV. Raised histamine concentrations in chronic cholestatic liver disease. *Gut* 1990; **31**: 96-99.

10. Fjellner B, Hägermark Ö. Potentiation if histamine-induced itch and flare response in human skin by the enkephalin analogue FK 33-824, β-endorphin and morphine. *Arch Dermatol Res* 1982; **274**: 29-37.

11. Thornton JR, Losowsky MS. Plasma methionine enkephaline concentration and prognosis in primary hiliary cirrhosis. *BMJ* 1998; **297**: 1241-1242.

12. Bergasa NV, Alling DW, Talbot TL, Swain MG, Yurdaydin C, Turner ML, Schmitt JM, Walker EC, Jones EA. Effects of naloxone infusions in patients with the pruritis of cholestasis. *Ann Int Med* 1995; **123**: 161-167.

13. Thornton JR, Losowsky MS. Opioid peptides and primary biliary cirrhosis. *BMJ* 1988; **297**: 1501-1504.

14. Wolfhagen FHJ, Sternieri E, Hop WLJ, Vitale G, Bertolotti M, Van Burren HR. Oral naltrexone treatment for cholestatic pruritus: A double-blind, placebo-controlled study. *Gasteroenterology* 1997; **113**: 1264-1269.

15. Bergasa NV, Alling DW, Vergalla J, Jones EA. Cholestasis in the male rat is associated with naloxone-reversible antinociception. *J Hepatol* 1994; **20**: 85-90.

16. Bergasa NV, Rothman RB, Vergalla J, Xu H, Swain MG, Jones EA. Central mu-opioid receptors are down-regulated in a rat model of acute cholestasis. *J Hepatol* 1992; **15**: 220-224.

17. Monroe EW. Efficacy and safety of nalmefene in patients with severe pruritus caused by chronic urticaria and atopic dermatitis. *J Am Acad Dermatol* 1989; **21**: 135-136.

18. Backs L, Parés A, Elena M, Piera C, Rodés J. Effects of long-term rifampicin administration in primary biliary cirrhosis. *Gastroenterology* 1992; **102**: 2077-2080.

19. Huet P-M, Deslauriers J, Faucher C, Charbonneau J. Fatigue, mental health and depression in patients with primary biliary cirrhosis. *Hepatology* 1996; **24**:A161.

20. Cauch-Dudek K, Abbey S, Stewart DE, Heathcote EJ. Fatigue and quality of life in primary biliary cirrhosis. *Hepatology* 1995; **22**:A6.

21. Huet P-M, Deslauriers J. Impact of fatigue on quality of life of patients with primary biliary cirrhosis. *Gastroenterology* 1996; **110**:A1215.

22. Jalan R, Gibson H, Lombard MG. Patients with PBC have central but no peripheral fatigue. *Hepatology* 1996; **24**:A162.

23. Clauw DJ, Chrousos GP. Chronic pain and fatigue syndromes: Overlapping clinical and neuroendocrine features and potential pathogenic mechanisms. *Neuroimmunomodulation* 1997; **4**: 134-153.

24. Swain MG, Maric M. Improvement in cholestasis associated fatigue with a serotonin receptor agonist using a novel rat model of fatigue assessment. *Hepatology* 1997; **25**: 291-294.

25. Kent S, Bluthe R-M, Dantzer R, Hardwick AJ, Kelly KW, Rothwell NJ, Vannice JL. Different receptor mechanisms mediate the pyrogenic and behavioural effects of interleukin 1. *Proc Natl Acad Sci USA* 1992; **89**: 9117-9120.

26. Swain MG, Le T. enhanced central sensitivity to IL-1β-induced "sickness behaviours" in cholestatic rats. *Hepatology* 1997; **26**:A1265.

27. Swain MG, Mogiakou MA, Bergasa NV, Chrousos GP. Facilitation of ACTH and cortisol responses to corticotropin-releasing hormone (CRH) in patients with primary biliary cirrhosis. *Hepatology* 1994; **20**:A197.

28. Swain MG, Patchev V, Vergalla J, Chrousos G, Jones EA. Suppression of hypothalamic-pituitary-adrenal axis responsiveness to stress in a rat model of acute cholestasis. *J Clin Invest* 1993; **91**: 1903-1908.

29. Swain MG, Maric M. Defective corticotropin-releasing hormone mediated neuroendocrine and behavioural responses in cholestatic rats: Implications for cholestatic liver disease-related sickness behaviours. *Hepatology* 1995; **22**: 1560-1564.

PRIMARY BILIARY CIRRHOSIS: ASSOCIATED MEDICAL CONDITIONS

James Neuberger

Liver Unit, Queen Elizabeth Hospital
Birmingham B15 2TH.

SUMMARY

Primary Biliary cirrhosis (PBC) is associated with a variety of extra-hepatic disorders which do not arise as a consequence of chronic liver disease.

Many of these disorders have a presumed autoimmune basis, in keeping with PBC being an auto-immune disorder.

The commoner associations include sicca syndrome, Raynaud's syndrome, thyroid disease and rheumatic disorders.

Coeliac disease may be found more commonly than in the general population and should be considered in any patient with PBC and diarrhoea.

There are no convincing data that patients with PBC are at greater risk of developing extra-hepatic malignancy. Despite the increase in blood lipids, there is no clear association between PBC and the consequences of atherosclerosis.

Although Primary Biliary Cirrhosis affects primarily the liver, the syndrome is associated with other extra-hepatic diseases which do not occur primarily as a consequence of liver disease. These associated diseases may occur from a common genetic cause or a common aetiologic factor. Reporting of another disease in a patient with PBC does not necessarily imply a true association. Patients with PBC, as with other forms of cholestatic cirrhosis, are at risk from gall-stones and primary liver cell cancer. In PBC the relatively low incidence of primary hepatocellular carcinoma is probably associated with the high female to male ratio.

Awareness and recognition of associated diseases is important since in many of these conditions respond to treatment.

Rheumatological disorders

PBC is associated with several rheumatological disorders which may occur together and in any combination; these include

- Sjogren's syndrome
- Calcinosis
- Raynaud's syndrome
- Sclerodactyly
- Telangiectasia
- Arthritis
- Polymyalgia rheumatica

A retrospective study of 558 patients with PBC identified 22 patients, all female, who had two or more symptoms of the CREST syndrome[1]: telangiectasia and Raynaud's syndrome were present in over 90% and sclerodactyly in 85%; calcinosis and oesophageal dysmotility were present in about 40%. In many cases, symptoms or signs of CREST ante-dated the diagnosis of PBC. Since the anti-centromere antibody is associated with sclerodactyly, the authors suggested that the syndrome should be named the PACK syndrome (Primary Biliary cirrhosis, anticentromere antibody, CREST syndrome and keratoconjunctivitis syndrome) but this acronym has not been adopted. Metcalf[2] found broadly similar results in a survey of 1000 patients with PBC that 1.2% had CREST syndrome; scleroderma was found in 2.7% and rheumatoid arthritis in 7.8%.

Sjogren's Syndrome

Sjogren's syndrome results from a lymphocyte-mediated destruction of the salivary, lachrymal and other exocrine glands leading to reduced or absent secretions. Several studies have shown that many patients with PBC have symptoms of Sjogren's syndrome; indeed the reported incidence in PBC varies between 60 and 100%.[3,4,5,6]

Patients with primary Sjogren's syndrome have circulating antibodies reacting with the 52kDa Ro protein (SSA). Dorner[7] found that, compared with primary Sjogren's syndrome, patients with PBC have a lower probability of having anti-Ro antibodies but these antibodies react with a more restricted number of epitopes within the target protein[8]. In patients with PBC, there is aberrant staining by AMA of the biliary epithelium, with prominent membrane staining of the luminal surface. Although using affinity purified antibodies to human AMA we were unable to find any aberrant staining of the salivary glands in PBC, with or without sicca syndrome[9], Tsuneyama[10], using different antibodies, found that two thirds of patients, with or without sicca syndrome had aberrant staining of the ductal epithelial cells. Although we cannot explain the discrepancy between the two observations, Tsuneyama's findings suggest a common disease process in the two conditions.

The diagnosis of Sjogren's syndrome is usually made just on the basis of a compatible clinical history of dry or gritty eyes or a dry mouth but confirmation depends on a number of investigations:

- Schirmer's test
- slit lamp examination of the eye (often after staining with Rose-Bengal)
- measurement of parotid flow (<0.5ml after 5 minutes)
- serum autoantibodies (anti Ro (SSA) and anti La (SSB))
- salivary gland histology

In practice, invasive investigations are rarely required as the treatment is symptomatic: there are several preparations of artificial saliva which are of neutral pH and contain a balance of electrolytes corresponding to normal saliva; the symptoms associated with dry eyes can be relieved by artificial tears which contain hypromellose and mucolytic agents. Vaginal dryness may cause problems, and women should be advised to take an appropriate lubricant.

Arthritis

Arthropathy has been reported in between 4 and 40% patients with PBC. There are many causes for the arthritis:

- Rheumatoid arthritis
- Chondrocalcinosis
- Hypertrophic osteodystrophy
- Immune complex disease
- arthropathy of systemic sclerosis and Sjogren's syndrome
- Secondary hyperparathyroidism

Treatment is primarily symptomatic.

Polymyalgia rheumatica

There have been case reports of polymyalgia rheumatica and giant cell arteritis occurring in patients with PBC[11,12].

Bone Disease

Bone disease is relatively common in patients with PBC and may be manifest as osteomalacia or osteopenia[13].

Osteomalacia

Osteomalacia is relatively rare in patients with PBC: although the initial report suggested a prevalence of 36%[14] subsequent studies have shown osteomalacia to be rare. Chronic steatorrhoea due to intraluminal bile salt deficiency or pancreatic hyposecretion, chelation of vitamin D by cholestyramine and poor intake may all contribute to the development of vitamin D maladsorption. The routine use of parenteral vitamin D supplementation in cholestatic patients and use of transplantation prior to the terminal phase have largely resulted in disappearance of osteomalacia in PBC.

Osteoporosis

The prevalence of osteoporosis in PBC is much higher than osteomalaga, with estimates ranging from 10 to 80% patients suffering with osteoporosis[15,16,17,18]; the average reported rate is about 30-40%. There are conflicting data whether the osteopenia in PBC results from decreased bone formation or increased bone resorption[19].

Osteoporosis may be detected by several methods

- X-ray of spine and other bones
- Bone biopsy and histomorphometry
- Bone densitometry

The last technique is probably the best for routine use since it is accurate, sensitive, reliable and non-invasive (Figure 1).

There are several reasons why patients with PBC are at risk of osteoporosis

- Female sex
- Calcium maladsorption
- Duration of cholestasis of liver disease
- Post-menopausal condition
- Treatment used to treat PBC or its symptoms (such as corticosteroids and cholestyramine)

Management of osteoporosis:

General measures: patients should be advised to take a healthy diet and calcium supplementation given, which is best taken last thing at night. Vitamin D supplementation is needed only where there is limited exposure to sunlight and when there is the probability of vitamin D maladsorption. Weight bearing exercise, such as walking or jogging but not swimming, are effective.

Estrogens: estrogen replacement therapy is effective in reducing bone loss in post-menopausal women.

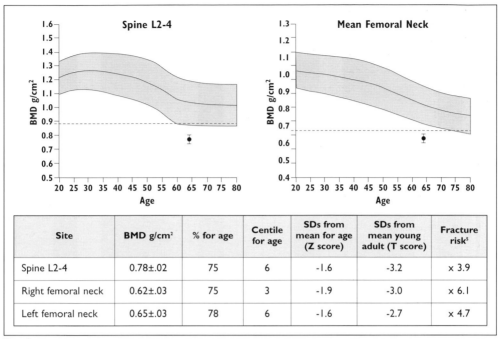

Site	BMD g/cm²	% for age	Centile for age	SDs from mean for age (Z score)	SDs from mean young adult (T score)	Fracture risk[5]
Spine L2-4	0.78±.02	75	6	-1.6	-3.2	x 3.9
Right femoral neck	0.62±.03	75	3	-1.9	-3.0	x 6.1
Left femoral neck	0.65±.03	78	6	-1.6	-2.7	x 4.7

Figure 1.
DEXA scan showing osteoporosis in a woman with PBC

Estrogens both inhibit bone resorption and stimulate bone formation. Although there are few clinical trials showing a significant benefit in PBC, estrogen (usually given as hormonal replacement therapy) is effective and usually well tolerated. There are, however, no prospective, controlled studies evaluating safety of these drugs in women with PBC.

Calcitonin: clinical trials of calcitonin show conflicting results in patients with PBC[20,21]. However, since the potential gain is less than with other therapies, calcitonin is rarely used in PBC.

Sodium fluoride: Sodium fluoride stimulates bone formation. Guanabens[22] showed that sodium fluoride at a dose of 50mg daily was associated with a minimal loss of bone density whereas the control group lost bone, suggesting a beneficial effect of the agent. There are concerns about its long term safety, particularly as fluoride may weaken bone strength even though bone density is increased.

Cyclical etridonate: Guanabens[18] undertook a randomised trial comparing oral etidronate (400mg/day for 2 weeks every 15 weeks) and sodium fluoride 50 mg daily. Etidronate was found to be more effective than fluoride in preventing bone loss.

Ursodeoxycholic acid: Lindor[16] found suggestive evidence that treatment with ursodeoxycholic acid may delay progression of osteopenia in PBC but long term results are needed to confirm the finding.

Liver transplantation: liver replacement is associated with a reduction in the rate of bone loss; in rare cases, in patients with moderate disease, transplantation may be indicated in patients with advancing osteoporosis.

Autoimmune disorders

PBC has been considered a paradigm for autoimmunity and many diseases associated with an autoimmune basis have been reported in association with PBC.

Thyroid disease

Up to 20% patients with PBC have thyroid disease [2,23]. Most patients have hypothyroidism but hyperthyroidism has been reported. Antibodies to thyroglobulin occur in about 20% and anti-microsomal antibodies in about 30%. Thyroid antibodies may be seen in up to one third of women but only 5% of men[24]. Abnormalities of thyroid function may pre-date the diagnosis of PBC or may develop either during the course of the disease or after transplantation. The usual clinical symptoms of hypothyroidism may be masked by the lethargy of PBC so it is recommended that patients with PBC should have serum TSH measured annually. Goitres are seen occasionally (Figure 2). One case report describes reversible jaundice associated with hyperthyroidism in a woman with PBC[25].

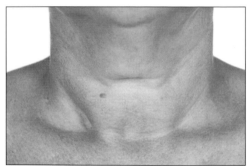

Figure 2.
Thyroid goitre may be found in patients with PBC.

Diabetes mellitus

Diabetes mellitus has been reported in up to 10% patients with PBC[2]; it remains uncertain whether this is an absolute failure of insulin secretion since some patients with PBC may have insulin intolerance rather than a true immune-mediated destruction of the pancreatic islet cells.

Pernicious anaemia

Pernicious anaemia has been reported in about 2% patients with PBC; the diagnosis may be difficult since patients with PBC may have increased red cell mean corpuscular volume because of the liver disease and serum B12 levels may be high since liver cell damage is associated with release into the circulation of B12. A high index of suspicion and measurement of anti-parietal cell antibody may lead to the diagnosis.

Addison's Disease

Addison's Disease is occasionally found in patients with PBC.

Gastrointestinal disorders

Patients with PBC, as with patients with other liver diseases, may have poor dietary intake and in those with weight loss, a full dietary history is helpful. The associated cholestasis may lead to fat intolerance, which should be managed with a low fat diet, supplemented by medium chain triglycerides; prolonged cholestasis may lead to maladsorption of the fat soluble vitamins (A,D,E and K) which may cause symptomatic disease.

Pancreatic disease

PBC has been considered a 'dry gland disease' and pancreatic hyposecretion is well described[26]. In clinical practice, pancreatic insufficiency is rarely a problem. In a careful prospective study, Nishimori[27] studied pancreatic function in patients with PBC and Sjogren's syndrome. One third of the patients with PBC had elevated serum pancreatic enzymes (either elastase-1, trypsin or lipase) and one quarter had reduced PABA excretion and 20% had abnormal pancreatograms demonstrated at ERCP, but these abnormalities were mild and limited to minimal changes in the branches of the pancreatic duct. Broadly similar findings were reported in those with Sjogren's syndrome.

Coeliac Disease

Since Logan's[28] initial report in 1978, there have been several reports of gluten senitive enteropathy in patients with PBC. It has been questioned whether this association was any more than chance. In 1998[29], Kingham reported an analysis of the prevalence of coeliac disease and PBC in a well-defined population of patients in South Wales. In the 143 patients with coeliac disease, the presence of PBC was detected using standard liver tests and in the 67 patients with PBC, coeliac disease was looked for by investigating maladsorption, positive antigliadin antibodies or a positive family history. One patient without these risk factors had coeliac disease detected on a routine duodenal biopsy. The prevalence of PBC in those with coeliac disease was 3% and of coeliac disease in PBC was 6%. The point prevalence of PBC was 20/100 000 and of coeliac disease 54/100 000, suggesting more than a chance association as the prevalence of coeliac disease in England and Wales is estimated to be about 27/100 000 and PBC about 20/100 000.

These findings have not been confirmed by all[30].

Low serum albumin in patients with PBC may be due to several factors but where the serum albumin is lower than might be expected from the serum bilirubin, coeliac disease should be considered. Indeed, we have seen three patients with PBC referred for transplantation because of lethargy and hypoalbu-minaemia: introduction of a gluten free diet corrected these abnormalities and allowed postponement of grafting. Elevated levels of IgA antibodies to gliadin is found in up to 20% patients with chronic liver disease but is not specific for coeliac disease[30] and is therefore of limited value in screening. Anti-endomysial antibodies should be measured and, when positive, the diagnosis confirmed by small bowel biopsy.

Ulcerative colitis has been reported to be associated with PBC, although there appear to be few cases described[31].

Dermatologic Associations

There are several dermatological abnormalities associated with PBC:

- excoriations are associated with itching

- pigmentation: this progresses with time and is most marked around the temples. The cause is not known but the pigmentation resolves after transplantation

- xanthomas and xanthelasmas: these are relatively uncommon but disappearance may be associated with progression of disease (Figure 3). There is no correlation with the serum cholesterol. Xanthomas are best left alone since there is often rapid recurrence after resection

- Vitiligo[32]

- Lichen planus[33]

- Bullous pemphigoid[34]

- Morphoea[33]

- Immune complex capillaritis

- Acanthosis nigricans[36]

Respiratory Problems

Patients with PBC, as with other chronic liver diseases, may develop respiratory disorders in association with the liver disease.

- The hepatopulmonary syndrome results in arterial hypoxaemia because of pulmonary vasodilatation and ventilation/perfusion mis-match, which may lead to intra-pulmonary arteriovenous shunting.

- Ascites may be so severe as to cause compression of the lungs and lead to a restrictive pattern of respiratory disorders.

- Pleural effusions may arise as a consequence of ascites.

- Plexigenic pulmonary hypertension may occur in association with portal hypertension.

- Finger clubbing (Figure 4).

Many of these, including clubbing, may resolve after transplantation[37].

Fibrosing alveolitis

Reduction in alveolar diffusion capacity is found in about 40% patients with PBC[38], and is unrelated to smoking habits, stage of disease or associated Sjogren's syndrome. However, it is found more commonly in association with the CREST syndrome and in association with anti-centromere antibodies.

Sarcoidosis

There is an overlap of PBC with sarcoidosis. Fagan[39] and colleagues described four patients with antimitochondrial antibodies and hepatic granulomas who had predominantly pulmonary signs and symptoms; three also had lung granulomas. Patients presented with cough, pleuritic pain and breathlessness; hepatomegaly was found incidentally, leading to further investigations. Maddrey had described similar cases[40]. Sarcoid can usually be distinguished readily from PBC since erythema nodosum, and the skin, eye and bone lesions of sarcoid do not appear in PBC and the Kveim test is negative. It remains uncertain whether co-existence is coincidental or reflects a common pathogenesis[40].

In addition, Chatte[42] has described one case of a woman with PBC who developed shortness of breath on exertion attributed to lymphocytic bronchitis and bronchiolitis which the authors suggest may be part of a generalised autoimmune process.

Neuropathy

Both peripheral and autonomic neuropathy are well recognised in patients with chronic liver disease[43,44]; Hendrickse and Triger[45] examined both autonomic and peripheral nerve function in 27 patients with PBC, of whom 15 had cirrhosis. Cardiovascular autonomic activity was studied using a battery of tests including change in heart rate on deep breathing, the Valsalva

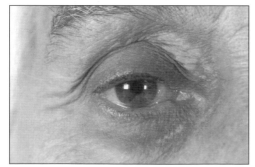

Figure 3.
Xanthelasma in a woman with advanced PBC

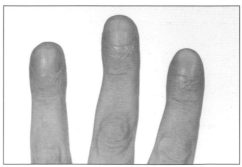

Figure 4.
Clubbing may be seen in association with lung disease in patients with PBC

ratio, changes in heart rate and blood pressure on standing, and heart rate variation at rest and in response to intravenous atropine. Peripheral nerve function was assessed both by symptoms and nerve conduction studies. Compared with controls (normal subjects without liver disease), they found that just under two thirds (63%) of patients with PBC had cardiovascular dysfunction compared with 7% controls; abnormal nerve conduction studies were found in 56% patients (73% of whom had signs or symptoms of a sensory neuropathy). There was a correlation between autonomic and peripheral nerve function.

Although there are many potential causes for autonomic neuropathy (such as vitamin deficiency, drug toxicity, malnutrition) it is probable that many of these changes are not associated with PBC itself but rather with the underlying liver disease. Mohammed and colleagues[46] showed that many of the abnormalities of neuropathy improve after liver transplantation.

Cardiovascular disease

Van Dam[47] did not find that patients with PBC had an excess mortality from cardiovascular compared with an age-matched population. Similar conclusions were reached by Crippen[48] who prospectively followed 312 patients for a median of 7 years. Cardiovascular disease (both ischaemic heart disease and deaths due to heart disease) are not over-represented in PBC compared with a matched population[2].

Serum lipids

The presence of xanthoma and xanthelasma in patients with PBC have focussed researchers' attention on serum lipids in patients with PBC. The xanthoma may rarely be associated with nerve compression.

In a detailed study of 50 patients with PBC, Crippen[48] concluded that in patients with PBC:

- serum cholesterol was markedly elevated with the highest levels in late stage disease.
- triglyceride levels were normal or slightly above normal in all patients.
- HDLs were elevated in all stages, especially stages 2 and 3.
- LDL were elevated in all patients, with highest levels in stage 4.
- Apoprotein A-I was elevated in all but stage 4 disease.

The effect of treatment with cholestyramine and with ursodeoxycholic acid is uncertain. In light of the lack of increased cardiovascular deaths, it remains uncertain whether the hyperlipidaemia of PBC should be treated.

Extra-hepatic malignancy

Early reports suggested that patients with PBC have an increased risk of extra-hepatic malignancy: thus in 1982, Mills[49] reported a retrospective analysis of 85 patients and found 10 (12%) who had extra-hepatic malignancies; there were three cases of carcinoma of breast, and one each of lung, uterus, ovary, stomach, kidney, cervix and larynx. Of the 10 who died, PBC rather than the tumour, was the cause of death in five. The observed number of malignancies was 3.5 times commoner than in the age- and sex matched population. Similarly, Wolke and colleagues[50] studied 208 patients with PBC followed for up to 16 years. Extra-hepatic malignancy developed in eleven patients: in six the malignancy was adeno-carcinoma of the breast; other tumours were papillary carcinoma of the thyroid, adenocarcinoma of the colon, renal cell carcinoma, lymphoma and mycosis fungoides. There was a 4 fold increase in the incidence of breast cancer compared with an aged matched population.

However, in a larger, retrospective analysis of 559 Swedish patients with PBC, Loof[51] could find no evidence of an increased incidence of either hepatic or extra-hepatic malignancy. In the whole cohort, there were 61 cancers identified in 57 patients: in sixteen, the cancer was diagnosed prior to the diagnosis of PBC. During follow-up, 45 malignancies were diagnosed in 42 patients at a mean time of 6 years after diagnosis of PBC. There was an overall increased risk of developing cancer of only 1.6 (95% confidence interval 0.3-2.1); the standardised increased risk for breast cancer was 0.9 (95% CI 0.3-2.1). In a more recent study, Floreani[52] reported a retrospective analysis of 179 Italian patients: extra-hepatic malignancies developed in 12, only 2 of whom had breast cancer. There was no increased risk for the development of breast cancer (proportional incidence ratio 0.7 and for other extrahepatic malignancies 1.0. There was no correlation between the development of extra-hepatic cancer and the presence of auto-immunity. Van Dam found that deaths related to extra-hepatic malignancies were not significantly increased in patients with PBC.

In conclusion, there are no convincing data to show that patients with PBC are at greater risk of developing extra-hepatic malignancy although most studies have involved relatively few patients; the close follow-up may mean that some cancers are detected when they would otherwise have been missed. The suggestion that breast cancer may be increased in patients with PBC is of interest since one study has shown that in immunosuppressed patients, all cancers except breast cancer are more common.

RENAL TRACT PROBLEMS

Urinary Tract Infection

The association of PBC with recurrent urinary tract infection and with bacteriuria has been an area of controversy. Burroughs[53] reported the findings of a prospective study where 87 women with PBC were studied over a 2 year period. Significant bacteriuria (defined as growth of 100 000 organisms/ml in pure culture) was found in 19% PBC patients compared with 7% in women with other chronic liver diseases. Furthermore, 35% developed bacteriuria over a 12 months follow-up and 57% developed recurrent bacteriuria. Over half (59%) of these episodes were asymptomatic. The most common isolates were E coli which did not show the normal adhesiveness to uroepithelial or buccal cells of normal or PBC women; there was no correlation between bacteriuria and age, serum bilirubin, drug therapy or urine pH. These findings, together with the demonstration that patients with recurrent urinary tract infection with E coli have low titer antimitochondrial antibodies have led to the hypothesis that such infections may lead to PBC.

However, conflicting findings were reported by Floreani and colleagues[54]; the prevalence of bacteriuria in patients with PBC (11%) was similar to that found in female patients with other chronic liver diseases (12%) and with Sjogren's syndrome (11%). The prevalence of bacteriuria was associated with the presence or absence of cirrhosis.

It is difficult to reconcile the two studies; differences in methodology or patient selection may be important but the specificity of the increased susceptibility to urinary tract infections in patients with PBC remains to be confirmed.

Glomerulonephritis

Glomerulonephritis is relatively uncommon in patients with PBC[55]; the cause is not clear but IgA nephropathy,

circulating immune complex deposition and the effects of complement activation may be implicated.

Renal tubular acidosis

Renal tubular acidosis occurs rarely and it usually causes no clinical problem. Deposition of copper in the distal renal tubule and the presence of antibodies to Tamm-Horsfall glycoprotein may be involved in the pathogenesis[56].

Isolated reports of diseases associated with PBC

There have been many case reports of rare conditions, many of which may have an immune basis, in association with PBC. Of course, the report of an association does not imply necessarily any more than a chance association. Many of these associated conditions are also presumed to have an autoimmune basis.

Polymyositis: There have been less than a dozen cases reported of polymyositis in patients with PBC; the clinical pattern and treatment is similar to polymyositis in women without PBC[57].

Idiopathic thrombocytopenia[58].

Haemolytic anaemia[59].

Autoimmune polyglandular syndrome (insulin-dependent diabetes mellitus, Hashimoto's thyroiditis, hypogonadism and PBC)[60].

Systemic lupus erythematosus[61]; in this case report, it was noted that the antimitochondrial antibody titer fell during exacerbation of SLE and rose again in remission.

Epidermolysis bullosa acquista[62]; this is probably an autoimmune disease associated with both circulating and tissue bound IgG autoantibodies to type VII collagen.

Myasthenia gravis: although myasthenia gravis has been associated with the use of d-penicillamine in the treatment of PBC, the two conditions may also occur without such treatment[63].

REFERENCES

1. Powell FC, Schroeter AL, Dickson ER. Primary biliary cirrhosis and the CREST syndrome: a report of 22 cases. Q J Med 1987; 62: 75-82

2. Metcalf J, James O. Vascular and autoimmune disease 'associations' with PBC. The best evidence available. Hepatology 1996; 24: A168 [abstract]

3. Tsianos E, Hoofnagle J, Fox P, Alspaugh M, Jones EA, Schafer D, Moutsopoulos H. Sjogren's syndrome in patients with primary biliary cirrhosis. Hepatology 1990; 11: 730-734.

4. Alarcon-Segovia D, Diaz-Jouanen E, Fishbein E. Features of Sjogren's syndrome in primary biliary cirrhosis. Ann Intern Med 1973; 79: 31-36.

5. Golding PL, Brown R, Mason AM, Taylor E. Sicca complex in liver disease. Brit Med J 1973; 79: 31-33.

6. Crowe J, Christensen E, Butler J, Wheeler P, Doniach D, Keenan J, Williams R. Primary biliary cirrhosis: the prevalence of hyperthroidism and its relationship to thyroid autoantibodies. Gastroenterology 1980; 78: 1437-1441.

7. Dorner T, Feist E, Wagenmann A, Kato T, Yamamoto K, Nishioka K, Burmester GR, Hiepe F. Anti-52 kDa Ro (SSA) autoantibodies in different autoimmune diseases preferentially recognise epitopes on the central region of the antigen. J Rheumatol 1996; 23: 462-468

8. Dorner T, Feist E, Held C, Conrad K, Burmester GR, Hiepe F. Differential recognition of the 52 kD Ro (SS-A) antigen by sera from patients with primary biliary cirrhosis and Primary Sjogren's syndrome. Hepatology 1996; 24: 1404-1407.

9. Joplin RE, Johnson g, Matthews J, Hamburger S, Lindsay JG, Hübscher, S, Strain A, Neuberger J. Distribution of pyruvate dehydrogenase dihydrolipoamide acetyl transferase and another mitochondrial marker on salivary gland and biliary epithelium from patients with primary biliary cirrhosis. Hepatology 1994; 19: 1375-1380.

10. Tsuneyama K, van der Water J, Yamazaki K, Suzuki K, Sato S, Takeda Y, Ruebner B, Yost BA, Nakanuma Y, Coppel RL, Gershwin ME. Primary biliary cirrhosis an epithelitis: evidence of abnormal salivary gland immunohistochemistry. Autoimmunity 1997; 26: 23-31.

11. Clarke P, Hamilton E, Williams R. Polymyalgia rheumatica and primary biliary cirrhosis. *Brit Med J* 1979; **1**: 125-126.

12. Gagnarie F, Taillan B, Eugler-Ziegler I, Ziegler G. Primary biliary cirrhosis, temporal arteritis and polymalgia rheumatica in a single patient. *Scand J Rheum* 1988; **17**: 231-232.

13. Cuthbert JA, Pak CYC, Zerwekh JE, Glass KD, Coombes B. Bone disease in primary biliary cirrhosis: increased bone resorption and turn-over in the absence of osteoporosis or osteomalacia. *Hepatology* 1984; **4**: 1-8.

14. Compston JE, Thompson RPH. Intestinal absorption of 25-hydroxyvitamin D and osteomalacia in primary biliary cirrhosis. *Lancet* 1977; **1**: 721-724.

15. Kehayoglou AK, Holdsworth CD, Agnew JE, Whelton M, Sherlock S. Bone disease and calcium absorption in primary biliary cirrhosis. *Lancet* 1968; **1**: 715-719.

16. Lindor KD, Janes CH, Crippen JS, Jorgensen R, Dickson ER. Bone disease in primary biliary cirrhosis: does ursodeoxycholic acid make a difference? *Hepatology* 1995; **21**: 389-392.

17. Mitchison HA, Malcolm AJ, Bassendine M, James O. Metabolic bone disease in primary biliary cirrhosis at presentation. *Gastroenterology* 1998; **94**: 463-470.

18. Guanabens N, Pares A, Monegal A et al. Etidronate versus fluoride for treatment of osteopenia in primary biliary cirrhosis: preliminary results after 2 years. *Gastroenterology* 1997; **113**: 219-224.

19. Rosen H. Primary Biliary Cirrhosis and Bone disease. *Hepatology* 1995; **21**: 253-255.

20. Floreani A, Zappala F, Fries W. A 3 year pilot study with 1,25 dihydroxyvitamin D, calcium and calcitonin for severe osteodystrophy in primary biliary cirrhosis. *J. Clin Gastroenterol* 1997; **24**: 239-244.

21. Camisasca M, Crosignani A, Battezzati P, Albisetti W, Grandinetti G, Pietrogrande L, Biffi A et al. Parenteral calcitonin for metabolic bone disease associated with primary biliary cirrhosis. *Hepatology* 1994; **20**: 633-637.

22. Guanabens N, Pares A, Del Rio L, Roca M, Gomez R, Munoz J, Rodes JI. Sodium fluoride prevents bone loss in primary biliary cirrhosis. *J Hepatol* 1992; **15**: 345-349.

23. Elta GH, Sepersky RA, Goldberg M, Connors CM, Miller KB, Kaplan MM. Increased incidence of hypothyroidism in primary biliary cirrhosis. *Dig Dis Sci* 1983; **28**: 971-975.

24. Crowe JP, Christensen E, Butler J, Wheeler P, Doniach D, Keenan J, Williams R. Primary Biliary Cirrhosis: the prevalence of hypothyroidism and its relationship to thyroid antibodies and sicca syndrome. *Gastroenterology* 1980; **78**: 1437-1438.

25. Thompson N, Leader S, Jamieson C, Burnham WR, Burroughs A. Reversible jaundice in primary biliary cirrhosis due to hyperthyroidism. *Gastroenterology* 1994; **106**: 1342-1343.

26. Epstein O, Thomas HC, Sherlock S. Primary biliary cirrhosis is a dry gland syndrome with features of chronic graft-versus-host disease. *Lancet* 1980; **1**: 1166-1168.

27 Nishimori I, Morita M, Kino J, Onodera M, Nakazawa M, Okazaki K, Yamamoto Y. Pancreatic involvement in patients with Sjogren's syndrome and primary biliary cirrhosis. *Int J Pancreatology* 1995; **17**: 47-54.

28. Logan RF, Ferguson A, Finlayson M, Weir DG. Primary biliary cirrhosis and coeliac disease: an association. *Lancet* 1998; 250-253.

29. Kingham J, Parker D. The association between primary biliary cirrhosis and coeliac disease: a study of relative prevalences. *Gut* 1998; **42**: 120-122.

30. Sjoberg K, Lindgren S, Eriksson S. Frequent occurrence of non-specific gliadin antibodies in chronic liver disease – endomysial but not gliadin antibodies predict coeliac disease in patients with chronic liver disease. *Scad J Gastroenterol* 1997; **32**: 1162-1167.

31. Kaplan M. Primary biliary cirrhosis. *New Engl.J.Med.* 187; **316**: 521-528

32. Enat R, Gilhar A. Vitiligo and primary biliary cirrhosis. *Am J Gastroenterol* 1984; **79**: 804-805.

33. Graham Brown RAC, Sarkany I, Sherlock S. Lichen planus and primary biliary cirrhosis. *Brit J dermatol* 1982; **106**: 699-703.

34. Hamilton DV, McKenzie AW. Bullous pemphigoid in primary biliary cirrhosis. *Brit J Dermatol* 1978; **99**: 447-450.

35. Natarajan S, Green ST. Generalised morphoea, lichen sclerosis et atrophicus and primary biliary cirrhosis. *Clin Exp Dermatol* 1986; **11**: 304-308.

36. Neuberger J, Primary Biliary Cirrhosis. *Lancet* 1997; **35**: 875-879.

37. Stoller JK, Moodie D, Schiavone W, Vogt D, Broughan T, Winkleman E, Rehm P, Carey WD. Reduction of intrapulmonary shunt and resolution of digital clubbing associated with primary biliary cirrhosis after liver transplantation. *Hepatology* 1990; **11**: 54-58.

38. Costa C, Sambataro A, Baldi S, Modena V, Todros L, Libertucci D, Coni F, Fusaro E, Revello F, Murgia A, Rizetto M, Recchia S, Bonino F, Verme G, Rosina F. Primary biliary cirrhosis – lung involvement. *Liver* 1995; **15**: 196-201.

39. Fagan EA, Moore-Gillon JC, Turner-Warwick M. Multiorgan granulomas and mitochondrial antibodies. *New Engl J Med* 1983; **308**: 572-575.

40. Maddrey WC, Johns CJ, Boitnott JK, Iber F. Sarcoidosis and chronic liver disease: a clinical and pathological study of 20 patients. *Medicine (Baltimore)* 1970; **49**: 375-395.

41. Maddrey WC. Sarcoidosis and primary biliary cirrhosis. Associated disorders? *New Eng J Med* 1983; **308**: 588-590.

42. Chatte G, Streichenberger N, Boillot O, Gille D, Loire R, Cordier JF. Lymphocytic bronchitis/bronchiolitis in a patient with primary biliary cirrhosis. *European Resp J* 1995; **8**: 176-179.

43. Lunzer M, Manghani KK, Newman SP, Sherlock S. Impaired cardiovascular responses in liver disease. *Lancet* 1975; **i**: 382-385.

44. Thuluvath PJ, Triger DR. Autonomic neuropathy and chronic liver disease. *Q. J. Med* 1989; **72**: 737-747.

45. Hendrickse MT, Triger MT. Autonomic neuropathy in primary biliary cirrhosis. *J Hepatol* 1993; **19**: 401-407.

46. Mohammed R, Forsey P, Davies M, Neuberger J. Effect of liver transplantation on QT interval prolongation and autonomic dysfunction in end-stage liver disease. *Hepatology* 1996; **23**: 1128-1134.

47. Van Dam GM, Gips CH. Primary Biliary Cirrhosis in the Netherlands - an analysis of associated diseases, cardiovascular risk and malignancy on the basis of mortality figures. *Scand J Gastroenterol* 1997; **32**: 77-83.

48. Crippen JS, Lindon K, Jorgensen R, Kottke B, Harrison J, Murtagh, P, Dickson ER. Hypercholesterolaemia and athersclerosis in primary biliary cirrhosis: what is the risk? *Hepatology* 1992; **15**: 858-862.

49. Mills PR, Boyle P, Quigley EMM, Birnie GG, Jarrett F, Watkinson G, MacSween R. Primary Biliary cirrhosis: an increased incidence of malignancies? *J Clin Pathol* 1982; **35**: 541-543.

50. Wolke AM, Schaffner F, Kapelman B, Sacks H. Malignancy in primary biliary cirrhosis: high incidence of breast cancer in affected women. *Am J Med* 1984; **76**: 1075-1078.

51. Loof L, Adami HO, Sparen P, Danielsson A, Eriksson L, Hultcrantz R, Lindgren S, Olsson R, Prytz H, Ryden BO, Sandberg-Gerten H, Wallerstedt S. Cancer risk in primary biliary cirrhosis: a population-based study from Sweden. *Hepatology* 1994; **20**: 101-104.

52. Floreani A, Chiaramonte M, Baragiotta A, Naccarato R. Incidence of hepatic and extrahepatic malignancies in primary biliary cirrhosis (PBC). *J Hepatol* 1998; **28**(suppl 1); 127 [abstract].

53. Butler PP, Valle F, Hamilton-Mille J, Brumtiff W, Bawm H, Burroughs. M2 mitochondrial antibodies and urinary rough mutant bacteria in patients with primary biliary cirrhosis and recurrent bacteria. *J. Hepatol* 1993; **17**: 408-414.

54. Floreani A, Bassendine MF, Mitchison H, Freman R, James O. No specific association between primary biliary cirrhosis and bacteriuria? *J Hepatol* 1989; **8**: 201-207.

55. Rai GS, Hamlyn AN, Dahl MGC, Sherlock S. Primary biliary cirrhosis, cutaneous capillaritis and IgM-associated membranous glomerulonephritis. *Brit Med J* 1977; **1**: 817.

56. Pares A, Rimola A, Bruguera M, Rodes J. Renal tubular acidosis in primary biliary cirrhosis. *Gastroenterology* 1981; **80**: 681-686.

57. Boki KA, Dourakis SP. Polymyositis associated with primary biliary cirrhosis. *Clin Rheum* 1995; **14**: 375-378.

58. Mizukami Y, Ohhira M, Matsumoto A, Murazumi K, Ohta H, Ohhira M, Ono M, Miyake T, Maekawa I, Khogo Y. Primary biliary cirrhosis associated with idiopathic thrombocytopenic purpura. *J Gastroenterol* 1996; **31**: 284-288.

59. Yoshida EM, Nantel SH, Owen DA, Galbraith PF, Dalal BI, Ballon HS, Kwan SY, Wade JP, Erb SR. Case-report - a patient with primary biliary cirrhosis and autoimmune haemolytic anaemia. *J Gastroenterol and Hepatol* 1996; **11**: 439-442.

60. Ko GTC, Szeto CC, Yeung VTF, Chow CC, Chan H, Cockram CS. Autoimmune polyglandular syndrome and primary biliary cirrhosis. *Brit J Clin Pract* 1996; **50**: 344-346.

61. Schifter T, Lewinski UH. Primary biliary cirrhosis and systemic lupus erythematosus: a rare association. *Clin Exp Rheum* 1997; **15**: 313-314.

62. Tsuji T, Fujimoto W, Tada J, Nagao Y, Arata J. Epidermolysis bullosa acquista and primary biliary cirrhosis. *Euro J Dermatol* 1997; **7**: 584-586.

63. Kiechl S, Kohlendorfer U, Willeit J, Pohl P, Vogel W. Myasthenia gravis and primary biliary cirrhosis – common immunological features and rare coincidence. *Acta Neurol Scand* 1996; **93**: 263-265.

64. Bissuel F, Bizollon T, Dijoud F, Bouletreau P, Cordier JF, Chazot C, Gouillat C, Trepo C. Pulmonary haemorrhage and glomerulonephritis in primary biliary cirrhosis. *Hepatology* 1992; **16**: 1375-1361.

PROGNOSTIC MODELLING IN PRIMARY BILIARY CIRRHOSIS

Erik Christensen

Clinic of Internal Medicine I, Bispebjerg University Hospital,
Bispebjerg Bakke 23, DK-2400 Copenhagen NV, Denmark.

SUMMARY

Prognostication is important in the evaluation of patients since the goal of doctors is to improve prognosis by therapy.

Patient characteristics (variables) being related to the survival hold prognostic information and can indicate prognosis.

Several prognostic variables can be combined into a prognostic model to improve prognostication.

In primary biliary cirrhosis (PBC) several prognostic variables have been identified, the most important being: high bilirubin, old age, low albumin, ascites or oedema, cirrhosis, GI bleeding or oesophageal varices, which all indicate a poor prognosis.

Using Cox regression analysis a number of prognostic models for PBC have been made.

Most models are time-fixed i.e. they predict survival on the basis of data at just one time (e.g. at diagnosis). They can indicate long-term prognosis.

A few models are time-dependent i.e. they also utilise follow-up data and can update short-term prognosis according to the status at the follow-up. They are well suited for monitoring the course of the disease. They can assist timing of liver transplantation.

Although the prognostic models can improve description of patient groups and be helpful in other ways, it is important to stress, that they are not precise and therefore only can indicate prognosis in individual patients. Thus prognostic models can assist in clinical decision making, but they cannot replace sound clinical judgement.

Introduction

In medicine prognosis or "fore-knowledge" is prediction of the probable course and outcome of a disease. Prognostication is an important aspect in the evaluation of any given patient since the primary objective of the doctor is to apply a therapy which improves the prognosis of the disease as much as possible. Therefore, it is highly relevant to study prognosis and its determinants. Patient characteristics (variables) being related to the course and outcome hold prognostic information and can indicate prognosis. Several prognostic variables can be combined into a prognostic model to improve prognostication.

Biologic variation

In principle prognostication seems simple but in practice it is difficult. The most important reason is the biologic diversity principle caused by the genetic recombination during the meiosis in all higher species including Homo Sapiens. This diversity increases adaptability and thereby the probability of survival of the species. In medicine this means that patients suffering from a certain disease, defined according to the state of the art, will show different manifestations giving a "spectrum" of variation between the patients. Furthermore, patients will present themselves to the doctor at various time-stages of the disease, they will present different combinations of symptoms and signs, different values of laboratory tests and different findings in paraclinical investigations.

Structure of patient data

The variation among patients with a given disease makes a complete description difficult and usually only a summarised description is made including for each variable the average (or proportion) and variation (e.g. range, standard deviation or standard error) and a survival curve giving the average survival probability for the patient group.

Since the characteristics of individual patients differ from the average, it cannot and does not describe individual patients. Furthermore, a given patient is poorly described by a single characteristic. Description is much improved by considering the particular combination of the characteristics presented by the patient. Thus, the task of the doctor may be described as one of pattern recognition i.e. recognising the certain combination or pattern in which the characteristics present themselves in the patient in order to identify the "type" or subgroup to which he/she belongs.

To attack this problem it is necessary to have access to a large data-base including for each patient the outcome variable and many descriptive variables. A fine setting for prospectively collecting data to a data-base is to perform a randomised clinical trial. Besides the prognostic aspect, the impact of therapy on prognosis can be studied in detail[1,2] and perhaps a therapeutic index can be obtained[2,3].

Identification of prognostic variables

The first step in the development of a prognostic model is to identify variables which covary with the survival. For example in patients with a high bilirubin, the survival may be found to be short, and in patients with a low bilirubin, the survival may be long. If the covariation (or correlation) between the level of bilirubin and the survival is large, the level of bilirubin may to some degree "explain" the variation in survival time between the subjects. In that case, the level of bilirubin in a new subject may to some degree be used to predict his/her survival time. Thus the simplest way to identify bilirubin as a prognostic variable is to divide the patients in subgroups (strata) according to different levels of bilirubin. In this way the prognostic influence of bilirubin in PBC was established[4,5].

COMBINATION OF PROGNOSTIC VARIABLES

Stratification

Normally, a single variable, even if it shows a strong covariation with survival, will not completely "explain" survival. Usually, it is to be expected that more variables in combination may "explain" survival to a higher degree. It is possible to stratify according to more than one variable at a time[1,5]. However, with an increasing number of strata, the number of patients in each stratum will rapidly decrease to such an extent that the corresponding survival curves will have too little "confidence" (the 95% confidence interval of the survival curves will be too wide) to be of any value. This puts a strong limitation on stratification. However, stratification may be used for a crude screening to identify prognostic variables which should be analysed further with more advanced methods.

Cox regression model

Methods have been developed by which the association of more variables with survival can be studied simultaneously. These include the Cox regression model for censored survival data[6,7], where the survival is modelled as a linear combination (function) of independent predictor variables taking into account the pattern of covariation (or correlation) between the variables. Generally the best model will tend to include variables which are correlated to survival but not strongly intercorrelated[7]. The coefficients in the model reflect their independent contribution in predicting survival. The model can be used in a given patient to calculate a prognostic index which can be transformed to a probability of surviving a given span of time[2,7].

Validation of results

Since such complex analyses are – to some degree – exploratory or heuristic, the results need some kind of validation before they can be considered "proved". Optimally the prognostic index should be validated using the data of independent patients to see if the prognostic index predicts prognosis correctly in these patients. If completely independent patients are not available, a validation in a more limited sense can be obtained by dividing the original patient data into a "model sample" used for the statistical development of the prognostic index and a "test sample" used for testing and validation of the prognostic index[2,7].

PROGNOSTIC VARIABLES IN PRIMARY BILIARY CIRRHOSIS (PBC)

Early univariate or stratified prognostic analyses

As PBC is an intrahepatic, chronic, nonsuppurative, destructive cholangitis ultimately leading to cirrhosis, indicators of cholestasis severity and cirrhosis would be expected to be associated with the survival.

In 1979 Shapiro et al.[4] reported the association between serum bilirubin and survival. They found that, after a relatively stable phase of varying length, the bilirubin showed an accelerative increase prior to death. This finding was confirmed in a larger study showing a marked increase in the incidence of jaundice prior to death from hepatic failure[5]. In addition similar course is seen in other types of cirrhosis as well[8]. Shapiro et al. found that after two successive bilirubin values above 2 mg per dl obtained 6 months apart, the patient lived on average 4.1 years (95% confidence interval 2.7 to 6.2 years); after two successive bilirubin values above 6 mg per dl, the average survival was 2.1 (1.6 to 2.7) years, and after two values above 10 mg per dl, the survival was 1.4 (1.1 to 1.8) years[4]. The paramount importance of bilirubin as a prognostic factor in PBC has been confirmed in all subsequent prognostic studies[9-17].

In 1980 in an early study using stratified analysis of the data from a large controlled clinical trial a high bilirubin, the presence of cirrhosis and old age were independently associated with a poor prognosis[5].

Time-fixed Cox regression models (overall prognosis)

The following models are all based on the association between the data at just one time (usually the time of diagnosis or the time of inclusion into a controlled clinical trial) and the subsequent survival. For this reason they are called time-fixed models.

In 1983, Roll et al. published the first Cox regression model for PBC[9]. They found that elevated bilirubin, old age, hepatomegaly and cirrhosis were associated with a poorer prognosis.

In 1985 a prognostic index[10] was devised from a Cox regression model developed using the data from a European trial of azathioprine versus placebo. The prognostic index included the following variables indicative of a poorer prognosis: increased serum bilirubin, old age, decreased serum albumin, cirrhosis, central cholestasis and placebo treatment (as opposed to azathioprine which had a beneficial effect on survival[10]). The prognostic index can easily be estimated using a pocket chart[2], and by applying simple diagrams, it can be transformed to a probability of surviving a given time or to an estimated median survival time[2,10]. Figure 1 shows the estimated survival curves corresponding to a patient with good, medium and poor prognosis. It was shown in a sample of independent

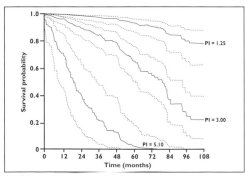

Figure 1.
Estimated survival curves with 95% confidence limits for 3 patients with prognostic index (PI) values = 1.25 (good prognosis), 3.00 (medium prognosis) and 5.10 (poor prognosis), respectively. These PI values corresponded to the 10th, 50th and 90th percentiles of the distribution of PI in the patients. From reference 10.

patients that survival predicted by the prognostic index corresponded closely to the observed survival in 3 groups with low, medium and high prognostic indices[10].

In 1989 Goudie et al.[11] from Glasgow found the following variables to be associated with a poor prognosis in Cox regression analysis: high bilirubin, high age, ascites, variceal bleeding, marked hepatic fibrosis, cholestasis, and Mallory's hyalin.

In 1989 Dickson et al.[12] from the Mayo Clinic reported a prognostic model including age, bilirubin, albumin, prothrombin time and peripheral oedema. They omitted the use of variables requiring a liver biopsy. The survival predicted by the model showed reasonable agreement with the observed survival in an independent sample of patients treated at the Mayo Clinic when divided into 3 groups with good, medium and poor prognosis.

In 1990 Biagini et al. from the Royal Free Hospital in London found the following variables to be independently associated with a poor prognosis: high bilirubin, high age, hepatomegaly, low albumin, oesophageal varices, ascites, pulmonary disease and high alkaline phosphatase[13]. They found, however, that the Cox model with these variables gave a poor prediction for survival of individual patients.

In 1990 Ryding et al. from Oslo found that in their PBC patients only bilirubin and GI bleeding had significant independent association with survival in Cox regression analysis[14].

In spite of the included variables being significant in the above time-fixed models, their predictive abilities are limited, especially for long periods of time. This is reflected in large confidence intervals for the survival predicted by the models[10] (see Figure 1). Thus the precision for survival in individual patients is poor, especially for longer time periods.

Time-dependent prognostic models (current updated prognosis)

To improve precision and to make the prognostic models more suitable for monitoring the course of the disease, models utilising follow-up data (so called time-dependent models or update models) have been developed.

In 1992 Hughes et al.[15] using data from the Royal Free Hospital in London published a model for prediction of short-term survival, (up to 2 years). The analysis was based on dividing the follow-up period of each patient in non-overlapping 2 years intervals each beginning at a time when data had been recorded. The analysis showed a decreased short term survival to be associated with high age, high bilirubin, low albumin and a history of ascites. The authors provided a chart presented in Figure 2 by which the predicted probabilities of surviving 6 months, 1 year and 2 years could be calculated in a simple way by using a pocket calculator[15]. The model was not validated in independent patients.

In 1993 a European time-dependent Cox model[16] for prediction of short-term survival was developed using the data of patients including in the European controlled clinical trial of azathioprine versus placebo[10]. Considering also histologic variables the final model found high bilirubin, central cholestasis, ascites, cirrhosis, GI bleeding, low albumin, low IgM, and old age to be independently associated with a decreased short-term (i.e. 6 months) survival probability. Excluding histology high bilirubin, old age, low albumin, ascites and gastro-intestinal bleeding were independently associated with poor 6 months survival probability. This model was also presented in a pocket chart (Table 1), by which a prognostic index for a given patient can be obtained by simple algebra. For example using Table 1 for a patient having the following variables: bilirubin 45 µmol/l, ascites, albumin 30 g/L, age 48 years and GI bleeding the following points are obtained: bilirubin 10, ascites 14, albumin -14, age 8, GI bleeding 7. The sum of these points is 10 + 14 -14 + 8 + 7 = 25. By dividing this number by 10 the prognostic index is found to be 2.5. The prognostic index can be transformed to a probability of surviving the following 1, 3 and 6 months by using Figure 3. For example for a prognostic index of 2.5 the estimated probability of surviving the next 6 months is only 82%. This prognostic model was validated in independent patients and it was found to predict more precisely than the previously developed time-fixed model[16].

TABLE I: POCKET CHART FOR CALCULATION OF PROGNOSTIC INDEX IN PBC USING EUROPEAN SHORT-TERM SURVIVAL MODEL			
Variable			**Points to add**
Serum bilirubin	mg/100ml	µmol/l	
	0.6	10	-6
	1.2	20	1
	2.0	34	7
	2.9	50	11
	4.1	70	15
	5.8	100	19
	8.8	150	23
	11.7	200	27
	17.5	300	31
	23.4	400	34
	29.2	500	37
Ascites		no	0
		yes	14
Serum albumin	g/l	µmol/l	
	20	304	-6
	30	456	-14
	34	517	-18
	40	608	-23
	50	760	-31
	60	912	-40
Age (years)		30	1
		40	5
		50	9
		55	11
		60	13
		70	17
		80	21
GI Bleeding		no	0
		yes	7

Sum of points S= Prognostic index PI(t) = S/10=
From reference 16.

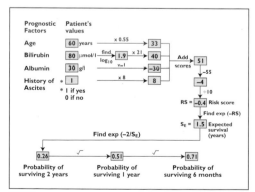

Figure 2.
Chart for calculating probabilities of surviving 6 months, 1 year or 2 years based on the exponential model for short-term survival presented in reference 15. The chart shows an example for a patient aged 60 years, with ascites and with a serum albumin of 30 g/l and a bilirubin value of 80 *mol/l.

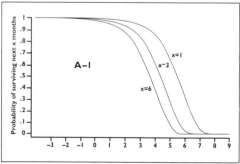

Figure 3.
Probability of surviving 1, 3 and 6 months as a function of the time-dependent prognostic index calculated using Table 1. Corresponding to a given prognostic index value at the horizontal axis one reads the survival probabilities on the vertical axis. For a prognostic index value of 2.5 the probability of surviving the following 1, 3 and 6 months can be read as 97%, 91% and 82%, respectively. From reference 16.

In 1994 Murtaugh et al.[17] from the Mayo Clinic published a new version of the Mayo model for prediction of short-term survival. For each patient the follow-up period was divided into short intervals, each interval corresponding to the time between one follow-up and the next. The median length of each interval was 1 year. The data from each interval was used as an independent set of information in the analysis. The resulting "update" model included the same variables as in the original Mayo model (age, bilirubin, albumin, prothrombin time and peripheral oedema) but the regression coefficients were different. The model was validated in independent patients. Like the European time-dependent model the update Mayo model could estimate survival probabilities with narrower confidence limits than the original Mayo model.

An overview of prognostic variables identified in the prognostic models presented above is shown in Table 2. The only variable common to all models is serum bilirubin; age is a significant variable in eight of the nine models. Thus a relatively large heterogeneity exists between the models. It is difficult to know which model is best. Probably the predictive abilities of the models within each of the categories (time-fixed or time-dependent) are not very much different[18], but a comprehensive comparative study has not been performed.

Some of the above models have been used to substantiate the value of liver transplantation by demonstrating that the survival observed after the procedure is better than without as predicted by the models[18-20]. Such evidence is markedly weaker than what could have been obtained in controlled clinical trials, but since such have not, and probably will not, be performed, the predictions provided by the prognostic

indices have become necessary in the evaluation of the transplantation procedure.

Furthermore, a prognostic model for prediction of survival after transplantation using the latest pre-transplant data has been devised for primary biliary cirrhosis[21]. Thus it is possible to predict survival time both with and without transplantation and the procedure would accordingly be justified only if the former were longer than the latter[22].

Why is the precision of prognostic models low?
Even when applying the time-dependent prognostic models which utilises the data much more efficiently and only predict for a smaller time period, the prediction is not very precise, the 95% confidence limits of the predicted survival probabilities being rather wide. The reasons for the imprecision include:

- *Statistical significance is different from predictive ability*
Variables are often included in a model if they are statistically significant. However, variables may be significant without being able to "explain" very much of the variation in survival, especially if the number of patients is large. It would be desirable to have better means of knowing how much variation a given prognostic models "explains" in analogy with the coefficient of determination R^2 of simple multiple regression analysis.

- *The prognostic variables are only weakly informative.*
The biologic variation is much larger then can be accounted for by the recorded variables. Many recorded variables are not central to the fundamental disease process but side events or epi-phenomena.

- *Too few variable recordings are being used*
Variables at diagnosis or at admission to hospital

TABLE 2: INDEPENDENT VARIABLES ASSOCIATED WITH A POOR PROGNOSIS IN PBC

Variable	Time fixed models						Time dependent models		
	Yale[9]	European[10]	Mayo[12]	Glasgow[11]	Oslo[14]	London[13]	European[16]	Mayo[17]	London[15]
high bilirubin	x	x	x	x	x	x	x	x	x
low serum albumin		x	x			x	x	x	x
low prothrombin index			x					x	
low immunoglobulin M							x		
high age	x	x	x	x		x	x	x	x
hepatomegaly	x					x			
peripheral edema			x					x	
ascites				x		x	x		x
esophageal varices						x			
GI bleeding				x	x		x		
cirrhosis	x	x		x			x	x	
histologic cholestasis		x		x			x		
Mallory bodies			x						

typically show short-term regression toward norma[18,16]. Later "steady-state" values may be more informative.

- *The changes during the course of the disease are not used*

The first course of the disease may indicate the following course. Information about the course of variables over time is not utilised in the time-dependent Cox model which only uses the current variable recordings, not their previous course.

- *Variables may interact in a highly complex manner*

The "linear" structure of the developed prognostic models may be too simple to give a complete description. The variables may interact in a complex way which may not be easy to identify. Neural networks[23] is a new methodology which can be used. However, since the number of parameters to fit in the neural network may be large, the necessary number of patient data sets must also be very large (thousands) to avoid over-fitting. Furthermore, the working of the trained neural network is hidden to the observer and thus no insight in the process can easily be obtained. These factors limit the use of neural networks.

- *Important prognostic variables may be unknown*

Our knowledge of many disease processes is not very detailed. Much needs to be discovered including better prognostic variables closely connected with fundamental disease processes. However, if new prognostic variables are to be useful in clinical practice, they should be easily obtainable.

What can prognostic models be used for?

- *Guides to prognosis*

Because prognostic models only explain a minor part of the variation in survival between the patients, they cannot predict prognosis precisely in individual patients. Thus for an individual patient the prognostic models can only give some guidance to prognosis, not more than that.

- *Monitoring of the course of the disease in the same patient*

When applied repeatedly in the same patient a time-dependent prognostic index may be useful in estimating the change in short-term prognosis during the course of disease. Such information may be valuable for the timing of special therapeutic options such as liver transplantation, especially if prognosis with and without the procedure can be compared[22]. In these cases the updated prognostic index can serve as a guide to therapy.

- *Summarised description of patient groups*

A prognostic index is a summarised description of the seriousness of the disease expressed in one number which is obtained as a combination of all the prognostic variables weighted according to their relative prognostic influence. Therefore the prognosis for a group of patients may be very well described by the average and distribution of their prognostic indices.

- *Improved comparison of patient groups*

The use of prognostic models and indices makes it possible to perform a more qualified comparison between different patient groups by adjusting for imbalance in prognostic variables between the groups. In this way it can be determined if any difference between the groups can be explained by different distribution in prognostic variables between the groups or must be attributed to other variables. This is of importance when patient groups from different centres are to be compared.

- *Illumination and inspiration of pathogenetic studies*

Because a prognostic index includes those variables which are strongly associated with the progression of the disease it can illuminate pathogenesis and inspire further pathogenetic studies.

- *Education*

For medical students and untrained doctors a prognostic index can have an educational value in describing which variables are important and which are not important as indicators of the course of the disease.

Future development

Until now a relatively large number of prognostic models in PBC have been published. Even if the models are the results of complex analyses, some are not difficult to use because they have been presented as pocket charts and diagrams, with which the prognosis can be estimated at the bedside.

The prognostic models vary somewhat in regard to the variables being included. This is to be expected because of differences in patient samples and because variables are often being selected according to statistical criteria and less often according to established knowledge. Attempts should be made to agree one or two prognostic indices in PBC. A commonly accepted prognostic model could be obtained by analysing a combined data base from various centres. Use of prognostic indices generally agreed upon would make comparison of results from different centres easier and would promote scientific progress[24].

Furthermore, the improved possibilities provided by modern information technology for systematic, continuous, prospective accumulation of consecutive patient data in large data bases should be utilised for the development of even better prognostic models in the future.

REFERENCES

1. Peto R, Pike MC, Armitage P, Breslow NE, Cox DR, Howard SV, Mantel N, McPherson K, Peto J, Smith PG. Design and analysis of randomised clinical trials requiring prolonged observation of each patient. II. Analysis and examples. *Br J Cancer* 1977; **35**: 1-39.

2. Christensen E. Individual therapy-dependent prognosis based on data from con-trolled clinical trials in chronic liver disease (thesis). *Dan Med Bull* 1988; **35**: 167-82.

3. Christensen E, Schlichting P, Andersen PK, Fauerholdt L, Juhl E, Poulsen H, Tygstrup N, CSL. A therapeutic index that predicts the individual effect of prednisone in patients with cirrhosis. *Gastroenterology* 1985; **88**: 156-65.

4. Shapiro JM, Smith H, Schaffner F. Serum bilirubin: a prognostic factor in primary biliary cirrhosis. *Gut* 1979; **20**: 137-40.

5. Christensen E, Crowe J, Doniach D, Popper H, Ranek L, Rodes J, Tygstrup N, Williams R. Clinical pattern and course of disease in primary biliary cirrhosis based on an analysis of 236 patients. *Gastroenterology* 1980; **78**: 236-46.

6. Cox DR. Regression models and life tables (with discussion) *J R Statist Soc B* 1972; **34**: 187-220.

7. Christensen E. Multivariate survival analysis using Cox's regression model. *Hepatology* 1987; **7**: 1346-58.

8. Christensen E, Schlichting P, Fauerholdt L, Juhl E, Poulsen H, Tygstrup N, CSL. Changes of laboratory variables with time in cirrhosis. Prognostic and therapeutic significance. *Hepatology* 1985; **5**: 843-53.

9. Roll J, Boyer JL, Barry D, Klatskin G. The prognostic importance of clinical and histologic features in asymptomatic and symptomatic primary biliary cirrhosis. *N Engl J Med* 1983; **308**: 1-7.

10. Christensen E, Neuberger J, Crowe J, Altman DG, Popper H, Portmann B, Doniach D, Ranek L, Tygstrup N, Williams R. Beneficial effect of azathioprine and prediction of prognosis in primary biliary cirrhosis. Final results of an international trial. *Gastroenterology* 1985; **89**: 1084-91.

11. Goudie BM, Burt AD, Macfarlane GJ, Boyle P, Gillis CR, MacSween RNM, Watkinson G. Risk factors and prognosis in primary biliary cirrhosis. *Am J Gastroent* 1989; **84**: 713-6.

12. Dickson ER, Grambsch PM, Fleming TR, Fisher LD, Langworthy A. Prognosis in primary biliary cirrhosis: a model for decision making. *Hepatology* 1989; **10**: 1-7.

13. Biagini MR, Guardascione M, Raskino C, McIntyre N, Surrenti C, Burroughs AK. Poor prognostication for survival of individual PBC patients with Cox models. *J Hepatol* 1990; **11** (Suppl 2): S7.

14. Rydning A, Schrumpf E, Abdelnoor M, Elgio K, Jenssen E. Factors of prognostic importance in primary biliary cirrhosis. *Scand J Gastroenterol* 1990; **25**: 119-26.

15. Hughes MD, Raskino CL, Pocock SJ, Biagini MR, Burroughs AK. Prediction of short-term survival with an application in primary biliary cirrhosis. *Stat Med* 1992; **11**: 1731-45.

16. Christensen E, Altman DG, Neuberger J, De Stavola BL, Tygstrup N, Williams R, PBC1 and PBC2 trial groups. Updating prognosis in primary biliary cirrhosis using a time-dependent Cox regression model. *Gastroenterology* 1993; **105**: 1865-76.

17. Murtaugh PA, Dickson ER, Van Dam GM, Malinchoc M, Grambsch PM, Langworthy AL, Gips CH. Primary biliary cirrhosis: prediction of short-term survival based on repeated patient visits. *Hepatology* 1994; **20**: 126-34.

18. Bonsel GJ, Klompmaker IJ, van't Veer F, Habbema JD, Slooff MJ. Use of prognostic models for assessment of value of liver transplantation in primary biliary cirrhosis. *Lancet* 1990; **335**: 493-7.

19. Neuberger J, Altman DG, Christensen E, Tygstrup N, Williams R. Use of a prognostic index in evaluation of liver transplantation for primary biliary cirrhosis. *Transplantation* 1986; **41**: 713-6.

20. Markus B, Dickson ER, Grambsch PM, Fleming TR, Mazzaferro V, Klintmalm GBG, Wiesner RH, et al. Efficacy of liver transplantation in patients with primary biliary cirrhosis. *N Engl J Med* 1989; **320**: 1709-13.

21. Neuberger J, Altman DG, Polson R, Buckels J, Rolles K, Elias E, Calne R, McMaster P, Williams R. Prognosis after liver transplantation for primary biliary cirrhosis. *Transplantation* 1989; **48**: 444-7.

22. Christensen E, Gunson B, Neuberger J. Optimal timing of liver transplantation for patients with primary biliary cirrhosis: Use of prognostic modeling. *Gut* 1997; **41** (Suppl 3): A77.

23. Hornik K. Multilayer feedforward networks are universal approximators. *Neural Networks* 1989; **2**: 359-66.

24. Christensen E. Prognostic models in chronic liver disease: validity, usefulness and future role. *J Hepatol* 1997; **26**: 1414-24.

CLINICAL TRIALS OF MEDICAL TREATMENT IN PBC

John Goulis, Andrew K Burroughs

Liver Transplantation and Hepatobiliary Medicine,
Royal Free Hospital, London, UK.

SUMMARY

The results of our meta-analysis have not shown any benefit in survival or survival free of transplantation from the use of UDCA. At present the data supporting a favourable effect of UDCA on these clinical meaningful end points are based mainly on the combined study of the three studies published recently[29]. We have pointed out several problems relevant to this analysis and do not believe it represents the real effect of UDCA. However we are convinced that there is still data that could be extracted from studies already published in order to clarify the efficacy of UDCA more precisely:

- A thorough reassessment of the effect of UDCA treatment on patients originally randomised to placebo, switched over to the active drug after the completion of the randomised phase is required. Studies of the extended follow-up did not provide the clinical and biochemical characteristics of the patients at the initiation of the open phase of UDCA treatment. Although some of the biochemical characteristics can be extrapolated from the original data obtained at the end of the randomised trials, information at the start of the cross-over phase is still necessary as only the 80% of the patients originally randomised to placebo were switched over to UDCA. This information should provide the clues to explain why in some studies the delay in the initiation of UDCA for 2 years was so unhelpful when the patients had not in fact deteriorated all that much after 2 years of placebo administration.

- Furthermore the same issue could also be clarified if the authors of the extended follow-up studies compared the efficacy of a 2 year UDCA treatment in patients originally assigned to the drug with those assigned to placebo. It is reasonable to anticipate that this effect should be similar if the analysis is started in both groups at the time of initiation of UDCA treatment and the comparison is adjusted for the same or similar prognostic indices (ie bilirubin etc).

- In the studies in which a combined end point is given (ie death or liver transplantation), the authors should specify the number of the events of each component of the end point. This would reveal the component that gives the statistical weight to the combined end point.

- The role of liver transplantation, as a valid end point, in clinical trials of treatment for PBC should be refined. Reporting of the general selection criteria for liver transplantation is very useful but not sufficient for the validation of this end point. The clinical and biochemical characteristics of the patients just before OLT should be also provided, in order to elucidate if similar criteria are used for both arms of each study and indeed between studies, especially during the unblinded cross-over phase of the trials. In addition this data could make clear if the decrease in bilirubin concentrations is accompanied by a respective decrease or stabilisation of the other markers of the prognostic index for PBC (ie albumin, prothrombin time, edema) or or whether UDCA simply has a wash-out effect on bilirubin. If the latter was proved to be true, it would be concluded that PBC patients on UDCA progress to the end stage of liver disease at the same rate as those taking placebo but simply with lower bilirubin levels. As a result UDCA would not reduce the need for liver transplantation and moreover the criteria for referral for liver transplantation in patients taking UDCA would need to be modified. A recently published report of the Mayo experience of liver transplantation for PBC during recent years, when UDCA was generally used, showed that end stage PBC patients were transplanted with a lower median bilirubin level of 6.7 mg/dL compared to 16mg/dL previously[34]. Is this trend due to an effect of UDCA on bilirubin levels or earlier referral from physicians, considering lengthening waiting times? It is apity that the authors did not examine the effect of UDCA in the analysis of their data.

Primary biliary cirrhosis (PBC) is a slowly progressive cholestatic liver disease which occurs almost exclusively in females with a male:female ratio of 1:9. The chronic cholestasis, due to immune-mediated destruction of small septal and interlobular bile ducts, can result in hepatic fibrosis, biliary cirrhosis and eventually liver failure in many cases[1]. Although liver transplantation offers very good results in patients with end-stage PBC, there is a great need for effective pharmacological treatment for patients in the earlier stages of the disease. Many therapies targeted at several points in the natural history of the disease have been tried in PBC, including azathioprine, D-penicillamine, corticosteroids, colchicine, cyclosporin-A, chlorambucil and methotrexate. Although some of these drugs have not yet been adequately evaluated, the results of most of the clinical trials have been largely disappointing either due to the lack of any effect on disease progression and survival or due to toxic drug side effects. As a result none of these agents is in routine clinical use. Moreover assessment of the efficacy of these therapies has been difficult to prove in view of the prolonged duration of PBC. The natural history of the disease is very long extending over decades. The onset of the disease probably occurs many years before the appearance of any symptoms as indicated by a recent paper[2]. Thus, although survival analysis should be the "gold standard" for evaluating response to treatment in clinical trials of PBC, it requires a large sample size, which can be only achieved with multicentre trials of long duration. To date this has never been done. We calculated the sample size that is needed for such studies. The average 2 year survival without liver transplantation in the published UDCA versus placebo trials (in which approximately 50% of the patients had stage III or IV histological disease) was 88%. To show an increase of 2 year survival free of liver transplantation from 85% to 95%, with an error of 0.05 and a power of 0.80, 300 patients would be needed and 30 events should be observed in a mean follow-up of 2 years. Furthermore if an increase from 90% to 95% was needed the study population should be 892 patients and 66 events observed.

Liver transplantation, which is the only effective treatment for the later stages of PBC, has been also used as a primary end point in clinical trials of therapy in PBC. However the lack of documentation of the criteria used for patient referral for liver transplantation, the possibility of transplantation for early but highly symptomatic disease, as well as the varying intervals on the waiting list between different transplant centres do confound the interpretation of this end point. Considering that in future years most patients with PBC will be transplanted rather than die without transplantation, more precise evaluation of this end point will be required.

Surrogate end points in the evaluation of treatment efficacy

The use of surrogate end points has been proposed to measure important treatment effects over much shorter periods of time[3]. A surrogate end point of a clinical trial is a laboratory measurement or a physical sign used as a substitute for a clinically relevant outcome[4]. Changes induced by a therapy on a surrogate end point can be expected to occur long before the onset of the clinical outcomes. This is particularly attractive considering the long natural history of PBC, so that a number of surrogate markers already have been used in clinical trials.

- **Symptoms:** The major symptoms of PBC namely fatigue and pruritus, could be important in this respect. Although they may fluctuate in time and they depend on a subjective assessment by the patient, they can be scored in a severity scale and there are standard patient questionnaires available for this purpose.

- **Liver histology:** This is another potential surrogate end point. However it is important to note that the assessment of this end point must overcome the problem of sampling variation, which is inherent in needle liver biopsies and estimated to occur more often in biopsy samples of PBC patients. The degree of sampling variation in PBC biopsy specimen reaches 40% even when end stage specimens obtained at transplantation are examined[5,6]. Patient refusal to undergo serial biopsies can further lessen the usefulness of this measure. In addition the staging criteria in PBC are mainly based on fibrosis which once is established rarely is reduced using any current treatment. It has been proposed that specific histological features (ie. cholestasis, bile duct inflammation, bile duct paucity, portal inflammation, piecemeal necrosis etc) could be used in the evaluation of the effects of treatment[7]. However this histologic approach needs standardization in order to provide a practical and better validated end point in future trials.

- **Serum markers of fibrosis:** The problems with the morphological evaluation of the liver biopsies could be avoided if serum markers of fibrosis were to be used as surrogate end points. The measurement of type III aminoterminal peptide of collagen (PNIIIP), and of the noncollageneous proteins hyalouronic acid and laminin have been proposed as promising markers of liver fibrosis and have been already evaluated in a few studies in PBC[8]. These markers may allow a serial and reproducible assessment of the fibrotic process of the liver that could not be achieved by the liver biopsy. Furthermore they could represent a dynamic indicator of fibrogenesis rather than a static indicator of the degree of fibrosis. However to date they have not been validated in PBC for survival or transplantation.

- **Serum biochemistry:** Alterations in serum biochemical variables are the most often used surrogate markers in therapeutic trials of PBC. Although serum transaminases have little prognostic value, increasing serum bilirubin levels are clearly associated with disease progression and worse prognosis in untreated patients[9]. Thus reduction of bilirubin concentrations have been widely used to assess treatment effects. Serum bilirubin together with age, serum albumin, prothrombin time and the presence of ascites/edema have been found to be independently predictive variables for survival using Cox multiple regression analysis[10,11]. These variables have been combined for the development of various prognostic models for the prediction of survival in patients with PBC (ie Mayo[10] and Royal Free Hospital[11] prognostic model). Hence the effect of treatment on every one of these prognostic important variables should be carefully evaluated in the clinical trials of PBC, but this has not always be the case so far.

This approach could overcome the problems associated with using a single surrogate end point - such as the bilirubin in PBC trials- as a substitute for more definite end points such as death and liver transplantation. Fleming and DeMets, in an excellent review of the use of surrogate end points in clinical trials[4], have pointed out that a surrogate must provide a high level of accuracy in predicting the treatment's effect on the true clinical end point, in order to be a valid replacement end point. The authors provide a large number of examples in which biological markers were correlates of clinical outcomes but failed to predict the effect of treatment on the clinical outcome (such as the count as surrogate of survival in HIV infection, blood pressure as surrogate of myocardial infarction and survival in antihypertensive treatment). A significant positive effect of a drug on the surrogate marker in these examples was interpreted as successful drug therapy, when in fact, the drug was associated with lower survival. The main explanation for this apparent paradox is the possibility that the disease process affects the clinical outcome through several causal pathways that are not mediated through the surrogate.

- **Disease remission as an end point:** Treatment efficacy has been also evaluated in chronic liver disease by the induction of disease remission. In the case of PBC a combination of clinical (ie. disappearance of symptoms and resuming of normal daily activities), biochemical (normalization of bilirubin. AST and IgM) and histological remission (inflammation absent or restricted to the portal tracts without bile duct destruction) has been suggested as a short-term target of PBC clinical trials[12]. However this end point has not been proven very useful as the achievement of a complete remission with the currently available drugs has only been reported in small series[13].

Use of Ursodeoxycholic Acid (UDCA)

We have evaluated the effect of ursodeoxycholic acid (UDCA) in randomised, placebo controlled trials in PBC as an example of the problems encountered in evaluating a therapeutic effect. At present UDCA is the drug that is widely prescribed by gastroenterologists and hepatologists as treatment for PBC[7]. UDCA can act in several ways in order to lessen the deleterious effects of cholestasis[14]. Firstly it leads to a replacement of the hydrophobic hepatotoxic bile acids by the hydrophilic and more cholesterol-solubilizing ursodeoxycholate in the bile acid pool. In addition it may directly decrease the toxicity of hepatotoxic bile acids as shown in cultured hepatocytes. Thirdly it has been shown in animals that UDCA could increase bile flow and stabilise hepatocyte membranes and it may do the same in humans. Finally, immunomodulatory properties have recently attributed to UDCA as it may inhibit the expression of cell surface HLA markers and lymphocyte activation and decrease cytokine production. Thus there is a good theoretical basis for the use of UDCA in PBC.

Following the initial report by Poupon et al in 1987[15] of a favorable response of PBC to UDCA, a large number of clinical trials of UDCA treatment in PBC have been reported. We have made a systematic review of these studies including the use of meta-analysis, when applicable, in order to clarify the clinical effect of UDCA on the progression of PBC.

Meta-analysis

Studies included in the systematic review had to fulfil the following criteria: (i) to be published as an abstract or article, (ii) to be randomised, prospective, (iii) to include patients with PBC according to established criteria, (iv) to include patients with a mean follow-up of more than 6 months (v) only placebo controlled comparisons were evaluated. Controlled trials without randomisation or comparing combined treatments were excluded.

Overall ten randomised double-blind placebo controlled trials met the inclusion criteria[16-25]. The extended follow-up, which has been published for 5 of the above studies, was evaluated separately as cross-over from placebo to UDCA, occurred after 2 years. These studies[26-29] were not included in the main analysis as they did not keep a double-blind design throughout the whole study period and they did not fulfil the inclusion criteria. Eight of the 10 studies included in the systemic review were published as peer-reviewed articles[16,18-24] and two in abstract form[17,25], involving 1211 patients. In order to improve the validity of the meta-analysis we have collected data from the principal authors of the abstracts to update information on the main end points. The study population is described in Table 1: 611 patients were randomised to UDCA and 601 to placebo. The mean age ranged from 49 to 57 years and

the mean follow-up, when specified, from 9 to 64 months. The daily dose of UDCA ranged from 7.7 mg/kg to 15 mg/kg. The Mayo risk score, when reported (18,20,23), did not differ significantly between the studies. In most of the studies patients with early (histological stages I and II) and advanced disease (histological stages III and IV) each accounted for approximately 50% of the patients.

- **Symptoms:** None of the studies except one showed any significant effect of UDCA on the predominant symptoms of PBC, pruritus and fatigue. Only Poupon et al[18] showed a beneficial effect of UDCA on the pruritus of PBC when they analysed the data of patients completing the study but not when the analysis was done on an intention to treat basis. Moreover UDCA has no effect on the PBC associated autoimmune phenomena (arthritis, CREST syndrome, Raynaud's phenomenon etc), in the only study which assessed this end point[18].

- **Biochemical values:** UDCA treatment resulted in a statistically significant decrease of serum levels of ALP, γ-GT, ALT and AST (Table 2). UDCA had also a beneficial effect on bilirubin levels in all studies except three[16,17,24] and in IgM levels in 6 studies[16,18,19,21,23,25]. However there was no statistically significant change in the prognostically important parameters of albumin and prothrombin time in any of the studies.

TABLE 1: BASELINE PATIENT CHARACTERISTICS IN RCT OF UDCA v PLACEBO							
First author (ref)	Patients No. UDCA/plac	Mean age (years) UDCA/plac	Duration of trial (months)	UDCA dose mg/kg/d	Mean baseline Bil (µmol/L)	Mayo score UDCA/plac	Histological stage (I/II-III/IV) UDAC/plac
Leuschner 1989[16]	10/10	ND	9	10	ND	ND	9/1-8/2
Hadziyannis 1989[17]	25/25	ND	Up to 24 (mean 19.5)	12-15	ND	ND	ND
Poupon 1991[18]	73/73	54/52	24	13-15	23.2/21.2	4.9/4.8	36/37-42/33
Battezzati 1993[19]	44/44	54/55	6-12 (med 9)	8.7	31.5/32.5	ND	23/21-22/22*
Lindor 1994[20]	89/91	54/52	Up to 48 (mean 24)	13-15	32.3/30.6	5.2/5.1	31/58-26/65
Heathcote 1994[21]	111/111	57.3/55.4	24	14	40/31	ND	50/57-47/60
Turner 1994[22]	22/24	57.5/57.7	24	10	17/17	ND	3/19-5/19
Combes 1995[23]	77/74	49.5/48.9	24	10-12	34/39.1	4.7/4.7	28/49-22/52
Eriksson 1997[24]	60/56	57/57	24	7.7	18.9/18.2	ND	ND
Pares 1997[25]	99/93	ND	Mean 63.6	15	ND	ND	ND
ND: not determined. plac: placebo. *(I/II/III-IV).							

TABLE 2: UDCA EFFECT ON SYMPTOMS AND BIOCHEMISTRY IN RCT OF UDCA v PLACEBO

First author (ref)	UDCA effect on symptoms	UDCA effect on Bilirubin	UDCA effect on ALP, γGT	UDCA effect on AST, ALT	UDCA effect on Albumin	UDCA effect on PT
Leuschner 1989[16]	None	None	Improvement	Improvement	None	None
Hadziyannis 1989[17]		None	Improvement	Improvement	None	ND
Poupon 1991[18]	None	Improvement	Improvement	Improvement	None	None
Battezzati 1993[19]	ND	Improvement	ND	ND	None	ND
Lindor 1994[20]	None	Improvement	Improvement	Improvement	None	ND
Heathcote 1994[21]	None	Improvement	Improvement	Improvement	ND	ND
Turner 1994[22]	None	Improvement	Improvement	Improvement	None	None
Combes 1995[23]	None	Improvement	Improvement	Improvement	None*	None
Eriksson 1997[24]	None	None	Improvement	Improvement	None	None
Pares 1997[25]	None	Improvement	Improvement	Improvement	ND	ND

ND: not determined. *improvement only in subgroup with Bil <2 mg/dL.

Only Combes et al.[23] reported a significant difference in albumin levels between UDCA and placebo but in a subgroup of patients with serum bilirubin of less than 2 mg/dL at baseline and not in their total population. Moreover serum albumin in this subgroup of patients with low bilirubin remained well within the normal values for both the UDCA and placebo treated patients at the end of the two-year study period.

- **Liver histology:** The evaluation of the effect of UDCA on liver histology is more complicated

(Table 3). The main reason is that the studies used different systems comprising various histological features in order to assess the histologic outcome. In some studies a statistically significant improvement of specific histological features (ie. bile duct paucity, ductular proliferation, polymorphonuclear infiltration etc) was reported but in 4 of 8 no improvement was noted[16,19,20,24]. It is also important to note that no study demonstrated any overall beneficial effect of UDCA on hepatic

TABLE 3: EFFECT OF UDCA ON HISTOLOGY IN RCT OF UDCA v PLACEBO

First author (ref)	UDCA effect on stage	UDCA effect on fibrosis	UDCA effect on other parameters
Leuschner 1989[16]	None	None	Beneficial for bile duct inflammation
Hadziyannis 1989[17]	ND	ND	ND
Poupon 1991[18]	None	None	Beneficial for bile duct paucity, lobular inflammation, piecemeal necrosis, parenchymal necrosis
Battezzati 1993[19]	ND	ND	ND
Lindor 1994[20]	None	None	ND
Heathcote 1994[21]	None	None	Beneficial for periportal hepatocellular balooning and Bile duct paucity
Turner 1994[22]	None	None	None
Combes 1995[23]	None	None*	Beneficial for piecemeal necrosis, portal inflammation and cholestasis in stratum 1 and cholestasis in stratum 2
Eriksson 1997[24]	None	None	ND
Pares 1997[25]	Beneficial	ND	ND

ND: not determined; stratum 1: pts with serum bilirubin < 2mg/dL and stage I or II histology; stratum 2: pts with serum bilirubin <2mg/dL and stage III or IV histology. *only in stratum 2.

fibrosis in PBC. Only in the study by Combes et al[23], it was reported that fibrosis was decreased (p= 0.003) in a subgroup of patients - ie. anicteric patients with stage III-IV PBC- but the numbers were small (26 patients on UDCA vs 33 on placebo) and the result is subject to type-2 error. Moreover no study achieved any prevention of the histological stage progression except the most recent one by Pares et al[25]. Although this study is currently published only as an abstract precluding a thorough evaluation, it is noteworthy that follow-up liver biopsy was performed in only 37.5% of the patients that took part in the study. Moreover clinically important end points death and/or liver transplantation were more frequent in the UDCA group despite the improvement in histology.

Results of meta-analysis

Three studies have used the term "treatment failure" as their main end point[18,20,23], while four other studies assessed directly the major clinical end points of death or liver transplantation[21,22,24,25], confounding further the overall evaluation of the efficacy of UDCA. The criteria used to define "treatment failure" varied among the former three studies, including voluntary withdrawal or inability to tolerate the drug (Table 4). However in all of these studies the criterion of an increase in serum bilirubin to a level greater than twice the value at entry was included. In the study by Combes et al.[23] this criterion was almost exclusively accountable for the reported improved outcome of the patients on UDCA (8 patients on UDCA versus 24 on placebo reported with a doubling of bilirubin, while the numbers for "treatment failure" were 43 versus 51 respectively).

For the meta-analysis we chose five clinically meaningful end points in order to estimate the clinical efficacy and morbidity of UDCA treatment: death, transplantation, death or transplantation, the development of complications of liver disease (ascites or GI bleeding) and the incidence of adverse events (Table 5). We also performed a meta-analysis for the end point of "treatment failure", as it was defined by the authors of the studies.

The following statistical techniques were used to analyse the data: the summary odds ratio (OR) and 95% confidence intervals (CI) were calculated from the raw data of the selected studies and heterogeneity tests were performed using the Peto method (fixed effect

TABLE 4: DEFINITION OF TREATMENT FAILURE IN RCT OF UDCA v PLACEBO

First author (ref)	Definition of treatment failure	Doubling of Bil UDCA/placebo	No of pts with treatment failure UDCA/placebo
Leuschner 1989[16]	ND	ND	ND
Hadziyannis 1989[17]	ND	ND	ND
Poupon 1991[18]	Doubling of Bil to >70µmol/L or Bil >200µmol/L – development of ascites/GI bleeding/encephalopathy – adverse effects	3/7	6/13
Battezzati 1993[19]	ND	ND	ND
Lindor 1994[20]	Death-liver transplantation-histological progression by 2 stages or to cirrhosis-developement of varices, ascites, encephalopathy-doubling of Bil (1.5mg/dL)-worsening of pruritus/fatigue-voluntary withdrawal – drug intolerence	2/11*	21/43
Heathcote 1994[21]	Death – Liver Transplantation	ND	12/19
Turner 1994[22]	Death – Liver Transplantation	ND	ND
Combes 1995[23]	Death-liver transplantation-histological progression by 2 stages/cirrhosis-development of varices, variceal bleeding, ascites encephalopathy-doubling of Bil (1.5mg/dL)-worsening of pruritus/fatigue-voluntary withdrawal – drug intolerence	8/24	43/51
Eriksson 1997[24]	Death – Liver Transplantation	ND	5/6
Pares 1997[25]	Death – Liver Transplantation	ND	17/11
ND: not determined; *UDCA (n=60); placebo (n=50).			

TABLE 5: NUMBER OF END POINTS IN RCT OF UDCA v PLACEBO						
First author (ref)	Death UDCA/plac	Transplant-ation UDCA/plac	Death/ Transplant-ation UDCA/plac	Development of ascites/GI bleeding UDCA/plac	Side effects UDCA/plac	Development of varices UDCA/plac
Leuschner 1989[16]	ND	ND	ND	ND	0/0	ND
Hadziyannis 1989[17]	ND	ND	ND	ND	ND	ND
Poupon 1991[18]	4/4	1/1	5/5	2/5	1/1	ND
Battezzati 1993[19]	ND	ND	ND	ND	4/1	ND
Lindor 1994[20]	4/7	3/5	7/12	1/5**	0/0	6/9**
Heathcote 1994[21]	5/9	7/12	12/19	ND	4/6	ND
Turner 1994[22]	1/3	2/1	3/4	ND	4/3	ND
Combes 1995[23]	ND	ND	12/11	15/8	1/1	6/3
Eriksson 1997[24]	1/1	2/3	3/4	1/0	3/0	ND
Pares 1997[25] **	10/4	7/7	17/11	9/12	0/0	ND
plac: placebo; *UDCA (n=60); placebo (n=50); **events by personal communication.						

model)[30] and the Der Simonian and Laird method (random effect model)[31]. Considering the lack of statistical power for heterogeneity testing for the detection and extent of clinically significant heterogeneity, we performed four sensitivity analyses according to: (i) the dose of the drug (two strata: daily dose < 13mg/kg and daily dose > 13 mg/kg), (ii) the duration of treatment (two strata: less than 4 years and equal or more than 4 years), (iii) the type of publication (two strata: full paper and abstract only) and (iv) the mean serum bilirubin level at entry (two strata: < 26 mmol/L and > 26 mmol/L). With regard to the potential mode of action of UDCA these sensitivity analyses are clinically very relevant.

Death

Six studies[18,20-22,24,25] including a total of 902 patients provided information on mortality. There was no statistical heterogeneity in the analysis of this end point. There was no difference in death rate between patients randomised to UDCA compared to those randomised to placebo by the Peto method (OR, 1.137 [95% CI, 0.653-1.981] and the Der Simonian and Laird method (OR, 1.140 [95% CI, 0.657-1.978] (Figure 1). The average number of patients needed to treat (NNT) with UDCA in order to avoid one death was 163 (NNT=163). Sensitivity analyses using the groups mentioned above did not reveal any statistical significance.

Liver transplantation

A total of 6 studies[18,20-22,24,25] involving 902 patients were available for this end point. There was no evidence of statistical heterogeneity in this analysis. The difference

between UDCA and placebo patients was not significant by the Peto method (OR, 1.263 [95% CI, 0.709-2.249] and the Der Simonian and Laird method (OR, 1.237 [95% CI, 0.711-2.152]) (Figure 2). The average number of patients needed to treat with UDCA in order to avoid one liver transplantation was 118 (NNT=118). The results of the four sensitivity analyses did not show any statistical significance.

Death or liver transplantation

Seven studies[18,20-25] involving 1053 patients were available to evaluate this end point. No statistical heterogeneity was identified in this analysis. The difference was not significant by the Peto (OR, 1.158 [95% CI, 0.797-1.685] and the Der Simonian and Laird method (OR, 1.145 [95% CI, 0.794-1.669]) (Figure 3). The average number of patients needed to treat with UDCA in order to avoid one death or liver transplantation was 61 (NNT=61). Sensitivity analyses according to the dose of the drug (excluding studies with daily dose < 13 mg/kg), the duration of treatment (excluding studies with a follow-up less than 4 years), the publication status (excluding studies published only in abstract form) and the mean serum bilirubin at entry (excluding studies with Bil < 26 μmol/L) did not reveal any significant difference. As a result we did not find any significant efficacy of UDCA in any specific subset of patients.

Development of complications (ascites or GI bleeding)

Five studies[18,20,23-25] involving 785 patients provide information for this end point. Considerable heterogeneity was identified in this analysis, although this was not statistically significant. There was no difference on the development of ascites or GI bleeding between the patients randomised to UDCA compared to placebo by the Peto (OR, 1.108 [95% CI, 0.639-1.919] and the Der Simonian and Laird method (OR, 1.187 [95% CI, 0.558-2.526])(Figure 4). From the four sensitivity analyses using the groupings mentioned above, heterogeneity was not present in the analysis including the studies with the high UDCA daily dose but the result was not statistically significant by the Peto (OR, 1.95 [95% CI, 0.957-3.977]) and the Der Simonian and Laird method (OR, 1.852 [95% CI, 0.9-3.787]).

Incidence of side effects

A total of 6 studies[18,19,21-24] involving 810 patients were available for this end point. No statistical heterogeneity was identified. There was no difference on the incidence of side effects between UDCA and placebo patients by the Peto method (OR, 0.685 [95% CI, 0.324-1.451]) and the Der Simonian and Laird method (OR, 0.785 [95% CI, 0.377-1.634])(Figure 5). The results of the four sensitivity analyses did not show any statistically significant difference.

Treatment failure

A total of 7 studies[18,20-25] involving 1053 patients were available for this end point. There was a considerable heterogeneity in this analysis but it was not statistically significant (p=0.12). This is not surprising as the components of treatment failure were different in the various studies (Table 6) and therefore it is questionable whether this end point so differently defined can be used in a meta-analysis. There was statistically significant difference in favour of UDCA on

the incidence of treatment failure by Peto (OR, 1.550 [95% CI, 1.119-2.147]) but not by the Der Simonian and Laird method (OR, 1.464 [95% CI, 0.941-2.278]), which is more robust for the meta-analysis of studies with considerable even not significant heterogeneity (Figure 6). From the four sensitivity analyses only the analysis according to type of publication (excluding the study published as an abstract) showed lack of heterogeneity (p=0.45). In this analysis there was a statistically significant difference in favour of UDCA by both Peto (OR, 1.842 [95% CI, 1.289-2.631]) and Der Simonian and Laird method (OR, 1.811 [95% CI, 1.261-2.601]).

The results of the above meta-analysis clearly showed no benefit in survival or survival free of transplantation from the use of UDCA studied in a population of more than 1000 patients. The number of patients needed to treat with UDCA to prevent one death or liver transplantation is large (NNT=61).

The current cost in the UK of two year UDCA treatment needed to avoid one death or liver transplantation in PBC is estimated to be £85,400 (calculations based on the treatment of a female patient of 60 kg with a dose of 15 mg/kg/d, ie £1,400 over 2 years). Moreover although most of the studies were not designed specifically to evaluate the development of complications of liver disease as an end point, there was no effect of UDCA on this outcome. However if one selects to evaluate the end point of "treatment failure" as it was reported in the studies the results are in favour of UDCA treatment. This discrepancy in the interpretation clearly shows that the results of a meta-analysis based on combined end points can be misleading, especially when the components of a composite end point are defined differently among the studies.

TABLE 6: DEATH AND/OR OLT IN TRIALS OD UDCA v PLACEBO SEPARATING THESE ENDPOINTS INOT RANDOMISED AND CROSS-OVER PHASES

First author	Trial phase	Mean baseline Bil[a] (µmol/L)	Death UDCA/Plac	OLT UDCA/Plac	Death+OLT UDCA/Plac
Poupon	RCT	23.2/21.2	4/4	1/1	5/5
	Cross over	21.2/35.6	2/6	2/13	4/19
Heathcote	RCT	19/18[b]	5/9	7/10	12/17
	Cross-over	13/22[b,c]	10/8	8/4	18/12
Lindor	RCT	32.3/30.6	4/7	3/5	7/12
	Cross-over	ND	ND	ND	ND
Combes	RCT	34/39.1	ND	ND	12/11
	Cross-over	ND	ND	ND	15/18
Eriksson	RCT	18.9/18.2	ND	ND	3/4
	Cross-over	ND	ND	ND	2/3

ND: not determined; [a] Baseline Bil at entry of the cross-over phase is estimated by Bil at the end of original randomised study; [b] Median Bil level; [c] Estimated from Fig 2, ref 19.

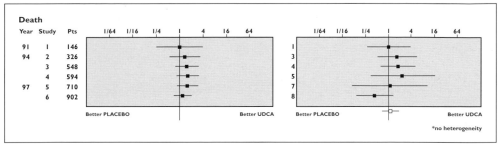

Figure 1.

Mortality in trials comparing UDCA with placebo in the treatment of primary biliary cirrhosis. Cumulative Plot standard (1A) and Plot Standard (1B) graphic representation of ORs (log scale) and CIs of the 6 studies (ranked in chronological order) based on fixed-effect model (Peto method).

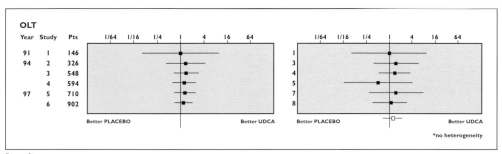

Figure 2.

Liver transplantation in trials comparing UDCA with placebo in the treatment of primary biliary cirrhosis. Cumulative Plot standard (2A) and Plot Standard (2B) graphic representation of ORs (log scale) and CIs of the 6 studies (ranked in chronological order) based on fixed-effect model (Peto method).

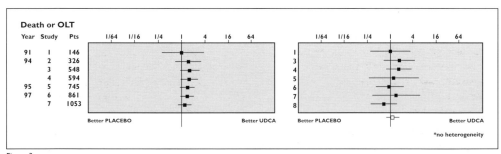

Figure 3.

Mortality or liver transplantation in trials comparing UDCA with placebo in the treatment of primary biliary cirrhosis. Cumulative Plot standard (3A) and Plot Standard (3B) graphic representation of ORs (log scale) and CIs of the 7 studies (ranked in chronological order) based on fixed-effect model (Peto method).

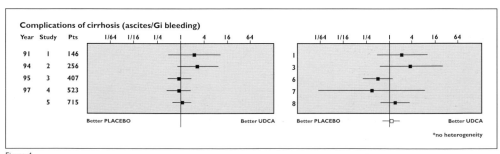

Figure 4.

Complications of cirrhosis (ascites/GI bleeding) in trials comparing UDCA with placebo in the treatment of primary biliary cirrhosis. Cumulative Plot standard (4A) and Plot Standard (4B) graphic representation of ORs (log scale) and CIs of the 5 studies (ranked in chronological order) based on fixed-effect model (Peto method).

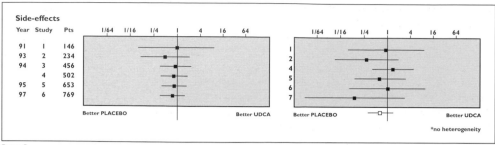

Figure 5.
Side effects in trials comparing UDCA with placebo in the treatment of primary biliary cirrhosis. Cumulative Plot standard (5A) and Plot Standard (5B) graphic representation of ORs (log scale) and CIs of the 6 studies (ranked in chronological order) based on fixed-effect model (Peto method).

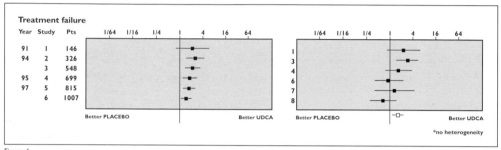

Figure 6.
Treatment failure in trials comparing UDCA with placebo in the treatment of primary biliary cirrhosis. Cumulative Plot standard (2A) and Plot Standard (2B) graphic representation of ORs (log scale) and CIs of the 6 studies (ranked in chronological order) based on fixed-effect model (Peto method).

Evaluation of cross-over period from placebo to UDCA in randomised trials

Four of the groups that conducted the above randomised placebo controlled studies have published reports of the extended follow-up of their study population[24,26-28]. In addition a combined report has been published recently of the extended follow-up of Poupon and Heathcote studies together with the original Mayo study has been published recently[29]. The design of all of these studies is similar: patients originally assigned to placebo switched over to UDCA after the completion of the randomised controlled trial and were followed up for another 2 to 3 years. However the results of these 5 reports are different (Table 6). Three studies[26,28,29] have reported a beneficial effect of UDCA on survival free of transplantation, while in two[24,27] there was no difference between the two treatment arms.

Poupon et al.[26] did not find any statistically significant difference in the rate of death but they reported a statistical significant difference in the rate of referral for liver transplantation. As an increase in serum bilirubin levels is one of the main criteria used in that study for referral for liver transplantation and the main effect of UDCA is a decrease of serum bilirubin levels this finding does not seem surprising. Moreover it seems odd that the UDCA treatment for 2 years was not

shown to be of particular help, for patients originally randomised to placebo. One way to evaluate efficacy given the unblinded design of this part of the study, is to compare the outcome of UDCA treatment in the two groups of patients starting the analysis in both groups from the time of initiation of UDCA treatment up to 2 years of follow-up, perhaps matched for the same or similar prognostic index, or just bilirubin concentration.

The same if not more serious problems occur with the interpretation of the combined analysis of three randomised controlled trials of UDCA[18,20,21] published recently[29]. The original study by Lindor et al.[20] together with the extended follow-up of two other studies[18,21] including their data obtained during the cross-over period were combined in that report. Moreover about 20% of patients originally randomised to placebo were not included in the open phase of the trials. In order to clarify further the issue of poor efficacy in the group of patients originally assigned to placebo, despite the subsequent two year treatment with UDCA, we calculated the incidence of death and liver transplantation during the open phase of the studies of Poupon et al and Heathcote et al. (Table 6). It is surprising that Poupon et al reported 2 deaths and 3 referrals for liver transplantation in the group of patients originally assigned to UDCA and 6 deaths and 12 referrals for liver transplantation in the group originally assigned to placebo during the two year open phase of UDCA treatment. The matter is further complicated by realising that the same group has reported an equal number of events (deaths and liver transplantations) between UDCA and placebo treated patients in their initial double-blind study[18]. The authors explain these results arguing that UDCA might be less efficacious when introduced at a later stage of the disease. However the patients on placebo had a relatively good liver function at the end of the two-year follow-up in their original study with a mean bilirubin level of 17.9 µmol/L, mean albumin 39.8 g/L and normal prothrombin time. On the other hand the results of Heathcote et al seem more plausible and understandable. In the cross-over period they had 10 deaths and 8 liver transplantations in the group originally assigned to UDCA and 8 deaths and 4 liver transplantations in the group originally assigned to placebo. Thus when looking at the combined results of the 3 studies it is obvious that the favourable effect of UDCA comes about solely because of the results of Poupon in the extended open phase part of his study[26]. It is very likely that these results are caused by a biased referral for liver transplantation (4 times as frequent in the patients originally assigned to placebo when given UDCA than when taking placebo) during the open phase of the latter study.

Lindor et al. have also published an extended follow-up report of their original study[28]. The number of events that occurred in the two treatment arms was not provided. This precludes the comparison of the results with those of the above studies. The authors published an efficacy and an intention to treat analysis – censoring the patients receiving placebo at the end of their original randomised study. They showed a statistically significant effect of UDCA on survival without liver transplantation with both analyses and for survival alone, only with the efficacy analysis. They used Cox models, which require that proportionality is maintained in follow-up. This was not so, as censoring occurred in all placebo treated patients at the time of their cross-over to UDCA. In any case because of that censoring of patients from the original placebo group very few events are likely to have occurred to give sufficient statistical power. It would be very helpful if the numbers of patients at risk and the confidence intervals of the survival curves at different time points had been presented. The results of this study require further evaluation.

In contrast to the above results, the extended follow-up of the studies by Combes[27] and Eriksson[24] did not show any difference in survival free of transplantation between the two groups. The first study, with a cross-over phase of three years, was only published in abstract form, which precludes a full evaluation[27]. The negative results of the study may make its publication more difficult. Eriksson et al have given information of both the randomised and cross-over phases of the trial in their recently published paper[24]. The lack of a statistically significant difference remained even when a subgroup analysis was done in both studies (patients stratified according to bilirubin level and histology in the first study and to symptoms in the latter).

Finally the evaluation of the cross-over period of all the above studies would be complete if the data about the clinical and biochemical characteristics of the patients at the initiation of the cross-over phase of UDCA treatment and at the referral for and just before liver transplantation were given.

Trials of UDCA combined with new therapies

The failure of UDCA treatment to show a major benefit on survival or histologic progression in PBC patients together with its failure to induce complete remission in most patients (less than 15% in randomised controlled trials) has prompted several groups to undertake trials of combined treatment of UDCA with either colchicine or methotexate (MTX). These trials are based on the premise that because the mechanisms of action of these drugs are different the potential beneficial effects could be additive. However the results of the first studies do not appear very promising. Poupon et al in a two-year study failed to show a significant imrovement of symptoms, laboratory findings and histological features in patients treated with UDCA-colchicine combination compared with those treated with UDCA alone[32]. Moreover in the case of combined MTX and UDCA treatment was not associated with evidence of symptomatic, biochemical, or histologic improvement over that seen with UDCA alone but in addition resulted in a substantial toxicity (mainly pulmonary toxicity)[33].

RECOMMENDATIONS FOR FUTURE TRIALS

- A large enough randomised, placebo controlled study should be planned to assess death or liver transplantation in PBC. As it will require approximately 1000 patients a multicentre and probably multinational basis will be required. Funding should be sought outside the biomedical industry to avoid bias or prejudice in the trial design, particularly as the average follow-up will be at least 4-5 years.

- It is usually suggested that the assessment of novel therapies for PBC should be in combination with UDCA, compared to UDCA alone. This approach is not justified by our analysis of the existing data on UDCA. Furthermore it could lengthen and thus make more expensive the proper evaluation of the new drug. Hence we believe placebo controlled trials are still justified, although we understand the reticence of clinicians and indeed patients following this course. If UDCA is still used in the control arm, then decrease in bilirubin levels should not be used as a marker of effectiveness as it has not been validated as a surrogate marker for improvement in prognosis.

- There is also a need, to define clinically meaningful end points in PBC trials, eg death, liver transplantation −the indications for the operation and the clinical characteristics of the patients must be stated- and development of complications of liver disease −ie ascites, variceal bleeding and encephalopathy.

- We also suggest the introduction and validation of two potential surrogate end points:

(a) serum markers of fibrosis (ie serum hyaluronate, laminin and type III procollagen, or others) as surrogates of hepatic fibrosis because these are probably as accurate as liver histology and should have less variation due to the possibility of repeated sampling. These factors have shown some predictive value for PBC in previous studies[8], although UDCA had no effect on their serum levels in small studies.

(b) hepatic venous pressure gradient that accurately reflects the portal pressure, as a surrogate for the progression from the presinusoidal to sinusoidal portal hypertension and the development of cirrhosis. This is a safe and simple technique[35] that can be applied and reproduced easily in any trial centre.

REFERENCES

1. Kaplan MM. Primary biliary cirrhosis. *N Engl J Med* 1987; **316**: 521-528.

2. Metcalf JV, Mitchison HC, Palmer JM, Jones DE, Bassendine MF, James OF. Natural history of early primary biliary cirrhosis. *Lancet* 1996; **348**:1399-1402.

3. Poupon RE, Balkau B, Guechot J, Heintzmann F. Predictive factors in ursodeoxycholic acid treated patients with primary biliary cirrhosis: role of serum markers of connective tissue. *Hepatology* 1994; **19**: 635-640.

4. Fleming TR, DeMets DL. Surrogate end points in clinical trials: are we being misled? *Ann Intern Med* 1996; **125**: 605-613.

5. Locke GR III, Therneau TM, Ludwig J, Dickson ER, Lindor KD. Time course of histological progression in primary biliary cirrhosis. *Hepatology* 1996; **23**: 52-56.

6. Garrido MC, Hübscher SG. Accuracy of staging in primary biliary cirrhosis. *J Clin Pathol* 1996; **49**: 556-559.

7. Lindor KD. Primary biliary cirrhosis: Questions and promises. *Ann Intern Med* 1997; **126**: 733-735.

8. Poupon RE, Balkau B, Guéchot J, Heintzmann F. Predictive factors in ursodeoxycholic acid-treated patients with primary biliary cirrhosis: role of serum markers of connective tissue. *Hepatology* 1994; **19**: 635-640.

9. Shapiro JM, Smith H, Schaffner F. Serum bilirubin: a prognostic factor in primary biliary cirrhosis. *Gut* 1979; **20**: 137-140.

10. Dickson ER, Grambsh PM, Fleming TR, Fischer LD, Langworthy A. Prognosis in primary biliary cirrhosis: model for decision making. *Hepatology* 1989; **10**: 1-7.

11. Hughes MD, Raskino CL, Pocock SJ, Biagini MR, Burroughs AK. Prediction of short-term survival with an application in primary biliary cirrhosis. *Stat Med* 1992; **11**: 1731-1745.

12. Beukers R, Schalm SW. Immunosuppressive therapy for primary biliary cirrhosis. *J Hepatol* 1992; **14**: 1-6.

13. Kaplan MM, DeLellis RA, Wolfe HJ. Sustained biochemical and histologic remission of primary biliary cirrhosis in response to medical treatment. *Ann Intern Med* 1997; **126**: 682-688.

14. Lim AG, Jazrawi RP, Northfield TC. The ursodeoxycholic acid story in primary biliary cirrhosis. *Gut* 1995; **37**: 301-304.

15. Poupon R, Chrétien Y, Poupon RE, Ballet F, Calmus Y, Darnis F. Is ursodeoxycholic acid an effective treatment for primary biliary cirrhosis. *Lancet* 1987; **1**: 834-836.

16. Leuschner U, Fischer H, Kurtz W, Guldutuna S, Hubner K, Hellstern A, Gatzen M, *et al.* Ursodeoxycholic acid in primary biliary cirrhosis: results of a controlled double-blind trial. *Gastroenterology* 1989; **97**: 1268-1274.

17. Hadziyannis S, Hadziyannis ES, Makris A. A randomised controlled trial of ursodeoxycholic acid (UDCA) in primary biliary cirrhosis (PBC). (Abstract) *Hepatology* 1989; **10**: 580.

18. Poupon RE, Balkau B, Eschwége E, Poupon R and the UDCA-PBC Study Group. A multicenter controlled trial of ursodiol for the treatment of primary biliary cirrhosis. *N Engl J Med* 1991; **324**: 1548-1554.

19. Battezzati PM, Podda M, Bianchi FB, Naccarrato R, Orlandi F, Surrenti C, Pagliaro L, Manenti F and the Italian Multicenter Group for the Study of UDCA in PBC. Ursodeoxycholic acid for symptomatic primary biliary cirrhosis. Preliminary analysis of a double-blind multicenter trial. *J Hepatol* 1993; **17**: 332-338.

20. Lindor KD, Dickson RE, Baldus WP, Jorgensen RA, Ludwig J, Murtaugh PA, Harrison JM, *et al.* Ursodeoxycholic acid in the treatment of primary biliary cirrhosis. *Gastroenterology* 1994; **106**: 1284-1290.

21. Heathcote JE, Cauch-Dudek K, Walker V, Bailey RJ, Blendis LM, Ghent CN, Michieletti P, *et al.* The Canadian multicenter double-blind randomised controlled trial of ursodeoxycholic acid in primary biliary cirrhosis. *Hepatology* 1994; **19**: 1149-1156.

22. Turner IB, Myszor M, Mitchison HC, Bennett MK, Burt AD, James OFW. A two year controlled trial examining the effectiveness of ursodeoxycholic acid in primary biliary cirrhosis. *J Gastroentrol Hepatol* 1994; **9**: 162-168.

23. Combes B, Carithers RL, Maddrey WC, Lin D, McDonald MF, Wheeler DE, Eigenbrodt EH, *et al.* A randomised, double-blind, placebo-controlled trial of ursodeoxycholic acid in primary biliary cirrhosis. *Hepatology* 1995; **22**: 759-766.

24. Eriksson LS, Olsson R, Glauman H, Prytz H, Befrits R, Rydén BO, Einarsson K, *et al.* Ursodeoxycholic acid treatment in patients with primary biliary cirrhosis. A Swedish multicentre, double-blind, randomised controlled study. *Scand J Gastroenterol* 1997; **32**: 179-186.

25. Parés A for the Spanish Association for the Study of the Liver. Long-term treatment of primary biliary cirrhosis with ursodeoxycholic acid: results of a randomised, double-blind, placebo controlled trial. (Abstract). *J Hepatol* 1997; **26**(Suppl 1): 166.

26. Poupon RE, Poupon R, Balkau B and the UDCA-PBC Study Group. Ursodiol for the long-term treatment of primary biliary cirrhosis. *N Engl J Med* 1994; **330**: 1342-1347.

27. Carithers Jr RL, Luketic VA, Peters M, Zetterman RK, Garcia-Tsao G, Munoz SJ, Combes B. Extended follow-up of patients in the U.S. multicenter trial of ursodeoxycholic acid for primary biliary cirrhosis. (Abstract). *Gastroenterology* 1996; **110**:A1163.

28. Lindor KD, Therneau TM, Jorgensen RA, Malinchoc M, Dickson RE. Effects of ursodeoxycholic acid on survival in patients with primary biliary cirrhosis. *Gastroenterology* 1996; **110**: 1515-1518.

29. Poupon RE, Lindor KD, Cauch-Dudek K, Dickson RE, Poupon R, Heathcote JE. Combined analysis of randomised controlled trials of ursodeoxycholic acid in primary biliary cirrhosis. *Gastroenterology* 1997; **113**: 884-890.

30. Yusuf S, Peto R, Lewis J, Collins R, Sleight P. Beta-blockers during and after myocardial infarction: an overview of the randomised trials: *Prog Cardiovasc Dis* 1985; **27**: 335-371.

31. Der Simonian R, Laird N. Meta-analysis in clinical trials. *Controlled Clin Trials* 1986; **7**: 177-188.

32. Poupon RE, Huet PM, Poupon R, Bonnand AM, Tran Van Nhieu J, Zafrani ES and the UDCA-PBC Study Group. A randomised trial comparing colchicine and ursodeoxycholic acid combination to ursodeoxycholic acid in primary biliary cirrhosis. *Hepatology* 1996; **24**: 1028-1103.

33. Lindor KD, Dickson RE, Jorgensen RA, Anderson ML, Wiesner RH, Gores GJ, Lange SM, *et al*. The combination of ursodeoxycholic acid and methotrexate for patients with primary biliary cirrhosis: the results of a pilot study. *Hepatology* 1995; **22**: 1158-1162.

34. Kim RW, Wiesner RH, Therneau TM, Poterucha JJ, Porayko MK, Evans RW, Klintmalm GB, *et al*. Optimal timing of liver transplantation for primary biliary cirrhosis. *Hepatology* 1998; **28**: 33-38.

35. Armonis A, Patch D, Burroughs A. Hepatic venous pressure measurement: An old test as a new prognostic marker in cirrhosis? *Hepatology* 1997; **25**: 245-248.

PRIMARY BILIARY CIRRHOSIS: TREATMENTS OTHER THAN URSODEOXYCHOLIC ACID

Ulrich Beuers

Department of Medicine II, Klinikum Grosshadern, University of Munich,
Marchioninistrasse 15, D-81377 München, Germany.

SUMMARY

Immunosuppressive and antifibrogenic therapies of PBC are of limited efficacy and/or may induce major side effects during long-term treatment. Therefore, they can not be recommended as a single drug treatment of PBC at present. Combination treatment with UDCA and immunosuppressive (e.g., glucocorticosteroids, methotrexate, azathioprine) and/or antifibrogenic (e.g., colchicine) drugs tailored to the stage of disease are being evaluated in controlled trials. Future therapy of PBC will include a combination of drugs with different mechanisms and sites of action. Further elucidation of the pathogenesis of PBC will be the key for the development of new therapeutic strategies.

During the last 25 years, numerous drugs have been evaluated for the medical treatment of primary biliary cirrhosis (PBC). Treatment strategies were aimed at stopping or retarding the progression of the disease on different levels in the pathogenesis of PBC (Table I). This chapter provides a brief overview on medical therapies other than ursodeoxycholic acid (UDCA) which have been evaluated so far for the treatment of PBC by randomised, controlled trials.

Immunosuppressive treatment of PBC

Azathioprine was one of the first drugs used to suppress the T-cell-mediated destruction of interlobular bile ducts in patients with PBC. Azathioprine exerts its immunosuppressive effect after cleavage and release of mercaptopurine, a purine analogue that inhibits DNA synthesis and clonal proliferation of lymphocytes in the induction phase of the immune response. Two randomised, controlled trials for the treatment of PBC with azathioprine have been published[1-3]. Heathcote *et al.* studied 45 symptomatic, but non-cirrhotic PBC patients of whom 22 received the drug in a dose of 2 mg/kg daily and the others were followed in parallel. Differences in symptoms, biochemical tests and histological features were not observed between the groups. The survival was similar during the first 5 years[1]. In a multicenter European trial which included 248 patients of whom 127 were treated with azathioprine at doses of 0.5-1.5 mg/kg daily Christensen and colleagues observed that survival was slightly,

TABLE I: PATHOGENESIS AND TREATMENT OF PRIMARY BILIARY CIRRHOSIS

Pathogenesis	Therapeutic strategy	Recommendation for long-term monotherapy
T-cell-mediated destruction of interlobular bile ducts	Azathioprine[1-3]	no
	Chlorambucil[5]	no
	Cyclosporin A[7-9]	no
	Glucocorticosteroids[11,12]	no
	Methotrexate[15,16]	no
	Thalidomide[18]	no
Retention of hydrophobic bile acids in hepatocytes	*Ursodeoxycholic acid*	yes
Liver cell damage, apoptosis, necrosis, liver fibrosis, cirrhosis	Colchicine[19-22]	no
	D-Penicillamine[23-30]	no
	Malotilate[31]	no
Liver failure	*Liver transplantation*	

but not significantly longer in the treatment group when a Kaplan-Meier analysis was performed[3]. As patients in the treatment group were sicker (as determined by higher serum bilirubin levels when included in the trial), adjustment for a slight imbalance in serum bilirubin levels at entry into the trial by using a Cox multiple-regression analysis revealed a slight, but significant improvement of survival by 20 months in patients treated with azathioprine. The study was flawed by a considerable drop-out rate: 25.4% of patients were lost to follow-up and 12.1% of patients had to be withdrawn because of putative side effects during the study period. The drug was generally well tolerated. However, its use as a long-term monotherapy of PBC was not generally recommended[4].

Chlorambucil is an alkylating agent which particularly inhibits clonal proliferation in lymphocytes. Chlorambucil was evaluated in one randomised, controlled, but unblinded trial which included 24 symptomatic patients with PBC[5]. The dose of chlorambucil was adjusted to 0.5-4 mg daily in order to keep the lymphocyte count to 50% of the pretreatment level. Under these conditions, a significant decrease of serum bilirubin levels, a strong prognostic marker in PBC[3,6], and of other serum liver tests was observed. In addition, a histomorphological analysis of liver specimens revealed a marked reduction of the inflammatory activity in patients treated with chlorambucil. However, treatment was stopped in 4 patients because of severe bone marrow suppression[5]. Thus, long-term treatment with chlorambucil can not be recommended in PBC.

Cyclosporin A is a cyclic fungal peptide with powerful immunosuppressive activity. It is unique in that it has a relatively selective action on T lymphocytes. It inhibits the transduction pathway for the synthesis of lymphokines, particularly interleukin-2 (IL-2), and impairs the expression of IL-2 receptors on T-cells. Cyclosporin A has been evaluated for the treatment of PBC in 2 short-term trials[7,8] and one large European multicenter trial[9]. This multicenter trial, the largest trial so far for the treatment of PBC, included 349 patients of whom nearly 82 % continued to take the drug or placebo during the follow-up period of 6 years until death, transplantation, or the final analysis. Pruritus improved in patients treated with cyclosporin A. Serum bilirubin levels and other serum liver tests worsened significantly during the trial period in the placebo group when compared to the group treated with cyclosporin A. Survival free of liver transplantation was similar in both groups when analyzed according to Kaplan-Meier. Similar to the large European azathioprine trial[3], however, a slight imbalance between the groups with regard to

disease severity at entry into the study was adjusted by use of a Cox regression analysis and led to a minor improvement in transplant-free survival over a period of 5 years for the group treated with cyclosporin A. However, serum creatinine levels increased significantly in the cyclosporin A group to above 150 µmol/L in 9% of patients and drug-induced arterial hypertension required dose reduction of cyclosporin A in 11% of patients[9]. Thus, these data barely justify the use of cyclosporin A for long-term treatment of PBC.

Glucocorticoids have been considered but assessed unsuitable (because of steroid-induced osteoporosis) for the treatment of PBC as early as 1960[10]. Prednisolone and other glucocorticoids exert a multitude of immunosuppressive effects which lead to a depression of clonal T-cell expansion by impaired interaction of resting T-cells with antigen presenting cells and depressed secretion of lymphokines such as IL2 by T-cells. Only one randomised, placebo-controlled trial on prednisolone monotherapy in PBC has been published so far[11,12]. This trial included 36 patients with PBC. It did not show significant differences but only a trend in favor of prednisolone between the groups for symptoms, serum liver tests, and liver histology[12]. A score for "overall hepatic assessment" which included criteria such as hepatic death, doubling of raised bilirubin, fall in albumin by more than 6g/L, new symptoms of portal hypertension, or new appearance of cirrhosis was in favor of the prednisolone group. A significant progression of osteoporosis was not observed in this trial, but osteodensitometry was not performed in the axial skeleton which is mostly affected by osteoporosis in patients with chronic cholestatic liver disease. Thus, it was recommended by others that glucocorticoids should be evaluated with caution and only in controlled clinical trials in which bone loss is closely monitored[4].

Vertebral bone loss during glucocorticoid treatment in PBC was assessed by a small controlled pilot study which compared patients with PBC treated with prednisone with those treated with prednisone and the bisphosphonate etidronate. A significant difference in change of vertebral bone density was observed betweeen the placebo and the etidronate group after one year of treatment[13].

Use of locally acting glucocorticoids with only limited systemic side effects such as budesonide or of combination treatments with glucocorticoids and bisphosphonates are under evaluation. At present, the use of glucocorticoids for long-term monotherapy of PBC can not be recommended.

Methotrexate is a folate antagonist which affects the immune response at different sites: it inhibits lymphokine secretion by T-cells and impairs lymphokine binding to receptors, and thereby reduces the clonal expansion of T-cells. It has been proposed for the treatment of PBC[14]. At present, however, only case studies, but no randomised, controlled trials have been published on the effect of methotrexate as a single drug treatment in PBC[15, 16]. Although some improvement in serum liver tests and liver histology was reported in a subgroup of patients during long-term treatment with low doses of methotrexate (15 mg/week), it needs to be mentioned that methotrexate may induce serious complications, for example pneumonitis may evolve in up to 15% of patients[17]. Controlled studies are awaited, and a large multicenter trial is comparing UDCA monotherapy with a combined treatment of UDCA and methotrexate in PBC at present.

Thalidomide has been reported to be an effective treatment of steroid-resistant graft-versus-host disease (GVHD). GVHD of the liver presents with histomorphological features similar to those observed in liver specimens of PBC. In a small double-blind, randomised, placebo-controlled pilot study, thalidomide did not affect serum liver tests and liver histomorphology in patients with PBC indicating that thalidomide is not effective in PBC[18].

Antifibrogenic treatment of PBC

Colchicine inhibits collagen synthesis and increases collagen degradation in vitro at high pharmacological concentrations. In addition, colchicine modulates lymphokine secretion of macrophages and lymphocytes, and inhibits endothelial adhesiveness of neutrophils. Four randomised, controlled trials in the treatment of PBC with colchicine have been published[19-22]. One of them reported significant beneficial effects of colchicine on serum liver tests including the prognostic marker bilirubin and a trend towards improved survival[19]. This trial, however, was flawed by exclusion from analysis of 2 deaths (unrelated to the liver disease) and one severely ill patient in the colchicine group. The other trials which followed more stringent statistical criteria were unable to observe a difference in survival between the groups although a trend towards improvement for serum liver tests was observed[20-22]. The drug was mostly well tolerated. Thus, some beneficial

effect of colchicine on serum liver tests may be expected in PBC. However, no clear effect has been shown for symptoms of disease, for histological features and for survival. Colchicine is, therefore, not recommended for long-term monotherapy in patients with PBC.

D-penicillamine was introduced to stimulate urinary copper excretion in patients with PBC as demonstrated before in the treatment of Wilson's disease. Livers of patients with chronic cholestatic liver disease are overloaded with copper due to impairment of biliary copper excretion, and hepatic copper accumulation was assumed to play a pathogenetic role in PBC. An additional antifibrogenic effect of D-penicillamine may be explained by impairment of crosslinking of collagen as observed in vitro. In addition, an immuno-modulatory effect has been described which is characterized by reduction of circulating T-cells and impairment of T-cell function. D-Penicillamine was tested in 8 controlled trials including 740 patients with PBC[23-30]. These trials did not observe beneficial effects of D-Penicillamine on symptoms, biochemical test, histological features, and survival. In contrast, severe side effects including proteinuria, allergic drug reactions, or bone marrow suppression were observed in a third of patients Thus, D-Penicillamine should not be used for treatment of PBC.

Malotilate was first introduced in Japan and had shown some antifibrotic and antisteatotic activity in experimental animals and improvement of serum liver tests in patients with cirrhosis of variable origin. In a randomised, double-blind, controlled multicenter trial, 101 patients with PBC were treated with 500 mg malotilate or placebo three times daily[31]. The drug was well tolerated in most patients and was withdrawn in 6 patients due to gastrointestinal complaints. After a mean follow-up of 28 months, symptoms were not affected by treatment, whereas some serum liver tests including alkaline phosphatase, AST and ALT improved significantly. There was improvement in a number of histological features including lymphocyte and plasma cell infiltration and piecemeal necrosis, but not fibrosis. The survival was not affected during the observation period. Thus, the observed benefits appeared limited and malotilate is not recommended for long-term treatment of PBC.

REFERENCES

1. Heathcote J, Ross A, Sherlock S. A prospective controlled trial of azathioprine in primary biliary cirrhosis. Gastroenterology 1976; 70: 656-660.

2. Crowe J, Christensen E, Smith M, Cochrane M, Ranek L, Watkinson G, et al. Azathioprine in primary biliary cirrhosis: a preliminary report of an international trial. Gastroenterology 1980; 78: 7005-1010.

3. Christensen E, Neuberger J, Crowe J, Altman DG, Popper H, Portmann B, et al. Beneficial effect of azathioprine and prediction of prognosis in primary biliary cirrhosis. Final results of an international trial. Gastroenterology 1985; 89: 1084-1091.

4. Wiesner RH, Grambsch PM, Lindor KD, Ludwig J, Dickson ER. Clinical and statistical analyses of new and evolving therapies for primary biliary cirrhosis. Hepatology 1988; 8: 668-676.

5. Hoofnagle JH, Davis GL, Schafer DF, Peters M, Avigan MI, Pappas SC, et al. Randomised trial of chlorambucil for primary biliary cirrhosis. *Gastroenterology* 1986; **91**: 1327-1334.

6. Dickson ER, Grambsch PM, Fleming TR, Fisher LD, Langworthy A. Prognosis in primary biliary cirrhosis: model for decision making. *Hepatology* 1989; **10**: 1-7.

7. Minuk GY, Bohme CE, Burgess E, Hershfield NB, Kelly JK, Shaffer EA, et al. Pilot study of cyclosporin A in patients with symptomic primary biliary cirrhosis. *Gastroenterology* 1988; **95**: 1356-1363.

8. Wiesner RH, Ludwig J, Lindor KD, Jorgensen RA, Baldus WP, Homburger HA, et al. A controlled trial of cyclosporine in the treatment of primary biliary cirrhosis. *N Engl J Med* 1990; **322**: 1419-1424.

9. Lombard M, Portmann B, Neuberger J, Williams R, Tygstrup N, Ranek L, et al. Cyclosporin A treatment in primary biliary cirrhosis: results of a long-term placebo controlled trial. *Gastroenterology* 1993; **104**: 519-526.

10. Hoffbauer FW. Primary biliary cirrhosis. Observation on the natural course of the disease in 25 women. *Am J Dig Dis* 1960; **5**: 348-383.

11. Mitchison HC, Bassendine MF, Malcolm AJ, Watson AJ, Record CO, James OF. A pilot, double-blind, controlled 1-year trial of prednisolone treatment in primary biliary cirrhosis: hepatic improvement but greater bone loss. *Hepatology* 1989; **10**: 420-429.

12. Mitchison HC, Palmer JM, Bassendine MF, Watson AJ, Record CO, James OF. A controlled trial of prednisolone treatment in primary biliary cirrhosis. Three-year results. *J Hepatol* 1992; **15**: 336-344.

13. Wolfhagen FH, van Buuren HR, den Ouden JW, Hop WC, van Leeuwen JP, Schalm SW, et al. Cyclical etidronate in the prevention of bone loss in corticosteroid-treated primary biliary cirrhosis. A prospective, controlled pilot study. *J Hepatol* 1997; **26**: 325-330.

14. Kaplan MM. The use of methotrexate, colchicine, and other immunomodulatory drugs in the treatment of primary biliary cirrhosis. *Semin Liver Dis* 1997; **17**: 129-136.

15. Kaplan MM, Knox TA. Treatment of primary biliary cirrhosis with low-dose weekly methotrexate. *Gastroenterology* 1991; **101**: 1332-1338.

16. Kaplan MM, DeLellis RA, Wolfe HJ. Sustained biochemical and histologic remission of primary biliary cirrhosis in response to medical treatment. *Ann Intern Med* 1997; **126**: 682-688.

17. Lindor KD, Dickson ER, Jorgensen RA, Anderson ML, Wiesner RH, Gores GJ, et al. The combination of ursodeoxycholic acid and methotrexate for patients with primary biliary cirrhosis: the results of a pilot study. *Hepatology* 1995; **22**: 1158-1162.

18. McCormick PA, Scott F, Epstein O, Burroughs AK, Scheuer PJ, McIntyre N. Thalidomide as therapy for primary biliary cirrhosis: a double-blind placebo controlled pilot study. *J Hepatol* 1994; **21**: 496-499.

19. Kaplan MM, Alling DW, Zimmerman HJ, Wolfe HJ, Sepersky RA, Hirsch GS, et al. A prospective trial of colchicine for primary biliary cirrhosis. *N Engl J Med* 1986; **315**: 1448-1454.

20. Warnes TW, Smith A, Lee FI, Haboubi NY, Johnson PJ, Hunt L. A controlled trial of colchicine in primary biliary cirrhosis. Trial design and preliminary report. *J Hepatol* 1987; **5**: 1-7.

21. Bodenheimer H, Jr., Schaffner F, Pezzullo J. Evaluation of colchicine therapy in primary biliary cirrhosis. *Gastroenterology* 1988; **95**: 124-129.

22. Vuoristo M, Farkkila M, Karvonen AL, Leino R, Lehtola J, Makinen J, et al. A placebo-controlled trial of primary biliary cirrhosis treatment with colchicine and ursodeoxycholic acid. *Gastroenterology* 1995; **108**: 1470-1478.

23. Triger DR, Manifold IH, Cloke P, Underwood JCE. D-penicillamin in primary biliary cirrhosis: two year results of a single center double-blind controlled trial (Abstract). *Gut* 1980; **21**: 919-920.

24. Epstein O, Jain S, Lee RG, Cook DG, Boss AM, Scheuer PJ. D-penicillamin treatment improves survival in primary biliary cirrhosis. *Lancet* 1981; **1**: 1275-1277.

25. Bassendine MF, Macklon AF, Mulcahy R, James OFW. Controlled trial of high and low dose D-penicillamine in primary biliary cirrhosis (Abstract). *Gut* 1982; **23**: 909.

26. Matloff DS, Alpert E, Resnick RH, Kaplan MM. A prospective trial of D-penicillamine in primary biliary cirrhosis. *N Engl J Med* 1982; **306**: 319-326.

27. Taal BG, Schalm SW, Tenkate FW, van Berge Henegouwen GP, Brandt KH. Low therapeutic value of D-penicillamin in a short-term prospective trial in primary biliary cirrhosis. *Liver* 1983; **3**: 345-352.

28. Neuberger J, Christensen E, Portmann B, Caballeria J, Rodes J, Ranek L, et al. Double blind controlled trial of d-penicillamine in patients with primary biliary cirrhosis. *Gut* 1985; **26**: 114-119.

29. Bodenheimer HC, Jr., Schaffner F, Sternlieb I, Klion FM, Vernace S, Pezzullo J. A prospective clinical trial of D-penicillamine in patients with primary biliary cirrhosis. *Hepatology* 1985; **5**: 1139-1142.

30. Dickson ER, Fleming TR, Wiesner RH, Baldus WP, Fleming CR, Ludwig J, et al. Trial of penicillamine in advanced primary biliary cirrhosis. *N Engl J Med* 1985; **312**: 1011-1015.

31. A European multicentre study group. The results of a randomised double blind controlled trial evaluating malotilate in primary biliary cirrhosis. *J Hepatol* 1993; **17**: 227-235.

PRIMARY BILIARY CIRRHOSIS: RATIONALE FOR THE USE OF URSODEOXYCHOLIC ACID

Gustav Paumgartner

Department of Medicine II, Klinikum Grosshadern,
Marchioninistrasse 15, D-81377 Munich, Germany.

SUMMARY

Ursodeoxycholic Acid (UDCA) is normally present in human bile in a low concentration. UDCA is a hydrophilic bile acid with little cytotoxic potential. The mode of action of UDCA in patients with PBC and other cholestatic conditions is not clear but may relate to protection of cell membranes against the detergent effects of more hydrophobic bile acids and to co-stimulation of biliary secretion of endogenous hydrophobic bile acids. It remains uncertain the extent to which these properties of UDCA are important *in vivo* and how they relate to the therapeutic effects of UDCA that have been observed.

The best rationale for the use of any drug is an effect on the cause of the disease. If the cause is not known, a rational therapeutic approach must be aimed at influencing later stages of the pathogenesis. In primary biliary cirrhosis the cause of the disease is not known. The disease presents with features of an autoimmune disease that lead to the destruction of interlobular bile ducts by an inflammatory bile duct lesion (small duct cholangiopathy) and small duct obstruction[1]. The further pathogenetic processes include aggravation of the bile duct lesion by endogenous hydrophobic bile acids, retention of bile acids in the hepatocytes, liver cell injury, apoptosis, necrosis, fibrosis and cirrhosis.

At least two of these processes appear to be *major therapeutic targets* of ursodeoxycholic acid (UDCA) therapy, namely i) the *aggravation of the bile duct lesion by hydrophobic bile acids,* and ii) the *retention of bile acids* in the hepatocytes.

Since injury of cholangiocytes by the detergent actions of endogenous hydrophobic bile acids is considered to be an important pathogenetic factor, one rationale for UDCA has been to enrich the bile acid pool with the hydrophilic non-toxic bile acid, UDCA. Another rationale has been to use the effect of UDCA on bile formation in order to stimulate bile acid secretion and by this way lower the levels of hydrophobic bile acids and other potentially toxic cholephils in the hepatocyte. A third rationale has been derived from experimental evidence that ursodeoxycholic acid therapy of cholestasis is followed by changes in the immune system which may be beneficial in primary biliary cirrhosis.

The following potential mechanisms of action of UDCA will be discussed:

1. Protection of cell membranes against the detergent effects of hydrophobic bile acids.

2. Stimulation of biliary secretion of endogenous hydrophobic bile acids and other cholephils.

3. Reduction of MHC expression.

Protection of cell membranes

UDCA is normally present in human bile, albeit in low concentration. It is a hydrophilic bile acid which practically lacks cytotoxic potential when compared to other bile acids of human bile. The cytotoxic potential of bile acids is related to their detergency which increases with relative hydrophobicity as estimated by reverse-phase high-pressure liquid chromatography in the order tauroursodeoxycholic acid < taurocholic acid < taurochenodeoxycholic acid < taurodeoxycholic acid[2]. It has, therefore, been postulated that enrichment of the bile acid pool with UDCA might be beneficial in chronic cholestasis.

Under ursodeoxycholic acid treatment, the biliary bile acid composition becomes enriched with ursodeoxycholic acid[3]. After six months of ursodeoxycholic acid treatment of patients with primary biliary cirrhosis, ursodeoxycholic acid in bile increases to nearly 40% of total bile acids, rendering the bile acid composition less detergent. This may reduce bile acid injury at the site of the bile duct lesion in primary biliary cirrhosis. Heuman et al.[4] have shown that the physicochemical disruptive effects of bile acids towards membranes are a function of both concentration and hydrophobicity. As an index of canalicular disruption, the solubilization of the structural canalicular ectoenzyme alkaline phosphatase under various *in vitro* conditions was studied[5]. The hydrophobic bile acid taurodeoxycholic acid caused a release of alkaline phosphatase from the canalicular membranes. This effect was inhibited by tauro-ursodeoxycholic acid. The magnitudes of these disruptive and protective effects were not only dependent upon the concentrations of the bile acids, but also on the concentrations of lipids. Lecithin: cholesterol vesicles at concentrations found in bile markedly reduced the disruption of canalicular membranes by taurodeoxy-cholic acid. This confirms previous findings that phospholipids can reduce the cytolytic effects of bile acids towards hepatocytes[6].

The mdr2 knock-out mouse has been an excellent model to study the protective effects of UDCA[7]. Normally, the cholangiocytes are protected against the detergent effects of bile acids by phospholipids, which are secreted by the mdr2 P-glycoprotein. This protection results from the incorporation of the bile acids into mixed micelles with phospholipids. In the mdr2 knock out mouse, phospholipid transport is defective and phospholipids in bile are practically absent. As a consequence, the biliary epithelium is not protected by phospholipids against the detergent actions of hydrophobic bile acids. A form of non-suppurative destructive cholangitis with chronic cholestatic liver disease develops. The liver histopathology is that of a non-suppurative destructive cholangitis, which results in a vanishing bile duct lesion[7].

Under a normal control diet, the cholestatic liver disease, evaluated by a histological score progressed with time[7]. When cholic acid was added to the diet, the histological progression of the disease was even more pronounced. By contrast, addition of UDCA to the diet prevented the progression of this cholestatic liver disease. UDCA feeding renders the biliary bile acid composition less hydrophobic and less detergent and thus diminishes the detergent actions of endogenous hydrophobic bile acids on the bile duct epithelium.

Stimulation of biliary secretion

Another important mechanisms of action of UDCA appears to be stimulation of biliary secretion of hydrophobic bile acids and other potentially toxic cholephils. This reduces the retention of potentially toxic bile acids in the hepatocyte. Kitani et al.[8,9] have shown that in the presence of ursodeoxycholic acid, the liver can secrete a hydrophobic bile acid such as chenodeoxycholic acid at a rate that would otherwise be toxic. When taurochenodeoxycholic acid was infused in the bile fistula rat at a high infusion rate bile flow decreased and cholestasis occurred. At the same time lactate dehydrogenase (LDH) excretion into the bile, a sign of toxic liver cell injury, increased. During simultaneous infusion of tauroursodeoxycholic acid

with taurochenodeoxycholic acid, secretion of bile acids and bile flow increased and LDH excretion into the bile was negligible. Thus, ursodeoxycholic acid can overcome the cholestasis caused by hydrophobic bile acids.

Jazrawi et al.[10] have shown that ursodeoxycholic acid increases the net hepatic excretion rate of 75 Se homocholic acid taurine in patients with primary biliary cirrhosis. Stiehl et al.[11] have recently measured the effect of ursodeoxycholic acid on bile acid secretion directly. By duodenal perfusion studies, they could demonstrate that ursodeoxycholic acid increases the hourly secretion rate of endogenous bile acids in patients with primary sclerosing cholangitis and elevated bilirubin. Phospholipid secretion also increased in these patients. This additional effect may be of importance in view of the role of phospholipids in protecting the biliary epithelium against the detergent effects of bile acids.

The increased biliary secretion of bile acids under UDCA treatment enhances the elimination of endogenous hydrophobic bile acids from the blood. Together with Poupon et al.[12] we could demonstrate that UDCA treatment decreased the serum concentration of chenodeoxycholic acid in patients with primary biliary cirrhosis while placebo had no effect.

Ursodeoxycholic acid stimulates not only the secretion of bile acids but also that of certain other cholephils. Colombo et al.[13] could demonstrate that in patients with cystic fibrosis the half-time of the hepatic washout of the biliary scintigraphic agent 99mTc-labelled trimethyl-bromo-iminodiacetic acid (TMBIDA) decreased after treatment with ursodeoxycholic acid. Organic anions like TMBIDA are transported into the bile by the multidrug resistance-associated protein 2 (MRP2).

It has been suggested that UDCA enhances the biliary secretion of bile acids and other organic anions by stimulation of exocytotic insertion of carrier molecules into the canalicular membrane of the hepatocyte[14]. The excretory transport capacity of the hepatocyte depends on the balance between the insertion into and retrieval of carrier molecules from the camalicular membrane. Beuers et al.[14-16] have shown that tauroursodeoxycholic acid increases cytosolic Ca++, translocates alpha-protein kinase C to the membrane, activates alpha-protein kinase C and, via these signalling pathways, stimulates hepatocellular exocytosis, a mechanism that is defective in cholestasis. Schliess et al.[17] have recently identified another signalling pathway, involving the activation of the MAP kinases Erk-1 and Erk-2, by which ursodeoxycholic acid could stimulate the exocytotic insertion of carrier proteins into the canalicular membrane. Via these mechanisms, canalicular carrier proteins such as the canalicular bile salt export pump

(BSEP), previously designated sister of P-glycoprotein (SPGP), the multidrug resistance-associated protein 2 (MRP2) and the chloride-bicarbonate anion exchanger 2 (AE2) may be directed towards and inserted into the canalicular membrane. This would increase the capacity of the hepatocyte for the secretion of both bile acids and other organic anions. Medina et al.[18] showed that the expression of the anion exchanger 2 (AE2), a carrier protein important for bile acid independent bile secretion which is diminished in primary biliary cirrhosis, increases under UDCA treatment.

Based on recent evidence, it may be speculated that UDCA also stimulates cholangiocellular bile secretion. Ursodeoxycholic acid stimulates Ca^{2+}-dependent Cl^- currents in a biliary cell line[19]. If these findings are relevant to native bile duct epithelial cells, ursodeoxycholic acid could, by increasing Cl^- efflux from bile duct epithelial cells into bile, stimulate cholangiocellular bile formation[20]. Thereby it could, by diluting hepatocellular bile, diminish cytotoxic effects of hydrophobic bile acids towards the bile duct epithelium.

Reduction of MHC expression

It has been suggested that the reduced expression of certain antigens of the major histocompatibility complex (MHC) observed under UDCA therapy contributes to the beneficial effects of UDCA. In primary biliary cirrhosis, MHC class I antigens are aberrantly expressed on hepatocytes and overexpressed on biliary epithelial cells, whereas MHC class II antigens are aberrantly expressed on biliary epithelial cells. Calmus et al.[21] showed that aberrant expression of MHC class I antigens on hepatocytes is considerably reduced in patients treated with ursodeoxycholic acid, while there is no detectable change of MHC class II antigens. MHC class I antigens are not only overexpressed on hepatocytes of patients with primary biliary cirrhosis, but also on hepatocytes of patients with extrahepatic cholestasis[22]. Therefore, the effects of ursodeoxycholic acid on MHC-expression in the liver of patients with primary biliary cirrhosis could be related to the improvement of cholestasis rather than to a direct effect of ursodeoxycholic acid on the immune system. Whatever the mechanism may be, the decrease of MHC expression may diminish immunologic attack by cytotoxic T-cells. It is unclear whether the effects of ursodeoxycholic acid on MHC expression contribute to the beneficial effects of ursodeoxycholic acid in primary biliary cirrhosis[23].

REFERENCES

1. Paumgartner G. Pathogenetic clasification of cholestasis. Proceedings of the International Symposium on Complications of Liver Cirrhosis. P. Gentilini, Ed., Elba 1998 (in press).

2. Heuman DM. Quantitative estimation of the hydrophobic – hydrophilic balance of mixed bile salt solutions. J Lipid Res. 1989; 30: 719-730.

3. Crosignani A, Podda M, Battezzati PM, Bertolini E, Zuin M, Watson D, Setchell KDR. Changes in bile acid composition in patients with primary biliary cirrhosis induced by ursodeoxycholic acid administration. Hepatology 1991; 14: 1000-1007.

4. Heuman DM, Bajaj RS. Ursodeoxycholic conjugates protect against disruption of cholesterol-rich membranes by bile salts: a possible physicochemical basis for the hepatoprotective action of ursodeoxycholate. Gastroenterology 1994; 106: 1333-1341.

5. Heuman DM. Disruptive and protective interactions of bile salts, cholesterol: lecithin vesicles, and canalicular membranes. In: Hofmann AF, Paumgartner G, Stiehl A, eds. Bile acids in Gastroenterology. Kluwer, Lancaster, 1995, 283-289.

6. Puglielli L, Amigo L, Arrese M et al. Protective role of biliary cholesterol and phospholipid lamellae against bile acid-induced cell damage. Gastroenterology 1994; 107: 244-254.

7. Van Niewkerk CMJ, Oude Elferink RPJ, Groen AK, Ottenhoff R, Tytgat GNJ, Dingemans KP, van den Bergh Weerman MA, Offerhaus GJA. Effects of ursodeoxycholate and cholate feeding on liver disease in FVB mice with a disrupted mdr2 P-glycoprotein gene. Gastroenterology 1996; 111: 165-171.

8. Kitani K, Ohta M, Kanai S. Tauroursodeoxycholate prevents the hepatocellular damage caused by other bile salts in the rat. Am J Physiol 1985; 248: G407-G417.

9. Kitani K. Hepatoprotective effect of ursodeoxycholate in experimental animals. In: Paumgartner G, Stiehl A, Barbara L, Roda E, Editors. Strategies for the treatment of hepatobiliary diseases. Kluwer, Dordrecht 1990, 43-56.

10. Jazrawi RP, de Caestecker JS, Goggin PM, Britten AJ, Joseph AEA, Maxwell JD, Northfield TC. Kinetics of hepatic bile acid handling in cholestatic liver disease: effect of ursodeoxycholic acid. Gastroenterology 1994; 106: 134-142.

11. Stiehl A, Rudolph G, Sauer P, Theilmann L. Biliary secretion of bile acids and lipids in primary sclerosing cholangitis. Influence of cholestasis and effect of ursodeoxycholic acid treatment. J Hepatol 1995; 23: 283-289.

12. Poupon RE, Chrétien Y, Poupon R, Paumgartner G. Serum bile acids in primary biliary cirrhosis: effect of ursodeoxycholic acid therapy. Hepatology 1993; 17: 599-604.

13. Colombo C, Castellani MR, Balistreri WF, Seregni E, Assaido ML, Giunta A. Scintigraphic documentation of an improvement in hepatobiliary excretory function after treatment with ursodeoxycholic acid in patients with cystic fibrosis and associated liver disease. Hepatology 1992; 15: 677-684.

14. Beuers U, Nathanson MH, Isales CM, Boyer JL. Tauroursodeoxycholic acid stimulates hepatocellular exocytosis and mobilizes extracellular Ca++, mechanisms defective in cholestasis. J Clin Invest 1993; 92: 2984-2993.

15. Beuers U, Nathanson MH, Boyer JL. Effects of tauroursodeoxycholic acid on cytosolic Ca++ signals in isolated rat hepatocytes. Gastroenterology 1993; 104: 604-612.

16. Beuers U, Throckmorton DC, Anderson MS, Isales CM, Thasler W, Kullak-Ublick GA, Sauter G, Koebe HG, Paumgartner G, Boyer JL. Tauroursodeoxycholic acid activates protein kinase C in isolated rat hepatocytes. Gastroenterology 1996; 110: 1553-1563.

17. Schliess F, Kurz AK, vom Dahl S, Häussinger D. Mitogen-activated protein kinases mediate the stimulation of bile acid secretion by taurourso-deoxycholate in rat liver. Gastroenterology 1997; 113: 1306-1314.

18. Medina JF, Martínez-Anso E, Vázquez JJ, Prieto J. Decreased anion exchanger 2 immunoreactivity in the liver of patients with primary biliary cirrhosis. Hepatology 1997; 25: 12-17.

19. Shimokura GH, McGill JM, Schlenker, T, Fitz JG. Ursodeoxycholate increases cytosolic calcium concentration and activates Cl- currents in a biliary cell line. *Gastroenterology* 1995; **109**: 965-972.

20. Roman R, Schlenker T, Fitz JG. Ursodeoxycholic acid activates Ca2+-dependent Cl- currents in a human biliary cell line. In: Paumgartner G, Stiehl A, Gerok W, Eds. Bile acids in hepatobiliary diseases: basic research and clinical application. Kluwer Academic Publishers, *Dordrecht* 1997, 219-223.

21. Calmus Y, Gane R, Rouger P, Poupon R. Hepatic expression of class I and class II major histocompatibility complex molecules in primary biliary cirrhosis: effect of ursodeoxycholic acid. *Hepatology* 1990; **11**: 12-15.

22. Calmus Y, Arvieux C, Gane R. *et al.* Cholestasis induces major histocompatibility complex class I in hepatocytes. *Gastroenterology* 1992; **102**: 1371-1377.

23. Neuberger J. Immune effects of ursodeoxycholic acid. In: Berg P, Lohse AW, Tiegs G, Wendel A, Eds. Autoimmune liver disease. Kluwer Academic Publishers, *Dordrecht* 1997, 93-103.

URSODEOXYCHOLIC ACID TREATMENT OF PBC: ALONE AND IN COMBINATION

Keith D Lindor

Mayo Clinic and Foundation
Rochester, MN, USA.

SUMMARY

- Ursodeoxycholic acid is an extremely safe drug for use in patients with primary biliary cirrhosis.

- A dose of 13-15 mg/kg/day seems like the best dose to be used.

- Patients of all stages of PBC are eligible for trial of treatment. Patients with far-advanced disease also need to be prepared for liver transplantation, but the use of ursodeoxycholic acid prior to transplantation is not detrimental.

- Ursodeoxycholic acid improves survival free of transplantation, reduces serum lipid level, particularly cholesterol, reduces the risk of developing varices, retards histologic progression to cirrhosis, and is a cost-effective therapy.

- There doesn't appear to be any obvious benefit to adding colchicine or methotrexate, although corticosteroids might be of potential advantage, particularly if their effects on inducing osteopenia can be avoided.

Ursodeoxycholic acid (UDCA) has recently taken its place as the only approved therapy for the treatment of primary biliary cirrhosis. This advance was brought about by investigators around the world working collaboratively in multi-centered trials. Progress was particularly sped along by the willingness of investigators to share data, providing a chance for analysis of a combined data set. In this section, individual studies will be discussed, the results of the combined analysis will be reviewed, other effects of ursodeoxycholic acid will be described, means of predicting response will be considered and efforts at enhancing this response using different doses of ursodeoxycholic acid or other drugs will be reviewed.

UDCA ALONE

There are several large studies each with over a 100 patients that have been reported using ursodeoxycholic acid. These are shown in Table 1.

These studies were generally of a duration of two years and included between 116 to 222 patients. The doses varied between an average of 7.7mg/kg/day to 15mg/kg/day of UDCA. All studies demonstrated improvement in biochemistries; histologic improvement was hinted at in two, and reduction in rate of treatment failure was noted in two of these studies. In all of these studies UDCA was well tolerated. Two of the studies had the follow-up extended and in these studies improvement in survival free of transplantation was noted after four to six years[6,7].

Three of the studies were combined that used a dose of between 13-15 mg/kg/day[8]. A significant improvement in survival free of transplantation was noted at 48 months. These results were even more impressive when its realised that on average the group initially randomised to placebo had received UDCA for an average of one year during this time as part of the study design.

TABLE 1: STUDIES OF PATIENTS USING URSODEOXYCHOLIC ACID				
Study	**Number**	**Dose (mg/kg/day)**	**Duration (years)**	**Results***
Poupon 1991[1]	145	13-15	2	B, TF
Heathcote 1994[2]	222	14	2	B, H
Lindor 1994[3]	180	13-15	5	B, TF
Combes 1995[4]	151	10-12	2	B, H
Eriksson 1997[5]	116	7.7	2	B
*B - biochemical, S - symptoms, TF - treatment failure, H - histology, D - death and/or OLT				

The improvement in survival free of transplantation was most marked in advanced stage disease. However, it is difficult to suggest that the drug should be reserved for those patients with more advanced disease. It is probable that the reason for this finding was that the endpoints of death of transplantation are unlikely to occur during a four-year period in patients with anything but advanced disease. However, it is unlikely at this time that long-term, placebo-controlled trials, reaching out over decades, will ever be performed with patients in early stage disease.

Ursodeoxycholic acid helps improve survival and reduces the need for liver transplantation; however, the question has been raised whether patients receiving ursodeoxycholic acid might have longer to develop other co-morbid conditions and might have a worse outcome after transplantation. A recent study based on the results of the combined analysis does not support this hypotheses. The outcome after transplantation in UDCA treated patients is at least as good as those patients who had received placebo prior to transplantation[9].

OTHER EFFECTS

Aside from the important effects of UDCA on survival and need for liver transplantation, ursodeoxycholic acid also improves serum lipids, reducing xanthomas and xanthelasma; helps improve pruritus; reduces the chance of developing varices; and retards progression to cirrhosis.

Lipids:

Ursodeoxycholic acids leads to a significant decrease in cholesterol levels. HDL and triglyceride levels are unchanged, although there is a significant decrease in LDL cholesterol (Figure 1). This is most prominent in patients with higher cholesterol levels[10].

Anecdotally, this has been associated with improvement in xanthomas or xanthelasma in number of patients.

Pruritus:

Clinically, the use of ursodeoxycholic acid has led to a reduction in pruritus in many patients. However, this was an inconsistent finding among various studies perhaps because of the difficulty in accurately quantifying pruritus in large scale trials. Recently, an abstract was reported based on the 222 patients who were entered into the Canadian multi-center trial. These patients performed weekly visual scale measurements of their pruritus. It was noted that in the ursodiol treated patients, pruritus was better in 59% verus 38% in the placebo and worse in 33% of the ursodiol patients versus 52% of the placebo treated patients; these differences were statistically significant[11].

Varices:

The use of ursodeoxycholic acid has led to a substantial reduction in the risk of developing varices in patients who did not have varices at the time of entry into study (Figure 2). Patients receiving placebo over the course of about five years are nearly four times as apt to develop varices as those patients receiving UDCA[12].

Cirrhosis:

Similarly, recent data suggests that risk of progressing to cirrhosis in noncirrhotic patients is substantially reduced by UDCA therapy. In a recent study from the Mayo Clinic, 16 patients who entered the UDCA trial without cirrhosis and who had been on UDCA for at least five years (mean 6.6 years) had progression to cirrhosis in only 13 % of patients. In contrast, among 51 patients in the placebo controlled penicillamine trial who had been in the study for at least five years and were noncirrhotic at entry, 51 % had progression to cirrhosis over a similar period of time (p< 0.009). These findings show clearly that the use of ursodeoxycholic acid long term delays histologic progression to cirrhosis[13].

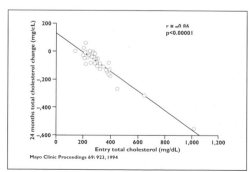

Figure 1. **UDCA for Primary Biliary Cirrhosis**[10].
Effects of UDCA therapy on serum total cholesterol level in patients with primary biliary cirrhosis.

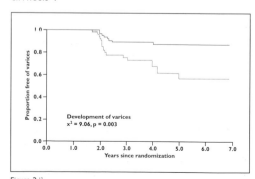

Figure 2.[12]
The effects of UDCA therapy on development of varices in patients without varices at the time of entry into the study.

Bone Disease:

Despite the above-mentioned beneficial effects of UDCA, bone disease does not appear to be beneficially affected. About one third of patients with PBC have bone densities below the fracture threshold. Early on, we had hoped that the use of UDCA would improve the bone disease in PSC, but it really leads to no improvement[14] (Figure 3).

PREDICTORS OF RESPONSE TO THERAPY

It is sometimes difficult to pick those patients who are responding to UDCA therapy. This becomes particularly true as investigators seek to develop newer therapies to be used in conjunction with UDCA.

A study by Jorgensen et al. identified the characteristics of patients achieving biochemical normalization with ursodiol therapy. This group with biochemical normalization is characterized by an extremely good clinical course and their response could be predicted by lower initial alkaline phosphatase and bilirubin levels and higher percent enrichment of biliary bile after two years of therapy[15].

During the course of therapy, the degree of improvement of alkaline phosphatase can be useful in predicting suboptimal responders. Patients who have an alkaline phosphatase that is less than 2 times normal after six months have about a 10 % chance of reaching treatment failure criteria after two years, whereas patients whose alkaline phosphatase levels remains greater than twice normal have nearly a 30 % chance of reaching treatment failure criteria[16].

The Mayo Risk Score is a valuable tool for predicting the prognosis in patients with untreated PBC. It has been found, however, that there is an excellent correlation when the Mayo Risk Score is recalculated six months after beginning UDCA therapy. The recalculated risk score has outstanding correlation with actual outcome in UDCA treated patients. In essence, the biochemical improvement induced by ursodiol therapy, particularly the effects on bilirubin, is a biologically important effect and the improvement of bilirubin levels with UDCA helps determine the prognostic scores[17].

MEASURES TO ENHANCE RESPONSE TO URSODIOL THERAPY

Patients with biochemical normalization had greater percent enrichment of bile with UDCA[18]. Other data show that there is a significant, although weak, correlation between UDCA in bile and improvement in AST and alkaline phosphatase. Because of these findings, measures to accomplish greater enrichment of

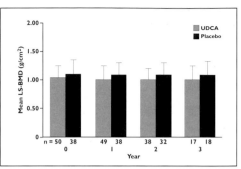

Figure 3. **Bone Mineral Density – UDCA vs Placebo**[14]
Effect of UDCA therapy or placebo on lumbar spine bone density in patients with primary biliary cirrhosis over time.

bile with ursodeoxycholic acid have been sought. Recently, this was attempted with cholylsarcosine, an inhibitor of endogenous bile acid production. When given with UDCA, cholylsarcosine was postulated to lead to substantial enrichment of the bile pool with UDCA. This in fact was the case in a small study, although biochemically and symptomatically no benefit was gained among a group of suboptimal responders to UDCA alone[19].

Another attempt at assessing this has been to vary the dose. As noted in the initial results, some of the patients receiving lower doses of UDCA had less obvious benefit. In a study from the Mayo Clinic, 150 patients were randomised to receive 5-7 mg/kg/day, 13-15 mg/kg/day, or 22-25 mg/kg/day of UDCA. All three doses were well tolerated. However, the lower dose had less enrichment of bile with UDCA, less biochemical improvement, and no influence on the Mayo Risk Score; whereas, more substantial improvement in Mayo Risk Score and biochemistries were seen with the two higher doses. There was no advantage to starting patients on the higher dose compared to the standard 13-15 mg/kg/day dose[20]. An unanswered question is whether increasing the dose in suboptimal responders would lead to benefit.

Ursodeoxycholic acid is a relatively expensive drug. The issue of cost-effectiveness is of increasing importance. Data from the Mayo and Canadian trials were combined looking at the incidence over time of developing complications of liver disease such as bleeding varices, ascites, encephalopathy, need for transplantation. The cost in U.S. dollars was calculated based on institutional and national data. In general, with a cost of $2,500/year for UDCA, ursodeoxycholic acid would save about $1,800 healthcare dollars per year per patient, primarily because of it effect on reducing the need for transplantation[21].

TABLE 2: STUDIES OF COMBINING WITH COLCHICINE			
Study	**Design**	**Number**	**Results***
Poupon 1996[22]	UDCA + colchicine or placebo	74	
Ikeda 1996[23]	UDCA + colchicine or non	22	B
Alamasu 1994 (A)[24]	UDCA + colchicine or placebo	90	TF
Raedsch 1991 (A)[25]	UDCA + colchicine or none	22	
*B - biochemically, TF - treatment failure, - negative			

UDCA IN COMBINATION

UDCA has been combined with colchicine, methotrexate, and corticosteroid in a limited number of studies. The studies combining with colchicine are shown in Table 2.

The results of these trials, two of which as yet are in abstract form only, are not very impressive. In one small study, biochemical improvement was seen. In a larger study, improvement in treatment failure was seen in patients with advanced disease; however, this study has not been reported in full form.

When ursodeoxycholic acid is combined with methotrexate, the results, particularly in the larger studies, have been unimpressive[26, 27, 28]. A much larger, multi-center, randomised trial is currently underway in the United States. The results of this trial should be

available in two to three years. In the trial at the Mayo Clinic with UDCA and methotrexate, substantial toxicity was seen, comparable to that reported from Boston using methotrexate alone. The large, multi-center, U.S. trial has reported a lower risk of toxicity, perhaps due to gradual initiation of the methotrexate.

Corticosteroids have been used in combination with ursodeoxycholic acid; although studies are small and of short duration. Two studies have shown improvement whether in symptoms, biochemistries, or histology[29, 30]. Bone disease is a concern in patients with PBC receiving corticosteroids. Etidronate, a bisphosphonate has been used to ameliorate the corticosteroid induced bone loss in these patients[31]. Other drugs, such as budesonide, with theoretically fewer side effects are currently of great interest and being evaluated in studies in combination with UDCA.

REFERENCES

1. Poupon RE, Balkau B, Escwege E, Poupon R, UDCA – PBC Study Group. A multicenter, controlled trial of ursodiol for the treatment of primary biliary cirrhosis. N Engl J Med 1991; **324**: 1548-54.

2. Heathcote EJ, Cauch-Dudek K, Walker V, Bailey RJ, Blendis LM, Ghent CN, Michieletti P, Minuk GY, Pappas SC, Scully LJ, Steinbrecher UP, Sutherland LR, Williams CN, Witt-Sullivan H, Worobetz LJ, Milner RA, Wanless IR. The Canadian multicenter double-blind randomised controlled trial of ursodeoxycholic acid in primary biliary cirrhosis. Hepatol 1994; **19**: 1149-56.

3. Lindor KD, Dickson ER, Baldus WP, Jorgensen RA, Ludwig J, Murtaugh PA, Harrison JM, Wiesner RH, Anderson ML, Lange SM, LeSage G, Rossi SR, Hofmann AF. Ursodeoxycholic acid in the treatment of primary biliary cirrhosis. Gastroenterol 1994; **106**: 1284-90.

4. Combes B, Carithers RL, Maddrey WC, Lin D, McDonald MF, Wheeler DE, Eigenbrodt EH, Muñoz SJ, Rubin R, Garcia-Tsao G, Bonner GF, West AB, Boyer JL, Luketic VA, Shiffman ML, Mills AS, Peters MG, White HM, Zetterman RK, Rossi SS, Hofmann AF, Markin RS. A randomised, double-blind, placebo-controlled trial of ursodeoxycholic acid in primary biliary cirrhosis. Hepatol 1995; **22**: 759-66.

5. Eriksson LS, Olsson R, Glauman H, Prytz H, Befrits R, Ryden BO, Einarsson K, Lindgren S, Wallerstedt S, Weden M. Ursodeoxycholic acid treatment in patients with primary biliary cirrhosis. Scand J Gastroenterol 1997; **32**: 179-186.

6. Poupon RE, Poupon R, Balkau B, UDCA–PBC Study Group. Ursodiol for the long-term treatment of primary biliary cirrhosis. N Engl J Med 1994; **330**: 1342-7.

7. Lindor KD, Therneau TM, Jorgensen RA, Malinchoc M, Dickson ER. Effects of ursodeoxycholic acid on survival in patients with primary biliary cirrhosis. Gastroenterol 1996; **110**: 1515-18.

8. Poupon RE, Lindor KD, Cauch-Dudek K, Dickson ER, Poupon R, Heathcote EJ. Combined analysis of French, American, and Canadian randomised controlled trials of ursodeoxycholic acid in primary biliary cirrhosis. Gastroenterology 1997; **113**: 884-90.

9. Heathcote EJ, Cauch-Dudek K, Stone J, Poupon R, Chazouilleres O, Lindor KD, Petz J, Dickson ER, Poupon RE. The effect of ursodiol therapy prior to transplantation on outcome of liver transplantation in patients with primary biliary cirrhosis. Hepatol 1997; **26**: 438A.

10. Balan V, Dickson ER, Jorgensen RA, Lindor KD. Effect of ursodeoxycholic acid on serum lipids of patients with primary biliary cirrhosis. Mayo Clinic Proceedings 1994; **69**: 923-29.

11. Heathcote EJ, Cauch-Dudek K, Stone J, Poupon R, Chazouilleres O, Lindor KD, Petz J, Dickson ER, Poupon RE. The effect of ursodiol therapy prior to transplantation on outcome of liver transplantation in patients with primary biliary cirrhosis. Hepatol 1997, **438**. A1239.

12. Lindor KD, Jorgesnsen RA, Therneay TM, Malinchoc M, Dickson ER. Ursodeoxycholic acid delays the onset of esophageal varices in primary biliary cirrhosis. Mayo Clinic Proceedings 1997; **72**: 1137-40.

13. Angulo P, Batts KP, Therneau TM, Jorgensen RA, Dickson ER, Lindor KD. Oral nicotine in the treatment of primary sclerosing cholangitis. Gastroenterol 1998; **114**: A1203.

14. Lindor KD, Janes CH, Crippin JS, Jorgensen RA, Dickson ER. Bone disease in primary biliary cirrhosis: does ursodeoxycholic acid make a difference? Hepatol 1995; **21**: 389-92.

15. Jorgensen RA, Dickson ER, Hofmann AF, Lindor KD. Characterization of patients with a complete biochemical response to ursodeoxycholic acid. Gut 1995; **36**: 935-8.

16. Pasha TM, Jorgensen RA, Dickson ER, Therneau T, Lindor KD. Early predictor of treatment failure in patients with ursodeoxycholic acid for primary biliary cirrhosis. Gastroenterol 1996; **110**: A1290.

17. Lindor KD, Therneau TM, Hermans JE, Dickson ER. Mayo risk score accurately predicts patient outcome with ursodeoxycholic acid treatment of primary biliary cirrhosis. *Hepatol* 1996; **24**: 167A.

18. Lindor KD, Lacerda MA, Jorgensen RA, Batta AK, Salen G, Dickson ER, Rossi SS, Hofmann AF. Relationship between biliary and serum bile acids and response to ursodeoxycholic acid in patients with primary biliary cirrhosis. *Am J Gastro*; in press.

19. Ricci P, Hofmann AF, Hagey LR, Jorgensen RA, Dickson ER, Lindor KD. Adjuvant cholylsarcosine during ursodeoxycholic acid treatment of primary biliary cirrhosis. *Dig Dis Sci* 1998; **43**: 1292-95.

20. Lindor KD, Jorgensen R, Therneau TM, Smith C, Mahoney SW, Dickson ER. Comparison of three different doses of ursodeoxycholic acid in the treatment of primary biliary cirrhosis. *Hepatol* 1997; **26**: 438A.

21. Pasha TM, Heathcote EJ, Cauch-Dudek K, Therneau T, Dickson ER, Gabriel S, Lindor KD. Cost-effectiveness of ursodeoxycholic acid in primary biliary cirrhosis. *Hepatol* 1996; **24**: 169A.

22. Poupon RE, Huet PM, Poupon R, Bonnand AM, Nhieu JTV, Zafrani ES, UDCA-PBC Study Group. A randomised trial comparing colchicine and ursodeoxycholic acid combination to ursodeoxycholic acid in primary biliary cirrhosis.

23. Ikeda T, Tozuka S, Noguchi O, Kobayashi F, Sakamoto S, Marumo F, Sato C. Effects of additional administration of colchicine in ursodeoxycholic acid-treated patients with primary biliary cirrhosis: a prospective randomised study. *J of Hepatol* 1996; **24**: 88-94.

24. Almasio P, Provenzano G, Battezzti PM, Podda M, Todros L, Tosina F, Saccoccio G, Manenti F, Floreani AR, Chiaramonte M, Ballardini G, Bianchi F, Pagliaro L, The Italian Multi-Centre PBC Study Group, Italy. The Italian multi-centre randomised controlled trial of ursodeoxycholic acid vs. ursodeoxycholic acid plus colchicine in symptomatic primary biliary cirrhosis. *Hepatol* 1994; **20**: A683.

25. Raedsch R, Stiehl A, Walker S, Theilmann L, Kommerell B. Double-blind pilot study on the efficacy of ursodeoxycholic acid versus urso plus colchicine in primary biliary cirrhosis. *Gastroenterol* 1991; **100**(2): A788.

26. Buscher HP, Zietzschmann Y, Gerok W. Positive responses to methotrexate and ursodeoxycholic acid in patients with primary biliary cirrhosis responding insufficiently to ursodeoxycholic acid alone. *J Hepatol* 1993; **18**: 9-14.

27. Lindor KD, Dickson ER, Jorgensen RA, Anderson ML, Wiesner RH, Gores GJ, Lange SM, Rossi SS, Hofmann AF, Baldus WP. The combination of ursodeoxycholic acid and methotrexate for patients with primary biliary cirrhosis: the results of a pilot study. *Hepatol* 1995; **22**: 1158-62.

28. González-Koch A, Brahm J, Antezana C, Smok G, Cumsille MA. The combination of ursodeoxycholic acid and methotrexate for primary biliary cirrhosis is not better than ursodeoxycholic acid alone. *J Hepatol* 1997; **27**: 143-149.

29. Leuschner M, Güldütuna S, You T, Hüber K, Bhatti S, Leuschner. Ursodeoxycholic acid and prednisolone versus ursodeoxycholic acid and placebo in the treatment of early stages of primary biliary cirrhosis. *J Hepatol* 1996; **25**: 49-57.

30. Wolfhagen FHJ, van Buuren HR, Schalm SW. Combines treatment with ursodeoxycholic acid and prednisone in primary biliary cirrhosis. *Nether J Med* 1994; **44**: 84-90.

31. Wolfhagen FHJ, van Buuren HR, Den Ouden JW, Hop WCJ, van Leeuwen JPTM, Schalm SW, Pols HA. Cyclical etidronate in the prevention of bone loss in corticosteroid-treated primary biliary cirrhosis. *J Hepatol* 1997; **26**: 325-330.

LIVER TRANSPLANTATION FOR PRIMARY BILIARY CIRRHOSIS

Suzanne Norris, John G O'Grady

Institute of Liver Studies, King's College Hospital,
Denmark Hill, London, England.

SUMMARY

- Primary biliary cirrhosis (PBC) is an excellent indication for liver transplantation.

- A rising bilirubin is associated with decreased patient survival in patients with PBC.

- A serum bilirubin of greater than 100 µmol/L should instigate referral to a liver transplant centre.

- Patients with Child-Pugh class B or C disease, should be referred to a liver transplant centre.

- Earlier referral is justified if symptoms or complications are prominent.

- Prognostic models have been developed to predict survival and aid in the timing of transplantation.

- A Mayo risk score of less than 8 is associated with better outcome following liver transplantation.

- One year survival figures for PBC after transplantation now routinely exceed 90%.

- A reduction in serum bilirubin with UDCA appears to parallel disease progression.

- Following UDCA therapy, bilirubin remains a good index of survival.

- PBC may recur after transplantation.

- The clinical significance of PBC recurrence after liver transplantation is unclear, as are the importance of maintenance immunosuppression regimens and UDCA in modifying this process.

Introduction

Liver transplantation is a well accepted modality of treatment for advanced primary biliary cirrhosis (PBC). It remains the only effective therapy for the disease as medical interventions have failed to significantly alter or prevent disease progression. The early experience of liver transplantation for PBC at the Mayo Clinic indicated a one year survival of 83%, based on 20 patients[1]. This has been validated by the European Liver Transplant Registry which has reported a one year survival for PBC of 81% for the period 1988-1996[2]. Furthermore, data from the Registry show that the eight year survival figures of patients transplanted for PBC compared favourably with transplantation for other liver disorders (Figure 1). With advanced surgical techniques and improvements in perioperative care, the one year survival of PBC patients following liver transplantation has been reported to be as high as 93%[3].

Once the 'bread and butter' of liver transplant programmes, PBC is now accounting for a much smaller proportion of patients being transplanted for chronic liver disease. PBC was the commonest indication for liver transplantation in Europe until 1987. However, during the decade 1988-97 it has fallen to third rank at 2135 cases behind virus related cirrhosis (6867 cases)

and alcoholic liver disease (4217 cases)[2]. While most of this change reflects an increase in activity for viral and alcohol related causes of cirrhosis, there is some evidence that the absolute numbers of patients transplanted for PBC has fallen. The number of cases transplanted for PBC in the King's College Hospital programme has fallen from a peak of 29 to a nadir of 11 in 1996 (Figure 2). The European Liver Transplant Registry data also suggest that the fall in absolute numbers may be a real phenomenon over the last

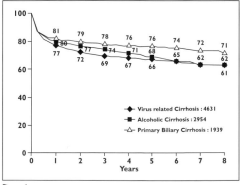

Figure 1.
Comparative survival curves for PBC, alcoholic cirrhosis and viral-related cirrhosis in Europe (from European Liver Transplant Registry).

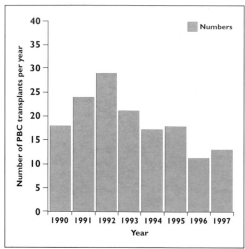

Figure 2.
PBC patients undergoing OLT at King's College Hospital 1990-1997.

few years[2]. If this observation is confirmed, it is debatable whether it represents an exhaustion of the pool of patients with PBC who were waiting transplantation or a change in the epidemiology or natural history of the disease. PBC accounted for 8% of transplant activity in the 15-45 age group, 15% in the 45-60 year olds and 28% of those over the age of 60 years[2].

Indications for Transplantation

The timing of liver transplantation is influenced by 4 considerations:

- natural history as assessed by prognostic models,
- the profile of life-threatening complications e.g. ascites, variceal bleeding, hepatorenal failure,
- the presence of other serious complications e.g. severe ostepdystrophy,
- quality of life issues especially relating to lethargy and intractable pruritus.

The success of liver transplantation is in part determined by the timing of the intervention. The natural history of PBC is more predictable than most of the other forms of chronic liver disease. It is characterised by prolonged periods of symptom-free survival, before the onset of jaundice usually accompanied by mild to moderate symptomatology and then a period when the serum bilirubin increases inexorably and life-threatening complications develop. There is no justification for liver transplantation during the asymptomatic phase of the disease. During the phase of the disease when the biochemical derangements are mild to moderate, liver transplantation may be required because of severe portal hypertension, accelerated osteodystrophy or poor quality of life. The prognostic models are most

useful as the disease progresses beyond this stage and the aim is to achieve transplantation before the onset of complications that would reduce the likelihood of a successful outcome. The role of the models is becoming increasingly important as the waiting times for transplantation increase and the physician is required to anticipate the clinical condition when a patient reaches the top of the waiting list, often after an interval in excess of a year.

Ideally, liver transplantation should be performed at a time when morbidity and mortality following transplantation are at their lowest but at a time when the liver disease has advanced sufficiently to warrant transplantation. One of the earliest attempts to identify factors predictive of survival in PBC followed 55 patients over a mean follow up period of 4.6 years[4]. All patients had an initial stable period with serum bilirubin levels less than 34μmol/L, the mean survival was 49 months. This fell to 25 months when the bilirubin was greater than 102 μmol/L (6.0mg/dL), and to 17 months when greater than 170 μmol/L (10.0 mg/dL). Another study from the 1980s found that amongst patients receiving transplants for PBC, those in the tertile with the best prognosis had a 78% one year actuarial survival rate, the middle tertile had a 63% survival rate and the worst tertile had only a 50% survival rate[5]. The same study gave one year survival rates on the basis of the serum bilirubin and these range from 75% for levels below 188 μmol/L, 63% for levels between 188-335 μmol/L and 45% for levels in excess of 335 μmol/L[5]. As a result of these studies, the majority of transplant centres have adopted a serum bilirubin of greater than 100 μmol/L as an indicator of when transplantation should be considered, with a view to achieving transplantation before the level exceeds 150 μmol/L.

Single tests have not be sufficient to generate accurate prognostic information and several investigators have used the Cox multiple regression analysis to generate prognostic models of survival for PBC in an attempt to optimise the timing of liver transplantation. The parameters demonstrated to predict survival are listed in table 1. The Yale Model[6], based on 280 patients, suggested that advanced age, bilirubin greater than 85 μmol/L (5.0 mg/dL), hepatomegaly, and fibrosis correlated with poor outcome. However, as a survival function was not determined, patient survival on an individual basis could not be estimated and this model is not particularly useful from the perspective of transplantation. The European trial of azathioprine as a treatment for PBC led to the generation of a survival model known as the European Model[7]. Factors which

TABLE 1: INDEPENDENT PARAMETERS PREDICTIVE OF SURVIVAL IN PBC			
Mayo Model	**European Model**	**Yale Model**	**Glasgow Model**
Age	Age	Age	Age
Albumen	Albumen	Bilirubin	Bilirubin
Bilirubin	Bilirubin	Hepatomegaly	Ascites
PT	Cirrhosis*	Fibrosis*	Variceal bleeding
Oedema	Cholestasis*		Cholestasis*
			Fibrosis*
			Mallory's bodies*
* based on histology			

independently predicted poor outcome included advanced age, high bilirubin, low albumen, the presence of cirrhosis and central cholestasis. In terms of decision making with regard to transplantation, this model did not particularly improve the value of serum bilirubin levels.

The same group subsequently devised a time-dependent model to estimate the effect of variables over time, thereby providing updated short-term survival estimates (ranging from 1-6 months) for an individual patient during the course of the disease[8]. Time-dependent variables indicating poor prognosis included high bilirubin, low albumin, ascites, gastro-intestinal bleeding, the presence of cirrhosis, central cholestasis and low IgM levels. A further model to predict patient survival was created at the Mayo Clinic, based on easily determined clinical parameters alone. This model (Mayo natural history model) was assessed in 312 patients with PBC enrolled in trials evaluating the use of D-penicillamine as a therapy for PBC[9]. Initially, 45 clinical parameters were included and stepwise selection subsequently limited the model to 5 variables: albumen, PT, bilirubin, age and oedema score (Table 2). This model predicts a relative risk score for individual patients with PBC, allowing estimation of the relative risk of death without transplantation. Other centres have established the general application of the Mayo Model[10,11], and, more recently, it has been updated[12] and reported to be superior in predicting short-term survival over a 2 year period. These models are likely to be more useful in clinical practice when determining the optimal time for transplantation.

While the prognostic models are useful in aiding decisions regarding the timing of liver transplantation, they are not without limitations. A subset of these patients with PBC develop portal hypertension early in the symptomatic phase and some of these with intractable variceal bleeding would benefit from transplantation considerably before the prognostic models suggest that this intervention is indicated. In addition, an increasingly recognised indication for transplantation in PBC is a poor quality of life due to pruritus or severe fatigue. These variables are also not accounted for in the Mayo model, yet they may precipitate referral for transplantation despite excellent predicted survival rates in the absence of transplantation. Other complications of PBC must be considered, in particular bone disease. While this complication does not always precipitate referral for transplantation, it is associated with significant morbidity and is to some degree reversed by transplantation.

Ursodeoxycholic acid (UDCA) is the most commonly used medical therapy for PBC and has been proven to improve biochemical indices of cholestasis[13,14]. In trials extending over four years, UDCA slows clinical progression by decreasing clinical treatment failure resulting in prolonged survival free of transplantation[13,14]. Combined analysis of the three largest UDCA trials (involving 548 patients) has indicated improved transplant-free survival particularly for moderate and severe disease[15]. Thus, UDCA delays liver transplantation in some patients with PBC. The major prognostic factor in all the models described above is serum bilirubin and this is significantly reduced with UDCA treatment. Therefore, the question arises as to whether the predictive value of the serum bilirubin or the models incorporating this parameter is altered by treatment with UDCA. In addition, might UDCA therapy lead to delayed referral when risk scores are higher (for

TABLE 2: MAYO NATURAL HISTORY MODEL FOR SURVIVAL WITH PBC
• Cox regression model

• Variables: age
       bilirubin
       PT
       albumen
       oedema score (0=none, 0.5=resolved with diuretics, 1=resistant to diuretics)

• Risk score = $0.871 \log_e$ bilirubin (mg/dL) $- 2.53 \log_e$ albumen (g/dL) $+ 0.039$ age (years) $+ 2.38 \log_e$ PT (seconds) $+ 0.859$ if oedema present

example, due to advanced age or lower albumen) resulting in poorer outcomes after transplantation? A trial of 222 PBC patients treated with UDCA or placebo used the Mayo model to identify low-, moderate-, and high-risk patients at baseline and after six months of treatment, and confirmed the value of serum bilirubin levels in determining prognosis even in those receiving UDCA[16]. Thus, despite clinical concerns, the currently available data suggest that UDCA therapy does not appear to eliminate the predictive power of the PBC models or deleteriously affect the timing of transplantation, provided for model when applied six months after initiation of therapy.

Outcome After Transplantation

The results of liver transplantation for PBC are excellent and are amongst the best achieved for a specific aetiological indication. In the European experience of 1988-97, the one year survival rate was similar for PBC, alcoholic cirrhosis and viral related cirrhosis, but at 8 years the survival rate in PBC patients was 70% and this was significantly higher than the equivalent figure of 62% for the other two aetiological groups[2]. The prognostic models provide valuable data regarding the factors influencing survival. To assess the efficacy of liver transplantation in improving survival, Markus and colleagues applied the Mayo model to 161 PBC patients undergoing liver transplantation in Pittsburgh and Dallas between 1980 and 1987[17]. The Kaplan-Meier survival probabilities three months following transplantation were significantly better than that predicted by the model, and this was true for patients at all risk levels (Figure 3, Table 3). At one year after transplantation, the actual survival probability was 0.76 compared to the predicted (using the model) survival probability of 0.45. Patients with a lower risk score had a better survival probability after transplantation and each unit increase in risk score increased the death rate by a factor of 1.3.

These results were validated by the King's College Hospital group after a retrospective analysis of actual survival compared to predicted survival of 29 patients

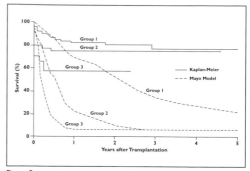

Figure 3.
Actual survival after transplantation in three risk groups of PBC patients and the estimated survival without transplantation predicted by the Mayo model. The risk groups were formed on the basis of pretransplantation risk scores, as listed in table 3 (Adapted from Markus et al, N Engl J Med 1989; **320**: 1709).

transplanted for PBC at that centre[18]. These studies, and a further review by Bonsel and colleagues, convincingly demonstrated the efficacy of transplantation as a therapeutic option for this disease[19]. The Mayo group have recently published the results of a further 143 PBC patients transplanted between 1987-1994 at Baylor University Medical Centre and the Mayo Clinic[3], reporting 1 and 2 year survival rates of 93% and 90%, respectively (Figures 4, 5). Compared to the earlier report by Markus et al, transplantation was performed at an early stage of disease (median risk score immediately prior to transplantation 7.5 v 8.3;p < 0.01), and the risk of death following transplantation remained low up to a risk score of 7.8, after which higher scores resulted in increased mortality. Furthermore, resource utilisation (days in hospital, days in ITU, intraoperative transfusion requirement) was significantly higher in recipients with risk scores greater than 7.8 compared to those with scores less than 7.8 (p < 0.001, 0.001, 0.006, respectively). These data indicate the effect of advanced disease on both survival and resource utilisation, emphasising the importance of early referral and transplanting prior to the development of advanced disease. The difficulty for transplant centres, therefore, will be the accuracy to

TABLE 3: VALUES FOR MAYO-MODEL VARIABLES IN 161 PATIENTS WITH PBC CLASSIFIED IN RISK SUBGROUPS. (ADAPTED FROM MARKUS *ET AL, NEJM* 1989; 320: 1709).			
Variable	**Low risk group 1 (n=98)**	**Mod risk group 2 (n=41)**	**High risk group 3 (n=22)**
Age	46.5 + 8.5	47.8 + 6.8	53.8 + 9.0
Bilirubin	12.1 + 8.2	24.1 + 12.1	27.8 + 11.7
Albumen	3.1 + 0.5	2.7 + 0.6	2.5 + 0.4
PT	13.4 + 1.4	15.1 + 2.5	19.5 + 5.7
Oedema score	0.4 + 0.4	0.8 + 0.4	0.9 + 0.4
Risk score	7.4 + 1.0	9.2 + 0.4	10.4 + 0.5

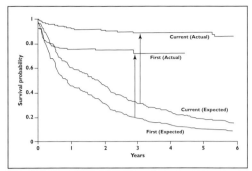

Figure 4.
Actual post-transplantation survival versus expected survival without transplantation in patients with PBC, in the first and current Mayo series. In both series, post-transplantation survival was better than that expected without transplantation by the natural history model. (Adapted from Kim et al, Hepatology 1998; 28: 33).

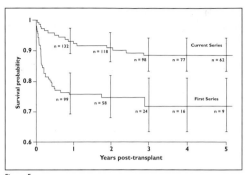

Figure 5.
Survival of patients with PBC. Current series (1987-1994) is compared to the first series (1980-1987). Numbers (n =) represent individuals being followed at each time point. (Adapted from Kim et al., Hepatology 1998; 23: 33).

predict from the time of evaluation ahead to when scores of greater than 8 may occur with a view to transplanting within that time frame. This is likely to be influenced by different waiting time on transplant lists across the transplant community with ensuing different thresholds for listing PBC patients.

Recurrent Disease

PBC recurrence after liver transplantation was first described in 1982 in three patients who developed a cholestatic illness with clinical, serological and histological similarities to PBC[20]. These patients were transplanted before the introduction of cyclosporine and had been maintained on prednisolone and azathiprine. The recurrence of disease was diagnosed 3.5-4.5 years after transplantation. Initially confirmatory studies were lacking and it was argued that alternative explanations existed for the various phenomena that had been observed[21,22]. The absence of a 'gold standard' for the diagnosis of PBC recurrence led to the debate being dominated by conviction rather than fact. A comprehensive Dutch study failed to find any confirmatory evidence of PBC recurrence but in retrospect it may be significant that these patients were maintained on relatively high doses of prednisolone[21]. Cases of possible recurrence of PBC remained scant during the period when cyclosporine dominated the maintenance immunosuppression regimens, but increased again following the introduction of tacrolimus[23,24]. Consequently, the evidence for recurrence of PBC needs to be considered in the context of the different immunosuppression regimens that have been used.

Antimitochondrial antibodies remained positive after liver transplantation in 72-100% of cases, although usually in lower titres than those seen before transplantation[25-28]. The persistence of antimitochondrial

does not establish the case for recurrence of the disease. However, the murine antibody C355.1 against the E2 component of pyruvate dehydrogenase, an early and sensitive marker of PBC, was found in 100% of cases with histological evidence of recurrence of PBC and in 0% of liver graft recipients for other indications[29]

Although this observation was not confirmed in a smaller study[30], it is the most engaging data to date to link antimitochondrial antibodies to disease recurrence. The other immunological marker, elevated serum IgM levels, tended to fall during the first two months after transplantation but increased again in some patients[25,31]. In one study, 80% of transplant recipients had serum IgM levels above the normal range[25].

Early histological evidence of PBC recurrence is associated with a normal profile of liver function tests. This is consistent with the equivalent stage of disease in the native liver. One study of 13 patients with histological evidence of recurrence found elevated alkaline phosphatase levels in 46% of cases, and mild elevations of transaminase and serum bilirubin levels in 23% each[31]. Biochemical parameters are, therefore, not a sensitive screen for PBC recurrence.

The difficulty with histological determination of possible PBC recurrence is that many of the individual features of PBC can be seen with other pathologies in the transplanted liver, particularly chronic rejection, biliary complications and hepatitis C infection. The histological features that overlap in these pathologies include ductular proliferation, portal lymphocytic aggregates, granulomas and paucity of bile ducts. Granulomatous destruction of bile ducts is considered pathognomonic of PBC. This feature was found in 8% of 60 patients followed for a mean of 3.3 years after transplantation[26]. This histological hallmark of PBC is transient and involves a minority of portal tracts. As a consequence it is easily missed through sample variation and the high specificity is tempered by a low sensitivity index. This suggests that it is likely to considerably underestimate the incidence of disease recurrence[26]. Although the other individual histological features lack specificity, particular combinations have been interpreted as suggestive of recurrence of PBC[24,25,31]. Adopting this approach, recurrent PBC was diagnosed in 16% of 83 patients followed-up for between 12-100 months, and similar appearances were not seen in 181 control biopsies from patients transplanted for other conditions[31]. The update of the original report of PBC recurrence showed that 70% of patients had stage 1 disease 1-3 years after transplantation and that the disease had progressed in 29% of these when followed up for up to nine years[25].

Immunosuppression policies may have influenced the apparent disparity between different studies. As indicated above, one careful study of liver biopsies from 19 patients followed for a median period of 4 years (range 1-11 years) found no histological evidence of PBC recurrence[21]. However, these patients had been maintained on relatively high doses of prednisolone (median doses of 17mg at 1 year and 12mg at 2 years), and this has been shown to modify histological appearances in PBC[32]. Two cases of florid granulomatous disease suggestive of PBC recurrence were reported a year after transplantation under tacrolimus immuno-suppression[23]. Subsequently, systematic prospective assessment of liver biopsies at one and two years found that 44% of patients randomised to immunosuppression with tacrolimus had histological appearances consistent with recurrent PBC, as compared with only 9% of cases randomised to cyclosporine[24]. This apparent increased susceptibility to recurrence with tacrolimus immuno-suppression could be due to the lower dose of

corticosteroids used, as compared with cyclosporine based immunosuppression. Alternatively, cyclosporine may be more effective than tacrolimus in preventing PBC recurrence in line with the beneficial effect documented in the non-transplant patients[33]. Current immunosuppression regimens using tacrolimus and cyclosporine tend to use similar concomitant doses of corticosteroids and as a result this issue should become clearer in the near future.

The majority of patients with recurrence with PBC have been asymptomatic as would be expected considering the relatively short follow-up periods that have been observed and the long pre-symptomatic period characteristic of the disease. Pruritus had developed in only one of 13 patients (8%) with histological evidence of PBC recurrence followed for up to 51 months after liver transplantation[31]. The incidence of pruritus increased to 22% in another study with longer follow-up[25]. Less data are available on progression to jaundice and the other clinical manifestations of PBC, although one patient with a progressive cholestatic syndrome leading to death at 9 years post-transplant has been reported[25]. Non-hepatic clinical phenomena associated with PBC have been documented to occur *de novo* after transplantation, including Raynaud's phenomenon, sicca syndrome, sclerodactyly and hypothyroidism[25]. There have only been anecdotal cases of patients coming to retransplantation for recurrence of PBC, and there is no evidence of any effect of recurrent disease on long-term survival rates. It is clear that possibility of PBC recurrence, while of great academic interest, should not influence the policy with respect to the use of liver transplantation in this condition.

REFERENCES

1. Krom RAF, Wiesner RH, Rettke SR, et al. the first 100 liver transplantations at the Mayo Clinic. *Mayo Clin Proc* 1989; **64**: 84.

2. Registry of the European Liver Transplant Association.

3. Kim WR, Wiesner RH, Therneau TM, et al. Optimal timing of liver transplantation for primary biliary cirrhosis. *Hepatology* 1998; **28**: 33.

4. Shapiro JM, Smith H, Schaffner F. Serum bilirubin: a prognostic factor in primary biliary cirrhosis. *Gut* 1979; **20**: 1371.

5. Neuberger JM, Gunson BK, Buckels JAC, Elias E, McMaster P. Referral of patients with primary biliary cirrhosis for liver transplantation. *GUT* 1990; **31**: 1069-72.

6. Roll J, Boyer JL, Barry D, et al. The prognostic importance of clinical and histologic features in asymptomatic and symptomatic primary biliary cirrhosis. *N Engl J Med* 1983; **308**: 1.

7. Christensen E, Neuberger J, Crowe J, et al. Beneficial effect of azathioprine and prediction of prognosis in primary biliary cirrhosis: final result of an international trial. *Gastroenterol* 1985; **89**: 1084.

8. Christensen E, Altman DG, Neuberger J, et al. Updating prognosis in primary biliary cirrhosis using a time-dependent Cox regression model. *Gastroenterol* 1993; **105**: 1865.

9. Dickson ER, Grambsch PM, Fleming TR, et al. Prognosis in primary biliary cirrhosis: model for decision making. *Hepatol* 1989; **10**: 1-7.

10. Grambsch PM, Dickson ER, Kaplan M, et al. Extramural cross-validation of the Mayo primary biliary cirrhosis survival model establishes its generalizability. *Hepatol* 1989; **10**: 846.

11. Van Dam GM, Verbaan V, Murtaugh PA, et al. Primary biliary cirrhosis: Dutch application of the Mayo model before and after orthotopic liver transplantation. *Hepato-Gastroenterology* 1997; **44**: 732-743.

12. Murtaugh PA, Dickson ER, Gooitzen MVD, et al. Primary biliary cirrhosis: prediction of short-term survival based on repeated patient visits. *Hepatol* 1994; **20**: 126.

13. Poupon RE, Poupon R, Balkau B, et al. Ursodiol for the longterm treatment of primary biliary cirrhosis. *N Engl J Med* 1994; **19**: 1342.

14. Lindor KD, Therneau TM, Jorgensen RA, et al. Effects of ursodeoxycholic acid on survival in patients with primary biliary cirrhosis. *Gastroenterol* 1996; **110**: 1515.

15. Poupon R, Lindor KD, Cauch-Dudek K, et al. Combined analysis in randomised controlled trials of ursodeoxycholic acid in primary biliary cirrhosis. *Gastroenterol* 1997; **113**: 884.

16. Kilmurry MR, Heathcote EJ, Cauch-Dudek K, *et al.* Is the Mayo model useful for predicting survival useful after the introduction of ursodeoxycholic acid treatment for primary biliary cirrhosis? *Hepatol* 1996; **23**: 1148.

17. Markus BH, Dickson ER, Grambsch PM, *et al.* Efficacy of liver transplantation in patients with primary biliary cirrhosis. *N Engl J Med* 1989; **320**: 1709.

18. Neuberger J, Altman DG, Christensen E, *et al.* Use of prognostic index in evaluation of liver transplantation for primary biliary cirrhosis. *Transplantation* 1986; **41**: 713.

19. Bonsel GJ, Essink-Bot M-L, Klompmaker UJ, *et al.* Assessment of the quality of life before and after liver transplantation. *Transplantation* 1992; **53**: 796.

20. Neuberger J, Portmann B, MacDougall B, Calne RY, Williams R. Recurrence of primary biliary cirrhosis after liver transplantation. *N Engl J Med* 1982; **306**: 1-4.

21. Gouw ASH, Haagsma EB, Manns M, Klompmaker UJ, Slooff MJH, Gerber MA. Is there recurrence of primary biliary cirrhosis after liver transplantation? A clinicopathologic study in long-term survivors. *J Hepatol* 1994; **20**: 500-7.

22. Van Thiel DH, Gavaler JS. REcurrent disease in liver transplantation: when does it occur and how can we be sure? *Hepatology* 1987; **7**: 181-3.

23. Wong PYN, Portmann B, O'Grady JG, *et al.* Recurrence of primary biliary cirrhosis after liver transplantation following FK506-based immunosuppression. *J Hepatol* 1993; 17: 284-7.

24. Dmitrewski J, Hübscher SG, Mayer D, Neuberger JM. Recurrence of primary biliary cirrhosis in the liver allograft: the effect of immunosuppression. *J Hepatol* 1996; **24**: 253-7.

25. Polson RJ, Portmann B, Neuberger J, Calne R, Williams R. Evidence for disease recurrence after liver transplantation for primary biliary cirrhosis: clinical and histological follow-up studies. *Gastroenterology* 1989; **97**: 715-25.

26. Balan V, Batts KP, Porayko MK, Krom RAF, Ludwig J, Wiesner RH. Histological evidence of recurrence of primary biliary cirrhosis after liver transplantation. *Hepatology* 1993; **18**: 1392-8.

27. Esquivel CO, Van Thiel DH, Demetris AJ, *et al.* Transplantation for primary biliary cirrhosis. *Gastroenterology* 1988; **94**: 1207-16.

28. Buist LJ, Hübscher SG, Vickers C, Michell I, Neuberger J, McMaster P. Does liver transplantation cure primary biliary cirrhosis? *Trans Proc* 1989; **21**: 2402.

29. Van de Water J, Turhcony J, Leung PSC, *et al.* Molecular mimicry in primary biliary cirrhosis. *J Clin Invest* 1993; **91**: 2654-64.

30. Neuberger J, Wallace L, Joplein R, Hübscher S. Hepatic distribution of E2 component of pyruvate dehydrogenase complex after transplantation. *Hepatology* 1995; **22**: 798-801.

31. Hübscher SG, Elias E, Buckels JAC, Mayer D, McMaster P, Neuberger JM. Primary biliary cirrhosis: histological evidence of recurrence after liver transplantation. *J Hepatol* 1993; **18**: 173-84.

32. Michison HC, Bassendine MF, Malcolm AJ, Watson AJ, Record CO, James OFV. A pilot double blind controlled 1 year trial of prednisolone treatment in primary biliary cirrhosis: hepatic improvement but greater bone loss. *Hepatology* 1989; **10**: 420-9.

MANAGEMENT OF THE PATIENT WITH PRIMARY BILIARY CIRRHOSIS

Martin Lombard

Royal Liverpool University Hospital & Hon. Senior Lecturer in Medicine, University of Liverpool.

SUMMARY

PBC is probably the commonest chronic progressive liver condition where a long-term therapeutic relationship can develop between doctor and patient. The different clinical phases and symptoms which arise during the disease represent a challenge in management. Over the last decade in particular, much progress has been made in understanding the pathogenesis, predicting prognosis and focusing on treatments which modify the pathology. For the future, we need to focus research activity on those aspects of care which remain major problems for patients with PBC and their carers: namely fatigue and pruritus in particular but also bone disease, recurrence (persistence) of disease, and the relationship of female hormones to its pathogenesis. Patients are as keen to address these issues as we are and this bodes well for a fruitful future of collaboration in managing this chronic liver disease.

Patients with primary biliary cirrhosis (PBC) are generally referred to gastroenterologists for investigation of abnormal liver enzymes. Many patients end up in specialist liver units either for management of complications or in transplant centres for liver replacement. Figures are not available for the numbers attending each type of service but as two thirds of patients are asymptomatic or have a slowly progressive disease[1,2], it is likely that most patients are managed for most of the duration of their illness by general gastroenterologists until the end-stage of the disease or complications ensue. Research activity in primary biliary cirrhosis has been concentrated at either end of the timescale for which a patient has this condition. This is not to say that the patient's life experience with the disease has been ignored, but there is a dearth of practical information for managing patients with PBC during the course of their illness. Several issues which commonly arise are discussed in this chapter concentrating on frequently asked questions (FAQ's) both from the patients and from the doctors and other health professionals who come into contact with patients who have PBC.

BACKGROUND

Prevalence and Diagnosis:

Epidemiological studies indicate a wide range in prevalence for this condition between 50 and 400 per million of the general population[3] depending on the criteria used for ascertainment. The annual incidence reported is also very variable but in larger studies is of the order of 10-15 per million with most studies

agreeing on a female: male ratio of 10:1. Thus a conservative estimate would suggest that there are at least 3000 patients with this condition in the UK. In each health district of 400,000 there should be up to 100 patients which seems to tally with many clinician's experience. General practitioners who service a list of approximately 2000 patients cannot therefore be expected to be experts in primary biliary cirrhosis. Indeed, the average gastroenterologist in a district general hospital in the UK may only have between 20 and 50 patients with PBC to look after. Gastroenterologists with special interests will see more, hepatologists in transplant units, though accumulating larger numbers of patients with PBC may see an entirely different clinical spectrum of PBC, and are likely to see patients with more advanced disease, with complications or requiring transplant.

Symptoms and Presentation:

Most patients with PBC are referred initially for investigation of abnormal liver enzymes. Liver enzymes may have been measured during investigations for fatigue or pruritus, or during the course of investigation for a different presentation. Occasionally, patients are referred because anti-mitochondrial antibodies have been detected during screening tests for arthralgia. There have been many studies over the last three decades in which symptoms of PBC have been documented. Despite drawing on different populations and referral patterns, the results of these surveys are remarkably consistent in the proportions who report different symptoms (Table 1). The most prominent

TABLE 1: PRESENTING SYMPTOMS IN PBC	
Presentation	**Prevalence (%)**
Asymptomatic (detected by AMA+, abnormal liver enzymes)	20%
Fatigue	70%
Pruritus	60%
RUQ pain	17%
Xanthoma	20%
Hypercholesterolaemia	50%
Features of Advanced Disease (Jaundice, Ascites, Variceal haemorrhage, Encephalopathy)	20% first presentation 20% within 5 years
Associated Features	
Thyroid dysfunction	15%
Osteoporosis	accelerated for age
Sicca syndrome	50% symptomatic 100% on testing
CREST syndrome	15%
RA	5% symptomatic 20% RA factor +ve
Coeliac disease	20%

symptoms are fatigue and pruritus. As these are the symptoms which are least well understood, they are often the most difficult to manage.

Increasingly patients are referred in the asymptomatic stage of the disease because of the availability of biochemical autoanalysers and the high specificity of mitochondrial antibodies. Follow up studies in this group indicate that about one third are not truly asymptomatic at presentation and another third develop symptoms over a five to ten year period. This has led to use of the term "presymptomatic PBC" for patients who are AMA positive perhaps with abnormal liver enzymes but absence of symptoms. Although these patients were thought to have a benign prognosis, once they develop PBC symptoms their prognosis is no different to the group who are symptomatic at presentation.

About 20% patients with PBC present at a late stage of the condition with complications such as bleeding from

oesophageal varices, ascites or encephalopathy. In addition, follow-up studies of patients after initial presentation indicate that those events which define advanced disease may be expected to occur in a further 20% within 5 years[4].

Presentation of PBC can thus be considered to be a continuum (Figure 1) with 20-40 % having few or no symptoms including a proportion of whom may never present, 20-40% are in a symptomatic phase of variable progression which may last about five to ten years and 20% will manifest features or complications indicating the terminal stages of disease.

PATIENT'S FAQ's

When a patient is thought to have liver disease, they invariably become anxious. Most patients seem to know people who have died with metastatic liver disease and all seem to be aware of the ravages of alcohol on the liver. Patients therefore need to be emphatically

FIGURE 1: PHASES OF PBC & PRESENTATION		
Asymptomatic or "Presymptomatic" Phase: AMA +ve	**Fatigue Pruritus Arthralgia**	**Jaundice, ascites Variceal haemorrhage Encephalopathy**
? 5-10 years	5-10 years	2-5 years

Figure 1.

Continuum of presentation in PBC. Time periods are estimates, particularly for the presymptomatic period. Median time to survival from presentation in two large studies was 7-12 years.

reassured that they do not have cancer, and that there are other causes of liver disease besides alcohol. Beyond these initial issues, there are a number of questions which patients commonly ask. Subsequently they tend to concentrate on their symptoms.

What causes PBC?

There have been great advances in our understanding of the immuno-pathogenesis of PBC in the last 10 years and these are reviewed elsewhere in this book. Yet in the final analysis we may conclude that at the present time we do not know what *causes* PBC. This is frustrating for doctors and patients alike. However, because we now understand the pathogenesis of the liver damage reasonably well, some explanation can be given to our patients. Over the past couple of decades, there has been much more attention paid to giving patients information about their diseases and we know from that experience that it is important to convey information in a way that they understand in order to allay anxiety.

The pathogenic mechanisms resulting in the syndrome of PBC have been discussed in detail elsewhere in this book and are summarised in Figure 2. The disease begins, as far as we understand it, with an immune-mediated response resulting in bile duct damage. Patients know what an immune system is (from publicity about AIDS) but most will not understand its cellular basis and a very brief and simple biology lesson is occasionally required. Thereafter, it is relatively easy to convey information about immune responses invoking the theories of molecular mimicry and cellular damage in militaristic terms... "the problem is one of recognising whose side the bile duct cells belong to"... The important point to convey is that the smaller bile ducts of the liver are damaged and lost, it taking a very long time indeed for enough to be lost to cause sufficient damage, preventing bile from flowing and interfering

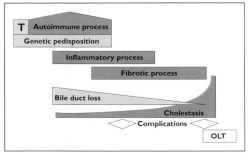

Figure 2.
Pathogenic mechanisms in PBC. An unknown trigger influenced possibly by genetic factors results in an "autoimmune process" possibly by molecular mimicry. The inflammatory process results in cell necrosis and fibrosis. The resultant bile duct loss results in cholestasis which causes localised secondary bile acid damage. The pathological processes are usually well established by the time of clinical presentation.

with all the other important functions of the liver. Usually some explanation about bile acids causing damage is also necessary particularly if treatment with ursodeoxycholic acid is being contemplated. Finally some explanation of the term "cirrhosis" is essential as the name of this condition is unfortunate in that it usually conveys misinformation to the patient about the state of their liver.

While this may seem the most naive explanation to appear in a medical text, a lack of simple-speak can often cause enormous anxiety to patients with PBC.

Why me and is my family at risk?

Patients can acquire PBC at any age but the vast majority present in the prime of their adult life. Inevitably there will be paranoia and even guilt. "Why me?" is a very common and most reasonable question to which we have no satisfactory answer as yet. If the initial trigger were an infective agent, that may be understandable and acceptable to patients but so far no agent has been identified. Undoubtedly, genetic factors play a role, probably in terms of conditioning the immune responsiveness. This leads on to the questions of heredity.

PBC is not a genetically determined condition. It is certainly familial and there are many reports of 2 or 3 first degree relatives being affected in combinations which transcend generations and gender[5]. The explanation could equally well be the familial exposure to a common trigger factor but so far this has not been identified.

Discussion of genetic-predisposition leads on to discussion of screening other family members. There is no information available on the risks and benefits of this at present. Indeed, the only test which may be suitable to use as a screening test is anti-mitochondrial antibody and its value for this purpose has not been studied. My own view is that this is a long-term, often progressive condition for which we know neither the cause nor have a proven strategy to prevent its progression and therefore it may be best to adopt an expectant approach and screen only those in whom investigation is warranted for other reasons. Patients should be strongly reassured that PBC is not a hereditary condition.

What causes the fatigue in PBC?

Fatigue is a symptom which is well recognised and has been experienced by everyone but is difficult to define, very difficult to understand and exceptionally difficult to measure objectively. It may be defined as a sensation or perception of having insufficient energy to undertake certain tasks. At the other end of the spectrum it has been defined as an inability to produce the required force to undertake a particular level of muscular activity.

These two definitions denote opposite ends of the biological spectrum of fatigue and have caused much confusion. The former relates to central fatigue and the latter to peripheral fatigue.

Information of the actions of muscle and the forces required to enact them are relayed through the spinal cord. The relays are modulated by such factors as motivation in the limbic system and perception at a cortical level. Undoubtedly, metabolic derangement can modulate relay of this information and thus affect perception of fatigue. Fatigue is often experienced very early in the course of PBC but sometimes not until end-stage disease is present.

Our own studies and those of others have demonstrated that there is no peripheral muscle fatigue in PBC and that central measures of fatigue are increased (Figure 3).

The modulated neurotransmitter theory has been explored in an animal model by looking at the adreno-cortical axis in cholestatic rats[6]. This is an important step in moving the problem of fatigue to centre stage but is likely to be only part of the mechanism and the model used by those investigators may have more to do with stress effects than central fatigue associated with chronic liver disease.

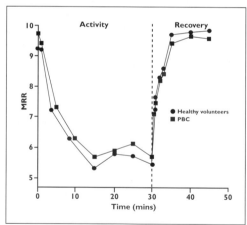

Figure 3.
Central and peripheral fatigue in PBC. The lower table shows that measures of central fatigue (FSA, VAS & MFQ) are increased in patients with PBC compared to controls as is depression score (CES-D). The upper graph shows data on muscle fatigueability and recovery rates obtained in the same patients and indicates there is no difference in peripheral fatigue in patients with PBC compared to controls.[15]

Other possibilities waiting to be explored are the effects of hypermetabolism on perception of fatigue. Patients with liver disease can be hypermetabolic[7] and it is not known whether this has an effect on perception of fatigue. Endogenous opioids may be increased in animal models of cholestasis and in PBC[8,9] and these may also modulate perception of fatigue. Finally, low levels of cholesterol esters have long been correlated with depression and fatigue in other groups of patients[10] and in PBC this fraction of LDL is depleted because of reduced lecithin cholesterol acyl transferase (LCAT) activity due to liver damage.

How can fatigue be managed?

Patients who complain of being "tired all the time" (TATT) are difficult to manage - mainly because doctors do not understand fatigue very well and cannot measure it. In primary biliary cirrhosis, the objective of management is to optimise the patient's quality of life and the long-term goal should be to ensure that they are in the best physical and mental state to withstand complications, should they arise, and to undergo OLT when considered appropriate. With these goals in mind, it is essential to motivate patients to remain active and adopt a positive attitude. As a group of patients, people with PBC often respond quite well to exhortation.

It is also important to optimise nutrition although we do not yet know how to do this in a way which may have a beneficial effect on the pathogenesis of their condition. Adequate protein-calorie intake is essential as subtle impairment of digestion and absorption can occur in PBC due to pancreatic exocrine dysfunction, fat or vitamin malabsorption in association with cholestasis, and perhaps malabsorption in association with undetected subtotal villous atrophy. Vitamin and trace element deficiency should be prevented by intermittent courses of multivitamin supplements. Patients with PBC do not usually drink excessive alcohol and should be discouraged from doing so.

Physical activity is important for well-being and fitness. A balance has to be struck between physical activity to maintain performance and rest to avoid exhaustion. A planned programme of regular exercise can be useful.

FIGURE 3: CENTRAL AND PERIPHERAL FATIGUE IN PBC			
Measure	**Controls**	**Patients**	**p-value**
Fatigue severity scale	2.30 (±1.6)	5.20 (±1.6)	<0.0009
Visual analogue scale	0.56 (±0.15)	0.36 (±0.1)	<0.003
Mental fatigue questions	4.30 (±2.8)	9.70 (±4.8)	<0.01
CES-D	15.30 (±3.3)	28.0 (±10.6)	<0.01

Depression scores are often high in PBC (Figure 3)[11], and may contribute to fatigue. It is important to consider treatment of depression although its optimal management in this context is not yet delineated. The depression which is measurable in PBC may be secondary to the predicament in which the patient perceived themselves. Nonetheless, as both fatigue and depression are mediated by neurotransmitter relays, they can be modified by neurotransmitter modulators such as anti-depressant medication. There have been no studies to determine which anti-depressants may be most effective in PBC and doctors are often reluctant to use them in the context of liver disease but they can produce dramatic effects on fatigue perception.

What causes the itching in PBC?

Traditionally it has been thought that bile salt deposition in the skin is responsible for the pruritus in PBC, possibly by irritating nerve endings. This notion lost some credence when it was demonstrated that the degree of itching did not correlate with the levels of hydrophobic bile salts in skin. It is possible that the absolute level of bile salts is less relevant than their metabolic availability i.e. the unbound fraction. It has been proposed that bile salts may also activate mast cells and cause release of histamine and kinins. More recently, it has been proposed that endogenous endorphins and enkephalins may play a role and evidence that morphine produces pruritus[8] which can be ablated by opiate antagonists is often cited in support of this hypothesis. The precise mechanism remains unclear and it is likely that a combination of central and peripheral mediators may be responsible.

How can pruritus be managed in PBC?

Pruritus can be a very difficult symptom to manage. It often does not correlate with stage of disease and can be very troublesome early on before clinical cholestasis is apparent. Treatment has generally been based on the ideas of causation prevalent at the time. Thus, cholestyramine has for many years been advocated on the basis of reducing the bile salt pool. It is not helpful in every patient but in my experience gives the most consistent relief. Colestipol is an alternative. Ursodeoxycholic acid replaces hydrophobic bile salt with a more hydrophilic compound. Reports of its efficacy for pruritus have been very variable although most evidence suggests that it helps more often than not. Antihistamines and mast cell stabilisers have not proved helpful in general and because of their adverse effects, predominantly sedation, are not much utilised. Rifampicin has been shown to be effective in relieving pruritus in PBC. It is thought to act by inducing cytochrome P450 which in turn increases hydroxylation of bile acids and may also act by interfering with their uptake. There have been concerns about using effective antibiotics for this purpose and it occasionally disconcerts patients because it turns their urine red. Opiate antagonists have been shown to be effective on an experimental basis but are not practical as they have to be administered parenterally.

Why do I get a pain underneath my ribs on the right hand side?

Abdominal pain in the right upper quadrant is reported by up to one fifth of patients with PBC. It is variously described as a "catch" or nagging sensation rather than a specific pain. It is not usually associated with nausea, vomiting or alteration in bowel habit and is unrelated to meals or posture.

The cause of this RUQ pain is unclear. Gallstones are more prevalent in patients with PBC and should be excluded by ultrasound scan. Their presence does not necessarily prove causation and it can be difficult to decide whether cholecystectomy is warranted. It is also important to exclude hepatoma by scan and alfa-fetoprotein level. If cholangiography is undertaken in patients with PBC, an indentation of the bile duct is commonly seen just below the hilar bifurcation (commonly referred to as a "PBC notch"). This is thought to represent an enlarged lymph node encroaching on the bile duct but its relationship to symptoms is not proven. The liver is normally enlarged in patients with PBC and it may be that capsular stretching best explains the sensations reported. Usually no specific treatment is necessary.

Why are my mouth and eyes are often dry?

Sicca syndrome, comprising xerostomia and xerophthalmia, occur in up to two thirds of patients with PBC. They are due to inflammatory destruction of lacrimal and salivary glands and histological changes can be found in these glands in one hundred percent of patients. No treatment to date has been reported to prevent this pathology.

Xerophthalmia is usually mild and can be managed in most patients by the use of hydrocellulose drops (artificial tears). Xerostomia can be more difficult to manage. There are a number of compounds available which improve lubrication in the mouth (e.g. Saliva Orthana) and occasionally dental consultation is necessary.

Where can I get information about PBC?

Access to information for patients has improved enormously in recent years. In some respects the quest for information may reflect a failure on the part of doctor's to inform their patients adequately. Nonetheless it provides an unparalleled opportunity to educate our patients about the problems of liver disease and the requirement to learn more together through their participation in research programmes.

Information is now readily available through national and local self-help groups and on the Internet. In the UK some of this information is co-ordinated by the British Liver Trust and the PBC Foundation and there are similar foundations in many other countries. The internet is the latest source of information for patients. Not all of the information is accurate and not all is easily understood so that it behoves us in consultation, and particularly when making a diagnosis, to explain PBC in terms which the patient will understand.

DOCTOR'S FAQ'S

How do I manage the hypercholesterolaemia in PBC?

Hypercholesterolaemia is common in PBC. With the advent of biochemical autoanalysers, cholesterol is frequently measured and found to be high. The link between hypercholesterolaemia and ischemic heart disease has prompted development of drugs to reduce it and general practitioners are bombarded with information and guidelines on the importance of using them - indeed this forms part of the strategy in the UK of preventing death from heart disease. It is not surprising against this background that patients and their doctors become concerned about high cholesterol levels (often very high) in patients with PBC.

Elevation of serum cholesterol in PBC occurs through a number of mechanisms including regurgitation of biliary cholesterol to plasma and an overall increase in its synthesis. In early PBC, cholesterol is largely contained in the HDL fraction and LDL is low. As cholestasis progresses, the LDL fraction increases and becomes predominant. It has been referred to as Lipoprotein-X because it differs from the LDL cholesterol commonly associated with increased risk of atherosclerosis. LP-X is virtually devoid of triglyceride and cholesterol ester because the activity of LCAT is markedly reduced when liver function is impaired. Cohort series have not shown any increased frequency of ischemic heart disease and it is generally thought that hypercholesterolaemia does not contribute in these patients but other factors such as smoking and family history still need to be addressed[12].

The newer cholesterol lowering drugs act by inhibiting HMG CoA reductase and occasionally cause elevation of liver enzymes even in the absence of liver disease. In my practice, cholesterol lowering drugs other than cholestyramine are not used.

Is it safe to prescribe HRT to patients with PBC?

PBC most commonly occurs in middle aged women. It has been reported to present in patients on anovulants, during pregnancy and following commencement of hormone replacement therapy and there have been reports of increased frequency of menstrual irregularities, hysterectomy and even breast cancer in these patients. These observations may well be due to the fact that such patients are closely supervised rather than represent a true causative association. Nonetheless, the female:male ratio of 10:1 for this condition, the fact that autoimmune diseases are more common in females and experimental evidence that oestrogens can modulate the immune response have implied that sex hormones may somehow be involved in its pathogenesis.

At the present time there is no proven link between the pathogenesis of PBC and pharmacologic doses of hormone replacement therapy. Symptoms of menopause can often be disabling and at present there seems no reason to deny patients with PBC this treatment if or when they require it. HRT has beneficial effects on bone abnormalities in post-menopausal women. It is not clear whether these benefits are preserved in patients with liver disease and there is an urgent need to acquire this information so that bone disease can be optimally managed in these patients.

How should arthritis in PBC be managed?

Arthralgia is common in PBC, particularly in the early stages. It may reflect generalised increase of cytokine activity to which joints seem especially susceptible. This non-specific arthralgia is usually self-limiting and can be controlled with paracetamol. (It is often necessary to reassure patients with PBC and other liver diseases that they can take paracetamol for pain in the recommended doses: it is an effective analgesic !). About 20% patients will have a positive rheumatoid factor but true rheumatoid arthritis is much less common. Non-steroidal anti-inflammatory agents can occasionally cause elevation of liver enzymes but can be used safely in patients with PBC who are well supervised. If rheumatoid disease develops, methotrexate is a useful disease modifying drug and has been claimed to have some benefit in the liver disease also.

Should patients with PBC be vaccinated?

This question commonly arises in patients who travel abroad on vacation. Concerns arise because many vaccines (and commonly used drugs) carry a cautionary warning about their use in liver disease. There is no evidence that patients with PBC are at special risk of contracting viral infections except following transplantation where they are taking immuno-suppressant drugs. There should be no problem exposing patients to killed or inactivated vaccines where these are indicated. Cholestatic patients who are elderly should be offered annual vaccination against influenza.

What treatment is available for PBC

PBC, of all liver disease, has attracted most attention in terms of clinical trials of treatment. We have learned much about design of trials and the course of PBC from these studies and most importantly, prognostic models have been developed. The development of orthotopic liver transplantation (OLT) as a viable treatment option for end-stage disease has clouded analyses in recent trials as to whether any treatment really prolongs survival particularly without adverse effects. Some trials have hinted that progression of fibrosis can be slowed.

Treatment can be considered as disease mollifying or disease modifying (Table 2). Mollifying treatments are directed at countering patients symptoms e.g. antidepressants for fatigue, cholestyramine for pruritus or preventing complications e.g. bisphosphonates for bone disease, propranolol to prevent variceal haemorrhage. Disease modifying drugs can be

TABLE 2: DRUGS USED IN PBC	
Disease Mollifying	**Effect**
Anti-pruritic	
Cholestyramine	relieves pruritus, may cause alteration of bowel habit
Cholestipol	alternative to cholestyramine
Antihistamines	not much effect on pruritus, may cause drowsiness
Opiate antagonists	effective in relieving pruritus in experimental conditions
Rifampicin	effective in relieving refractory pruritus: turns urine red
Bone disease	
Calcium Suppl.	useful in ensuring adequate nutritional intake
Vitamin D analogues	may help overcome subtle malabsorption due to cholestasis
Bisphosphonates	reduce bone loss, may be better given parenterally in PBC
Others	
Spironolactone	Mainstay of diuretic treatment for ascites in liver disease
Propranolol	Used for primary & secondary prevention of variceal haemorrhage
HRT	Alleviates menopausal symptoms, may benefit bone disease
Disease Modifying	**Effect**
Corticosteroids	Reduce inflammatory activity in the liver; uncertain effect on longevity; exacerbate osteoporosis.
Azathioprine	Statistical improvement in longevity; problems with marrow suppression
Cyclosporin A	Statistical improvement in longevity; problems with renal impairment and hypertension
Penicillamine	No benefit; very poorly tolerated
Chlormabucil	No benefit; marrow toxicity
Methotrexate	No proven benefit; theoretical advantages over other immunosuppressants; well tolerated
Colchicine	May ameliorate fibrosis but unlikely to affect course of disease; may cause diarrhoea.
Ursodeoxycholic acid	Predictable & repeatable beneficial effects on biochemistry; uncertain effect on longevity or pathology; well tolerated.

considered in three categories: immune modulating, fibrosis-modulating or against the effects of cholestasis.

Corticosteroids have been studied in small groups of patients with PBC but despite initial promising results, are not used because of concerns over accelerated osteoporosis in particular. Azathioprine and Cyclosporin A have also shown promise in a number of studies and have been included in the two largest and longest-running controlled therapeutic studies in PBC to date. These two trials[13,14] revealed much about the great difficulties encountered in studying this condition and improving survival. Despite the positive statistical analyses, neither treatment has been widely adopted because the risk of adverse effect over a prolonged period of time is unacceptable. Likewise, chlorambucil and penicillamine have proved much too toxic with even less therapeutic benefit. Methotrexate has been reported to be well tolerated with positive effect but has not been evaluated in a controlled trial. At present, immuno-modulatory agents are not widely used for treatment of PBC. Studies are on-going to determine whether use of low dose methotrexate or corticosteroid in combination with other treatments may retain some benefit with minimal adverse effect.

The anti-fibrogenic drug colchicine has been studied in PBC and other forms of cirrhosis. It has been shown in at least two trials to have beneficial effects and seems to be well tolerated. Diarrhoea is occasionally a problem. The data has not convinced many hepatologists sufficiently to recommend its widespread adoption.

Ursodeoxycholic acid is thought to act by replacing the hydrophobic, more toxic bile acids such as cholic acid and lithocholic acid, with a more hydrophilic species. By so doing, it abrogates the secondary bile acid damage associated with cholestasis. Studies have also shown that it may indirectly have immuno-modulatory effects. All studies to date have shown consistent and marked improvement in biochemical parameters. The same studies have shown variable effects on symptoms and possibly positive effects on histology. Survival has not been adequately studied but use of ursodeoxycholic acid may delay requirement for transplantation by perhaps 18-24 months. To date it is the only agent to have a predictable, repeatable effect on measurable parameters of disease in individual patients with PBC and this, in combination with its safety profile, has convinced most hepatologists to adopt it as primary treatment for their patients.

When do I start treatment?

Mollifying treatments are commenced on a symptomatic basis as the need to control symptoms arises. Prophylactic treatment should be used as soon as assessment of the patient has been completed e.g. calcium supplements to prevent osteoporosis, β-blockers for primary or secondary prevention of variceal haemorrhage.

Disease modifying treatments are more contentious. All trials in PBC have required entry criteria which usually include a high proportion of patients with later stage (histological stage 4) disease when modifying drugs are likely to be least effective. Conversely, if drugs are used at a much earlier stage where they are more likely to be effective, they will also be used for longer and may be more likely to produce adverse effects. It is mainly for this latter reason that immunomodulatory drugs have not found favour in PBC despite encouraging results in some trials. As discussed above, ursodeoxycholic acid has been shown to be effective in improving biochemistry and probably in delaying the requirement for OLT. Accordingly it tends to be used, outside the trial situation, in patients with a bilirubin which is rising above normal levels or with significantly elevated liver enzymes. There is a reasonable case to be made for ursodeoxycholic acid being considered the standard treatment in these circumstances. It is more difficult to justify its use in asymptomatic patients with normal bilirubin levels - indeed a biochemical response will be difficult to observe in such patients. There has also been concern that modulating biochemistry with ursodeoxycholic acid may "dupe" the clinician into thinking that disease is not sufficiently advanced to consider referral for OLT. However, it has a remarkable safety profile and is the only agent shown to have objective and repeatable effect in this condition. For maximum benefit ursodeoxycholic acid should probably be prescribed to all patients once their assessment has been completed.

Managing complications

Late complications such as those of portal hypertension, ascites and encephalopathy are managed by standard practice and there is nothing special about PBC in this respect. Females with PBC are still at risk of developing hepatoma and often regular screening with AFP or ultrasound is omitted, although no screening algorithm has been proven to be effective in picking up early hepatoma in any chronic liver disease.

There is a much greater awareness about osteoporosis in PBC. All patients should have their bone densitometry measured in their fifth decade. All should be given advice on diet and exercise and there are grounds for recommending calcium supplements to most. Any patient with reduced bone density should be treated with bisphosphonates and because of concerns about suboptimal absorption, it is our practice to use these intravenously. Women with PBC should be encouraged to participate in mammography and cervical smear screening programmes.

When to refer for OLT

There are three reasons to refer patients with PBC for OLT: intolerable symptoms, progression of disease and development of complications.

Patients have been transplanted for intractable pruritus and fatigue which interfere with quality of life. These are uncommon indications because, despite the excellent results of transplantation, most patients in this situation are better off with their own livers and without immunosuppression.

The commonest reason for referral is progression of disease. All studies have shown consistently that serum bilirubin is probably the best single predictor of progression and survival. As a rule of thumb, serum bilirubin persistently greater that 100 umol/l on average predicts a 50% 2 year survival and should be a prompt for consideration of OLT. Occasionally patients with lower levels of bilirubin with symptoms should be considered sooner and occasionally patients will tolerate this level of hyperbilirubinaemia very well for a long time. When considering referral for OLT, it is important to bear in mind that patients often have to wait three or six months for a suitable graft.

Development of complications such as those of portal hypertension, ascites, encephalopathy or hepatoma are harbingers of poor prognosis and serious consideration of OLT should be given to these patients regardless of biochemistry or symptoms.

Chronological age is not a bar to consideration of transplantation so much as biological fitness. There are many septuagenarians who are more fit than their younger counterparts. Concomitant disease such as respiratory or cardiac disease is an important consideration. The optimum management of patients with PBC should include the establishment of close working relationships between referring physicians and transplant centres.

Optimising the patient's condition for OLT

There has been no comparative study, but in my experience the patients with PBC who do best are those with "attitude". It is essential that patients see OLT as a positive step in management of their disease and not their last chance of survival. In this respect, patients should be told from an early stage in their illness that OLT is a possibility. As they become more confidant with their disease and their physician, this can become a probability, a matter of time and ultimately a

reality. It is very useful for patients to have contact with other patients who have had an OLT for PBC. Again, a close working relationship between referring physicians and transplant centres is very positive for management of patients and reinforces the notion of continuity of care.

Avoidance of osteoporosis, maintaining physical fitness and nutrition are important aspects of care. Variceal haemorrhage is a serious complication which clearly jeopardises survival and fitness for subsequent transplantation. Prevention with β-blockers and adequate control of bleeding by TIPS if necessary are essential. If possible it is best to avoid abdominal surgical operations, particularly portal vascular shunts as these may jeopardise the chance of a successful outcome at transplantation.

Managing the patient following orthotopic liver transplantation

Whether patients are referred to a transplant centre or within a transplant centre, most will be looked after by the same physician who looked after their PBC pre-transplant. Following uncomplicated transplantation, aftercare eventually settles into a similar routine to pre-transplant care. Monitoring involves clinical and biochemical vigilance for complications of transplantation, complications of immunosuppression and recurrence of disease.

MANAGING COMPLICATIONS

Bone disease

If bone density is suboptimal pretransplant, there is a risk of vertebral collapse with the high doses of corticosteroids used at time of transplantation. In those patients it may be important to assess bone densitometry after transplantation and treat with bisphosphonates as discussed.

Prevention is the best strategy. Calcium supplements and exercise are important. At time of referral, it is not too late to embark on a programme of treatment with bisphosphonates.

Nephrotoxicity

Cyclosporin A has been the mainstay of immuno-suppression post transplantation for the last decade. One of its most significant adverse effects is nephrotoxicity. Tacrolimus has similar side-effects. Attempts at monitoring this by plasma levels are probably less important than regularly checking blood pressure and serum creatinine and these should be routine measures every three months following the immediate post-transplantation period. Any rise in creatinine may require reduction in dose of immunosuppression or conversion onto an alternative regimen such as mycophenolate or azathioprine.

Headaches and neurological problems are less common for patients with OLT on CyA than for renal transplant recipients who often require higher doses of immuno-suppression.

Carcinoma & other medical conditions

It has been claimed that patients with PBC have an increased risk of carcinoma of breast and of hepatoma. Whilst the risk of the latter should be significantly reduced following transplantation, the risk of other cancers and lymphoma may be increased because of immunosuppression. Unfortunately, there is insufficient data at the present time to recommend specific screening programmes for particular cancers but eternal vigilance is the price for freedom from liver disease. Regular clinical review with enquiry about symptoms, physical examination and measurement of biochemistry and full blood count are important.

Abnormal Liver Enzymes

Regular follow-up of patients in clinic after transplantation must include measurement of liver enzymes. These should be normal. Rising enzymes may be an indication of biliary problems which can occur in up to 15% patients, graft rejection or recurrence of PBC.

The pattern of enzyme rise together with parameters of liver function (prothrombin time, bilirubin, albumen)

may give an indication of the cause and should be supplemented by ultrasound of liver to exclude bile duct obstruction with doppler studies if problems with the vascular anastomosis are suspected.

Recurrence (persistence) of disease and Rejection

Rejection may be manifest by subtle abnormalities of bilirubin or liver enzymes but usually and fortunately is easily managed by high dose coricosteroids. Recurrence of primary biliary disease is an accepted phenomenon and can often be more difficult to manage. As this may be considered to be a multisystem disease an alternative view contends that the disease persists and its manifestations are slowed by immunosuppression. Whichever is the case, PBC with all of its attendant complications can recur. One of the most difficult aspects of treating such patients is loss of the emotional stake they have invested in OLT as a cure. Recurrence in this situation can have a devastating effect on their morale and affect quality of life disproportionately to the effects of their liver condition. A long-term therapeutic relationship with patients is important in this context. Ursodeoxycholic acid should be added to immunosuppression from the outset if recurrence is suspected although there is no study in this context at the present time.

REFERENCES:

1. Long RG, Scheuer PJ, Sherlock S. Presentation and course of asymptomatic primary biliary cirrhosis. *Gastroenterology* 1977; **72**: 1204-7.

2. Mitchison HC, Bassendine MF, Hendrick et al. Positive anti-mitochondrial antibody but normal alkaline phosphatase: is this Primary Biliary Cirrhosis? *Hepatology* 1986; **6**: 1279-84.

3. Metcalf J, James O. The geo-epidemiology of primary biliary cirrhosis. *Seminars in Liver disease* 1997; **17**: 13-22.

4. Neuberger J, Lombard M, Galbraith R. Primary Biliary Cirrhosis. *GUT Supplement* 1991; S73-78S.

5. Jaup BH, Zettergren LSW. Familial occurrence of primary biliary cirrhosis associated with hypergammaglobulinaemia in descendents: a family study. *Gastroenterology* 1980; **78**: 549-555.

6. Swain MG, Maric M. Defective corticotropin-releasing hormone mediated neuroendocrine and behavioural response in cholestatic rats: implications for cholestatic liver disease-related sickness behaviour. *Hepatology* 1995; **22**: 1560-4.

7. Heymsfield SB, Waki M. Are patients with liver disease hypermetabolic? *Hepatology* 1990; **11**: 502-5.

8. Thornton JR, Losowsky MS. Opioid peptides and primary biliary cirrhosis. *Br Med J* 1988; **297**: 1501-4.

9. Swain MG, Rotham RB, Xu H, Vergalla J, Bergasa NV, Jones EA. Endogenous opioids accumulate in plasma in a rat model of acute cholestasis. *Gastroenterology* 1992; **103**: 630-5.

10. Boston PF, Dursun SM, Phelan M. Cholesterol and mental disorder. *Br. J. Psych* 1996; **169**: 682-9.

11. Huet PM, Des;airoers J. Faucher C, Charbonneau J. Fatigue, mental health and depression in patients with primary biliary cirrhosis.

12. Crippin JS, Lindor KD, Jorgensen R, Kottke BA, Harrison JM, Murtaugh PA, Dickson ER. Hypercholesteromaemia and athero-sclerosis in primary biliary cirrhosis: what is the risk? *Hepatology* 1992; **15**: 858-62.

13. Christensen E, Neuberger J, Crowe J et al. Beneficial effect of azathio-prine and prediction of prognosis in primary biliary cirrhosis: final results of an international trial. *Gastroenterology* 1985; **89**: 1084-91.

14. Lombard M, Portmann B, Neuberger J et al. Cycosporin A treatment in primary biliary cirrhosis: results of a long-term placebo controlled trial. *Gastroenterology* 1993; **104**: 519-26.

15. Jalan R, Gibson H, Lombard M. Patients with PBC have central but no peripheral fatigue. *GUT* 1996; Supple I: T119.

PRIMARY BILIARY CIRRHOSIS: THERAPIES OF THE FUTURE

Elmar Jaeckel, Christian P Strassburg, Michael P Manns

Medizinische Hochschule Hannover, Department Gastroenterology & Hepatology, Carl Neuberg Str. 1, D-30625 Hannover, Germany.

SUMMARY

Future therapies of PBC will largely depend on identification of the underlying aetiology of the disease. As long as the aetiology is unknown empirical therapies with immunosuppressants, antifibrotics and anti-cholestatic agents have to be improved. Combination therapies and new immunosuppressants will certainly be tested in the future.

If PBC is caused by an infectious agent such as bacteria, mycobacteria, yeast or viruses, future therapies will also include antibiotics, antimycotics or anti-viral therapy.

If PBC is an autoimmune disorder gene-therapy and tolerance induction might be new promising treatment approaches. Exciting results from animal models and clinical trials of multiple sclerosis, experimental autoimmune encephalomyelitis, diabetes and rheumatoid arthritis have paved the way in this direction.

As the aetiology of primary biliary cirrhosis (PBC) is still unknown, therapies are nowadays still symptomatic and empirical, although some symptomatic approaches might also influence the pathophysiology of an undefined cause. Symptomatic therapeutic options have already been discussed in previous chapters. Therefore it is the aim of this article to focus on possible future therapeutic options. Therapies of the future will largely depend on the underlying aetiology of PBC. Up to now there are three major pathophysiological aspects, which might play a role in the process of the disease. PBC might either be the consequence of an unknown infectious agent, might be a truly autoimmune disorder of the biliary tract or might be caused by genetic disorders with the result of a defective immunoregulation or abnormal antigen presentation.

PBC caused by infectious agents

There are several indirect hints supporting the theory of an infectious agent as the cause of PBC. There seems to be a specific geographical distribution with the highest incidence of the disease in northern Europe and a very low incidence in Asia. A clustering of cases in areas of a certain water reservoirs in Sheffield has also been reported[1]. Furthermore, the incidence of the disease seems to increase and a marked regional variation has been shown within 7 adjacent health districts in the UK. The increasing incidence seems not just be attributable to a more accurate diagnosis of previous unknown cases[2]. Some familial clustering of the disease has been described. The histological finding of granulomas also suggests an infectious agent,

although, as in sarcoidosis, a specific agent has not been shown within these lesions.

Another important hint for PBC as an infectious disease is provided by the recurrence of PBC after orthotopic liver transplantation. There has been a big controversy whether PBC recurs post-OLT[3-7] or not[8-11], but during the last few years there is growing evidence supporting the hypothesis of the recurrence of the disease. The reason for the controversy may be, that many parameters used for establishing the diagnosis of PBC are not helpful in the posttransplant setting. Cholestatic liver enzymes and histologic damages to bile ducts can have multiple reasons after liver transplantation.

Aetiologies like rejection, cholangitis, arterial hypoperfusion and drug treatment may cause similar changes as seen in PBC. Anti-mitochondrial antibody-titres (AMA) have been reported in some patients to stay elevated after OLT whereas in others titres fall. Nevertheless AMAs are also found in asymptomatic relatives of PBC-patients and they are not even correlated with disease activity before OLT. The same holds true for elevation of serum IgM, which rather seems to be an immunological B-cell defect, probably not cured by OLT, but masked by immunosuppression.

Therefore, careful histological evaluation seems to be the only method to prove disease recurrence. As many histologic lesions are not pathognomonic in the post-OLT setting, one has to look rather to the spectrum of changes and to exclude other reasons for the lesions by clinical means[4]. Many groups are reporting about disease recurrence rates between eight and 16% of patients within 5 years of follow-up[3-7]. These findings are supported by recent immunohistological findings of early PBC specific staining patterns in 73% of patients post OLT. Therefore disease recurrence might rather be the rule than the exception[11].

Nevertheless, OLT must be also seen as a therapy of the future. PBC is one of the three most common indications for OLT in most transplant centres. Five year survival can be as high 95% in some series[3] and is clearly superior to the estimated survival without OLT. Many surveys report about clear benefit for patients in quality of life despite bone disease, the main disease specific complication post OLT.

Several infectious agents have been reported to be associated with PBC. Several hypotheses are deriving from cross reactivities on immunoblots between AMAs and antigens of Escherichia coli, Staphylococcus aureus, Klebsiella pneumoniae and Mycobacterium tuberculosis[12-15]. Cross reactive epitopes seem to be evolutionary highly conserved, as two yeast antigens of 40 and 60kD, which are recognised by AMAs, are expressed on the surface of prokaryotic and eukaryotic cells[16]. Other groups are reporting about an increased frequency of rough (R)-mutants of enterobacteria. There is an increased number of aerobic gram negative bacteria in faeces of patients with PBC[13] and another group is describing a strong proportion of R-forms in urinary tract infections of patients with PBC[17]. These clinical data are supported by experiments in rabbits where injection of a lysate of Salmonella minnesota R-mutant lead to antibodies against mitochondrial antigens of 50 to 70kD[18]. Cross reactivities of AMAs have also been observed with mycobacterial antigens and liver biopsies of PBC patients were found to be positive for mycobacterial DNA by PCR[19, 20].

Molecular mimicry is the common pathophysiological idea behind these findings. It is suggested that certain components of enterobacterial antigens could be trapped by the liver, metabolised and excreted into the bile. This idea is supported by immunohistochemical studies showing the presence of lipid A in liver tissue and biliary endothelial cells of patients with PBC[13]. It is interesting to note that lipid A promotes IgM production and complement activation. In PBC these infections might be established by defects in macrophage activity or deficits of the C4 component of the complement system[21]. Just very recently more evidence for an infectious aetiology has been provided by elegant studies of Joplin and co-workers: Explanted lymph nodes of PBC patients stimulated biliary epithelial cells of healthy livers to produce PDH-E2 and PDH-X. Expression was also seen on the cell surface of the biliary epithelial cells[22]. If PBC is indeed caused by bacteria, mycobacteria or yeast then the therapy of the future is likely to contain antibiotics, tuberculostatics or antimycotics.

Several classical autoimmune[23] disorders like diabetes mellitus[24], multiple sclerosis[25] and Sjögren's syndrome[26] have been reported to be associated with viruses and especially retroviruses, and animal studies are supporting the possible importance in inciting and maintaining the autoimmune process[27]. An increased prevalence of positive immunoblot reactivities for HIV p24 protein and immunoblot reactivity against human intracisternal A-type particles of endogenous retroviruses have also been reported for PBC patients[28], although these results have to be confirmed as similar reactivities have also been seen in various other disease thereby questioning their specificity. We also have to be aware of the fact that with highly sensitive PCR methods more and more fragments of endogenous retroviruses will be amplified, which probably lack specificity, because nearly 2% of each human genome consists of endogenous retroviruses[29]. If PBC would be caused by viruses, then future therapies might also contain antiviral treatment strategies like various forms of interferons, nucleoside analogues, therapeutical vaccines and strategies of adoptive immune transfer.

PBC as an autoimmune disease

Several drugs have been tested for treatment of PBC (Table 1), but ursodeoxycholic acid (UDCA), and perhaps colchicine or methotrexate (MTX) are the only ones with proven benefit. The drugs interfere with different pathophysiological mechanisms involved in PBC, namely immune mediated mechanisms, fibrogenesis and cholestasis. In the future, combination therapies of these drugs have to be evaluated especially for those patients not responding properly to UDCA. Some preliminary data suggest an additive effect of a combination of UDCA, colchicine and MTX on liver function tests[30], although these approaches have to be evaluated in larger cohorts of patients and with other treatment endpoints. Future therapies might also include new immunosuppressive agents like budenoside or mycophenolate mofetil. New immunosuppressants might be especially tested for their ability to act on the biliary tree. Immunomodulators like interferon-beta, which have been successfully used in autoimmune disorders like multiple sclerosis[31], might also be an option for treatment of PBC.

Gene therapy of PBC

Gene therapy of PBC might either be symptomatic by immunomodulation or help of tissue regeneration

TABLE I: MEDICAL TREATMENT OF PBC			
Toxicity	**Efficacy**		
	0	**+/-**	**+**
0	Thalidomide	Malotilate	Colchicine*
		FK 506	Ursodeoxycholic acid*
		Azathioprine*	
+/-	Cyclosporine A*		Corticosteroids
+	Penicillamine*		Chlorambucil
	Levamisol		Methotrexate

* larger randomised trials

or it might aim directly at correcting genetic defects leading to PBC (Table 2). As none of these approaches has been investigated so far for PBC, most of our knowledge originates from other autoimmune disorders like diabetes mellitus or multiple sclerosis. The investigations of these approaches in PBC are hampered by the lack of an animal model for the disease.

In gene therapy the target cells of autoimmunity are modified to downregulate the autoimmune response. This approach has been proven to be protective for beta-cells of the pancreas in nonobese diabetic (NOD) mice. Transgenic mice with the Th2 cytokine interleukin (IL) 4-gene under the control of the insulin promotor expressed IL4 in a tissue specific way and were protected from diabetes[32]. This form of gene therapy might be used in PBC by tissue specific expression of IL4 or IL10 under the control of tissue specific promotors like the UGT 1A10 promotor[33]. An alternative approach is to modify tissue specific expression of Fas-ligand (FasL) in biliary epithelial cells. Expression could delete autoreactive CD4 and CD8 cells thereby inhibiting the local autoimmune response. Such experiments have been successfully undertaken in animal models of chronic arthritis: To upregulate FasL expression in the arthritic joints, a recombinant

TABLE 2: GENE THERAPY OF PBC

Symptomatic Therapy

Immunomodulation
1. Target tissue gene therapy
2. T-cell mediated gene therapy

Regenerative
1. Target tissue gene therapy
2. T-cell mediated gene therapy

Causative Therapy

Hepatocyte / Stem-cell transplantation
Gene transfer by different vectors

replication-defective adenovirus carrying FasL gene has been generated; injection of the FasL virus into inflamed joints conferred high levels of FasL expression and ameliorated collagen-induced arthritis in DBA/1 mice. The Fas-ligand virus also inhibited production of interferon-gamma by collagen-specific T-cells[34].

Another approach to target tissue gene therapy in PBC would use the production of antisense-RNA or ribozymes against structures like intercellular adhesion molecule (ICAM)-1 and vascular adhesion molecule (VCAM)-1, which are upregulated in biliary epithelium of PBC patients[35]. Inhibition of pro-fibrotic factors might also be tried with these approaches. The transfer into the biliary epithelium might be achieved by viral vectors via ERCP or by transplantation of hepatocytes or stem cells.

The T-cell mediated gene-therapy uses autoreactive T-cells as a vehicle for tissue specific expression of immunomodulatory cytokines like IL4 or IL10. The cytokine genes should be under the control of inducible promotors like the IL2-promotor, which ensures that the gene will be just expressed at the site of inflammation. A construct of the IL10 gene under the control of the IL2 promotor has been transferred in T-lymphocytes specific for myelin proteolipid protein. These cells could prevent and treat experimental autoimmune encephalomyelitis in mice[36]. These experiments demonstrate that immunomodulatory gene therapy could even be effective across the blood-brain barrier.

The T-cell mediated gene therapy can not just be used for the inhibition of the autoimmune response but also for promoting tissue regeneration after the damage has already occurred. It has been demonstrated that neurogenic T-lymphocytes expressing the mouse nerve growth factor were able to attenuate experimental autoimmune neuritis in mice[37]. T-cells with expression of anti-fibrotic factors might be used in PBC or other liver diseases.

Finally, gene therapy can also substitute a defective gene. Although a major genetic defect has not been found in PBC so far and although there is only a weak clustering of the disease within families, the link with HLA DR8-DQB1*0402 and DPB1*0301 alleles[38] and the defect for the complement factor C4[21] are at least pointing to some genetic predisposition for development of PBC. As long as no more genes are identified the correction of the C4 defect would be one therapeutic approach. The idea of a genetic contribution to autoimmune disease is further supported by mouse models with inherited defects in either FasL or Fas-receptor, which show a marked lymphoproliferative autoimmune syndrome[39,40]. Furthermore, a defective zinc-finger like transcription factor has been recently identified as the cause of the autoimmune polyglandular syndrome in humans[41]. It should be tried to identify similar defects in humans by pooling larger cohorts of PBC patients.

Tolerance induction as a therapy for PBC

Tolerance induction, especially tolerance induction of already activated T-cells, is a complicated immuno-logical process, which is not fully understood so far. Nevertheless there are several examples for the use of tolerance induction in autoimmune diseases and some clinical phase I studies using this approach have already been performed in multiple sclerosis. Table 3 shows the mechanisms by which peripheral tolerance can be established.

Although the mechanisms leading to oral tolerance are not completely understood, oral administration of autoantigens can lead to deletion of autoreactive T-cells, induction of T-cell anergy, shift of the T-cell response from Th1 to Th2 and to the development of active suppression. Oral tolerance induction has been successfully used in animal models of diabetes mellitus[42] and autoimmune encephalomyelitis. Furthermore, there are ongoing clinical trials in multiple sclerosis[43], which have shown that oral tolerance induction generates antigen specific transforming-growth factor (TGF)-beta1 secreting Th3 cells of presumed mucosal origin that represent a distinct lineage of T-cells. Since antigen-

specific TGF-beta1 secreting cells localise to the target organ and then suppress inflammation in the local microenvironment, oral tolerisation with self antigens may provide a therapeutic approach for the treatment of cell-mediated autoimmune disease. Regular supply of autoantigen might be obtained by transgenic plants expressing the autoepitope as shown in the non obese diabetic mouse[44]. But we should also be beware that autoimmunity might be aggravated by oral tolerisation[45].

Some tolerisation protocols use the administration of peptides, DNA-vaccines or monoclonal antibodies to induce tolerance, whereby autoreactive T-cells are the targets of the activated immune response. These approaches are aiming to restore the anti-idiotypic network around the autoreactive T-cells. As autoreactive T-cells are often exhibiting a certain Vβ-subtype of their T-cell receptor (TCR), peptides from this region have been successfully used in models of experimental encephalomyelitis[46] and clinical trials of multiple sclerosis[47]. Similar results have been obtained with DNA-vaccination encoding Vβ-specific structures. Interestingly these protocols are not completely deleting the autoreactive T-cells, but they are rather shifting their cytokine profile from Th1 to a Th2 type[49]. After vaccination the immune system recognises the autoreactive T-cell not just by direct interaction, but also in the context of MHC class II molecules. These findings indicate that activated T-cells can process and present their own TCR in the context of major histocompatibility complex class II molecules and, furthermore, that such peptides can be recognised by TCR variable gene-specific T cells[48].

Monoclonal antibodies against OX40, a protein selectively upregulated on encephalitogenic myelin basic protein specific T-cells, have also been used in animal models to suppress the autoimmune process in experimental autoimmune encephalomyelitis[50].

Like in many autoimmune diseases the cellular autoepitope is not known in PBC. Therefore T-cell vaccination might offer an opportunity to control autoreactive T-cells. The number of autoreactive T-cells is augmented by stimulating the cells with defined subsets of protein fractions of the target cells. Subsequently the activated T-cells are irradiated and re-injected to promote an immune response against these cells thereby restoring the anti-idiotypic network of T-cells (Figure 1). T-cell vaccination has been used with success in experimental autoimmune myelitis[51] and in clinical trials of multiple sclerosis[52]. In the context of future therapies of PBC it is interesting to note that T-cell vaccination has also been used in an animal model of autoimmune hepatitis, another liver specific autoimmune disease[53].

TABLE 3: TOLERANCE INDUCTION OF ACIVATED T-CELLS
Oral autoantigen administration
Vaccines – Peptide vaccines – DNA vaccines
T-cell vaccination / Immune-cell vaccination
Reconstitution of the immune system – Bone marrow transplantation

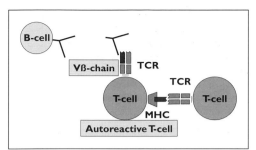

Figure 1.
Anti-Idiotypic Network

REFERENCES:

1. Triger DR. Primary biliary cirrhosis: an epidemiological study. *Br Med J* 1980 Sep 20; **281**: 772-5.

2. Metcalf J, Howel D, Bhopal R, OFW James. PBC prevalence is increasing. Geographic vaiations are probably real. *J Hepatol* 1998; **20**:138.

3. Knoop M, Bechstein WO, Schrem H, Lobeck H, Hopf U, Neuhaus P. Clinical significance of recurrent primary biliary cirrhosis after liver transplantation. *Transpl Int* 1996; **9** Suppl 1: S115-S119.

4. Hübscher SG, Elias E, Buckels JAC, Mayer AD, McMaster P, Neuberger JM. Primary biliary cirrhosis: Histological evidence for disease recurrence after liver transplantation. *J Hepatol* 1993; **18**: 173-184.

5. Neuberger J, Portmann B, MacDougall BRD, Calne RY, Williams R. Recurrence of primary biliary cirrhosis after liver transplantation. *N Engl J Med* 1982; **306**: 1-4.

6. Polson RJ, Portmann B, Neuberger J, Calne RY, Williams R. Evidence for disease recurrence after liver transplantation for primary biliary cirrhosis. *Gastroenterology* 1989; **97**: 715-25.

7. Dietze O, Vogel W, Margreiter R. Primary biliary cirrhosis after liver transplantation. *Transpl Proc* 1990; **22**: 1501-2.

8. Esquivel CO, Van Thiel DG, Demetris AJ et al. Transplanation for primary biliary cirrhosis. *Gastroenterology* 94: 1207-16.

9. Haagsma EB, Manns M, Klein R et al.. Subtypes of antimitchondrial antibodies in primary biliary cirrhosis before and after liver transplantation. *Hepatology* 1987; **7**: 129-33.

10. Demetris AJ, Markus BH, Esquivel C et al. Pathologic analysis of liver transplantation for primary biliary cirrhosis. *Hepatology* 1988; **8**: 939-47.

11. Van de Water J, Gerson LB, Ferrel LD, Lake JR, Coppel RL, Batts KP, Wiesner RH, Gershwin ME. Immunohistochemical evidence of disease recurrence after liver transplantation for primary biliary cirrhosis. *Hepatology* 1996; **24**: 1079-1084.

12. Flannery GR, Burroughs AK, Butler P. Antimitochondrial antibodies in primary biliary cirrhosis recognize both specific peptides and and shared epitopes of the M2 familiy of antigens. *Hepatology* 1990; **10**: 370.

13. Hopf U, Moller B, Stemerowicz R, Lobeck H, Rodloff A, Freudenberg M, Galanos C, Huhn D. Relation between Escherichia coli R(rough) forms in gut, lipid A in liver,and primary biliary cirrhosis. *Lancet* 1989; **2**: 1419-22.

14. Klein R, Wiebel M, Engelhart S, Berg PA. Sera from patients with tuberculosis recognize the M2a-epitope (E2-subunit of pyruvate dehydrogenase) specific for primary biliary cirrhosis. *Clin Exp Immunol* 1993; **92**: 308-16.

15. Lindenborn-Fotinos J, Baum H, Berg PA. Mitochondrial antibodies in primary biliary cirrhosis: species and nonspecies specific determinants of M2 antigen. *Hepatology* 1985; **5**: 763-9.

16. Ghadiminejad I, Baum H. Evidence for the cell-surface localization of antigens cross-reacting with the "mitochondrial antibodies" of primary biliary cirrhosis. *Hepatology* 1987; **7**: 743-9.

17. Buuroughs AK, Butler P, Valle F et al. M2 antibodies and rough (R)-mutants in uirine of normal woman with bacteriuria and woman with PBC. *J Hepatol* 1990; **11**: 13.

18. Stemerowicz R, Hopf U, Moller B, Wittenbrink C, Rodloff A, Reinhardt R, Freudenberg M, Galanos C. Are antimitochondrial antibodies in primary biliary cirrhosis induced by R(rough)-mutants of enterobacteriaceae? *Lancet* 1988; **2**: 1166-70.

19. Vilagut L, Pares A, Vinas O, Vila J, Jimenez de Anta MT, Rodes J. Antibodies to mycobacterial 65-kD heat shock protein cross-react with the main mitochondrial antigens in patients with primary biliary cirrhosis. *Eur J Clin Invest* 1997; **27**: 667-72.

20. Klein R, Wiebel M, Engelhart S, Berg PA. Sera from patients with tuberculosis recognize the M2a-epitope (E2-subunit of pyruvate dehydrogenase) specific for primary biliary cirrhosis. *Clin Exp Immunol* 1993; **92**: 308-16.

21. Manns MP, Bremm A, Schneider PM, Notghi A, Gerken G, Prager-Eberle M, Stradmann-Bellinghausen B, Meyer zum Buschenfelde KH, Rittner C. HLA DRw8 and complement C4 deficiency as risk factors in primary biliary cirrhosis. *Gastroenterology* 1991; **101**: 1367-73.

22. Joplin R, Sadmoto T, Wallace L, Carman W, Mason A, Neuberger JM. Evidence for a transmissible factor in primary biliary cirrhosis. *J Hepatol* 1998; **20**: 51.

24. Krieg AM, Gourly MF, Perl A: Endogenous retroviruses: potential etiologic agents in autoimmunity. *FASEB J* 1992; **6**: 2537-2544.

25. Perron H, Garson JA, Bedin F, Beseme F, Paranhos-Baccala G et al.: Molecular identification of a novel retrovirus repeatedly isolated from patients with multiple sclerosis. The collaborative Research group on multiple sclerosis. *Proc Natl Acad Sci* 1997; **94**: 7583-7588.

26. Garry RF, Fermin CD, Hart DJ, Alexander SS, Donehower LA, Zhang HL: Detection of a human intracisternal A-type retroviral particle antigenically related to HIV. *Science* 1990; **250**: 1127-1129.

27. Von Herrath MG, Holz A, Homann D, Oldstone MB: Role of viruses in type I diabetes. *Semin Immunol* 1998; **10**: 87-100.

28. Mason AL, Xu L, Guo L, Munoz S, Jaspan JB, Bryer-Ash M, Cao Y, Sander DM, Shoenfeld Y, Ahmed A, Van de Water J, Gershwin ME, Garry RF. Detection of retroviral antibodies in primary biliary cirrhosis and other idiopathic biliary disorders. *Lancet* 1998; **351**: 1620-4.

29. Jaeckel E, Heringlake S, Berger D, Brabant G, Hunsmann G, Manns MP. No Evidence for Association Between IDDMK1,222, a Novel Isolated Retrovirus, and Insulin-Dependent Diabetes Mellitus (IDDM). Diabetes in print.

30. PA Bonis, MM Kaplan. The effects of colchicine and methotrexate are additive to ursodeoxycholic acid for patients with primary biliary cirrhosis who respond incompletely to Urso. *Hepatology* 1997; **26**:438A.

31. The IFNB Multiple Sclerosis Study Group. Interferon beta-1b is effective in relapsing-remitting multiple sclerosis. I. Clinical results of a multicenter, randomised, double-blind, placebo-controlled trial. *Neurology* 1993; **43**: 655-61.

32. Mueller R, Krahl T, Sarvetnick N. Pancreatic expression of interleukin-4 abrogates insulitis and autoimmune diabetes in nonobese diabetic (NOD) mice. *J Exp Med* 1996; **184**: 1093-9.

33. Strassburg CP, Oldhafer K, Manns MP, Tukey RH. Differential expression of the UGT1A locus in human liver, biliary, and gastric tissue: identification of UGT1A7 and UGT1A10 transcripts in extrahepatic tissue. *Mol Pharmacol* 1997; **52**: 212-20.

34. Zhang H, Yang Y, Horton JL, Samoilova EB, Judge TA, Turka LA, Wilson JM, Chen Y. Amelioration of collagen-induced arthritis by CD95 (Apo-1/Fas)-ligand gene transfer. *J Clin Invest* 1997; **100**: 1951-7.

35. Yasoshima M, Nakanuma Y, Tsuneyama K, Van de Water J, Gershwin ME. Immunohistochemical analysis of adhesion molecules in the micro-environment of portal tracts in relation to aberrant expression of PDC-E2 and HLA-DR on the bile ducts in primary biliary cirrhosis. *J Pathol* 1995; **175**: 319-25.

36. Mathisen PM, Yu M, Johnson JM, Drazba JA, Tuohy VK. Treatment of experimental autoimmune encephalomyelitis with genetically modified memory T-cells. *J Exp Med* 1997; **186**: 159-64.

37. Kramer R, Zhang Y, Gehrmann J, Gold R, Thoenen H, Wekerle H. Gene transfer through the blood-nerve barrier: NGF-engineered neuritogenic T lymphocytes attenuate experimental autoimmune neuritis. *Nat Med* 1995; **1**: 1162-6.

38. Underhill JA, Donaldson PT, Doherty DG, Manabe K, Williams R. HLA DPB polymorphism in primary sclerosing cholangitis and primary biliary cirrhosis. *Hepatology* 1995; **21**: 959-62.

39. Watanabe-Fukunaga R, Brannan CI, Copeland NG, Jenkins NA, Nagata S. Lymphoproliferation disorder in mice explained by defects in Fas antigen that mediates apoptosis. *Nature* 1992; **356**: 314-7.

40. Takahashi T, Tanaka M, Brannan CI, Jenkins NA, Copeland NG, Suda T, Nagata S. Generalized lymphoproliferative disease in mice, caused by a point mutation in the Fas ligand. *Cell* 1994; **76**: 969-76.

41. The Finnish-German APECED Consortium. Autoimmune Polyendocrinopathy-Candidiasis-Ectodermal Dystrophy. An autoimmune disease, APECED, caused by mutations in a novel gene featuring two PHD-type zinc-finger domains. *Nat Genet* 1997; **17**: 399-403.

42. Friedman A, Weiner HL. Induction of anergy or active suppression following oral tolerance is determined by antigen dosage. *Proc Natl Acad Sci USA* 1994; **91**: 6688-92.

43. Fukaura H, Kent SC, Pietrusewicz MJ, Khoury SJ, Weiner HL, Hafler DA. Induction of circulating myelin basic protein and proteolipid protein-specific transforming growth factor-beta1-secreting Th3 T-cells by oral administration of myelin in multiple sclerosis patients. *J Clin Invest* 1996; **98**: 70-7.

44. Ma SW, Zhao DL, Yin ZQ, Mukherjee R, Singh B, Qin HY, Stiller CR, Jevnikar AM. Transgenic plants expressing autoantigens fed to mice to induce oral immune tolerance. *Nat Med* 1997; **3**: 793-6.

45. Blanas E, Carbone FR, Allison J, Miller JF, Heath WR. Induction of autoimmune diabetes by oral administration of autoantigen. *Science* 1996; **274**: 1707-1709.

46. Howell MD, Winters ST, Olee T, Powell HC, Carlo DJ, Brostoff SW. Vaccination against experimental allergic encephalomyelitis with T-cell receptor peptides. *Science* 1989; **246**: 668-70.

47. Vandenbark AA, Chou YK, Whitham R, Mass M, Buenafe A, Liefeld D, Kavanagh D, Cooper S, Hashim GA, Offner H. Treatment of multiple sclerosis with T-cell receptor peptides: results of a double-blind pilot trial. *Nat Med* 1996; **2**: 1109-15.

48. Broeren CP, Lucassen MA, van Stipdonk MJ, van der Zee R, Boog CJ, Kusters JG, van Eden W. CDR1 T-cell receptor beta-chain peptide induces major histocompatibility complex class II-restricted T-T cell interactions. *Proc Natl Acad Sci USA* 1994; **91**: 5997-6001.

49. Waisman A, Ruiz PJ, Hirschberg DL, Gelman A, Oksenberg JR, Brocke S, Mor F, Cohen IR, Steinman L. Suppressive vaccination with DNA encoding a variable region gene of the T-cell receptor prevents autoimmune encephalomyelitis and activates Th2 immunity. *Nat Med* 1996; **2**: 899-905.

50. Weinberg AD, Bourdette DN, Sullivan TJ, Lemon M, Wallin JJ, Maziarz R, Davey M, Palida F, Godfrey W, Engleman E, Fulton RJ, Offner H, Vandenbark AA. Selective depletion of myelin-reactive T-cells with the anti-OX-40 antibody ameliorates autoimmune encephalomyelitis. *Nat Med* 1996; **2**: 183-9.

51. Lohse AW, Mor F, Karin N, Cohen IR. Control of experimental autoimmune encephalomyelitis by T-cells responding to activated T-cells. *Science* 1989; **244**: 820-2.

52. Zhang J, Medaer R, Stinissen P, Hafler D, Raus J. MHC-restricted depletion of human myelin basic protein-reactive T-cells by T-cell vaccination. *Science* 1993; **261**: 1451-4.

53. Lohse AW, Dienes HP, Meyer zum Buschenfelde KH. Suppression of murine experimental autoimmune hepatitis by T-cell vaccination or immunosuppression. *Hepatology* 1998; **27**: 1536-43.